CATARACT SURGERY

THE STATE OF THE ART

CATARACT SURGERY
THE STATE OF THE ART

James P. Gills, MD
St. Lukes Cataract & Laser Institute
Tarpon Springs, Florida

Robert Fenzl, MD
St Lukes Cataract & Laser Institute
Tarpon Springs, Florida

Robert G. Martin, MD
Carolina Eye Associates
Southern Pines, North Carolina

Project Coordinators
Myra Cherchio
Marsha Raanan, MS

Medical Editor
Michelle Van Der Karr

SLACK INCORPORATED, 6900 GROVE ROAD, THOROFARE, NJ 08086

Publisher: John H. Bond
Editorial Director: Amy E. Drummond
Creative Director: Linda Baker

Printed in the United States of America

Gills, James P.
      Cataract surgery: the state of the art/James P. Gills.
            p. cm.
      Includes bibliographical references and index.
      ISBN 1-55642-362-4 (alk. paper)
      1. Cataract--Surgery.
I. Title.
      [DNLM: 1. Cataract Extraction. WW 260 G484c 1998]
RE451.G55 1998
617.7'42059--dc21
DNLM/DLC
for Library of Congress   97-31712

Published by: SLACK Incorporated
               6900 Grove Road
               Thorofare, NJ 08086-9447 USA
               Telephone: 609-848-1000
               Fax: 609-853-5991
               World Wide Web: http://www.slackinc.com

Last digit is print number: 10 9 8 7 6 5 4 3 2 1

To others - my patients and fellow ophthalmologists

-James P. Gills, MD

ACKNOWLEDGMENTS

We wish to acknowledge the kind assistance of:

Lynda Antman
Bill Earle
Mark Erickson, CRA, COT
Jason Evangelista
Geordie Frei
Soni Richardson

TABLE OF CONTENTS

Contributing Authors

JUAN F. BATTLE, MD
Chief of Ophthalmology,
Elias Santana Eye Center
Consultant, Christoffel Blindenmission
and Medical Ministries International
Santo Domingo, Dominican Republic

DAVID BROWN, MD
The Eye Centers of Florida
Fort Myers, Florida

MYRA CHERCHIO, COMT
St. Lukes Cataract & Laser Institute
Tarpon Springs, Florida

ROBERT CIONNI, MD
Cincinnati Eye Institute
Cincinnati, Ohio

AKEF EL-MAGHRABY, MD
Medical Director,
El-Maghraby Eye Hospital
Jeddah, Saudi Arabia

ROBERT FENZL, MD
St Lukes Cataract & Laser Institute
Tarpon Springs, Florida

I. HOWARD FINE, MD
Clinical Associate Professor of
Ophthalmology
Oregon Health Science University,
Portland Oregon
Co-Founder Oregon Eye Surgery
Center
Eugene, Oregon

JOHN R. FISH, MD
Fish Ophthalmology Clinic
Big Spring, Texas

HIDEHARU FUKASAKU, MD
Director, Fukasaku Eye Centre
Yokohama, Japan

JOHNNY L. GAYTON, MD
EyeSight Associates of Middle Georgia
Warner Robins, Georgia

JAMES P. GILLS, MD
Director and Founder,
St. Lukes Cataract & Laser Institute,
Clinical Professor of Ophthalmology,
University of South Florida
Tarpon Springs, Florida

HOWARD V. GIMBEL, MD, FACS
Gimbel Eye Centre
Clinical Associate Professor,
Department of Surgery
University of Calgary
Calgary, Alberta, Canada

HARRY B. GRABOW, MD
Sarasota Cataract Institute
Sarasota, Florida
Clinical Assistant Professor
University of South Florida
Tampa Florida

RICHARD S. HOFFMAN, MD
Eugene, Oregon

JACK T. HOLLADAY, MD, FACS
McNeese Professor of Ophthalmology,
University of Texas
Medical School at Houston
Houston Eye Associates
Houston, Texas

FELIX K. JACOBI, MD
Justus-Liebig-Universitat Giessen
Germany

MAURICE JOHN, MD
The Maurice and Vivian Jean John
Research Foundation, Inc.
Jeffersonville, Indiana

MANUS C. KRAFF, MD
Professor of Clinical Ophthalmology,
Northwestern University
Chicago, Illinois

WILLIAM MALONEY, MD
Eye Surgery Associates
Vista, California

ROBERT G. MARTIN, MD
Director, Medical Care International
Ophthalmic Research and Training
Institute
Founder, Carolina Eye Associates
Southern Pines, North Carolina

ROBERT H. OSHER, MD
Medical Director,
Cinicinnati Eye Institute
Cincinnati, Ohio

MARSHA RAANAN, MS
Director of Research
Center for Clinical Research
Elmhust, Illinois

JOHN R. SHEPHERD, MD, FACS
Clinical Professor of Ophthalmology,
University of Utah
Director, Shepherd Eye Center, Las
Vegas, Nevada

JACK A. SINGER, MD
Assistant Professor of Ophthalmology,
Dartmouth Medical School
Hitchcock Associates
Dartmouth Hitchcock Medical Center
Randolph, Vermont

MICHAEL E. SNYDER, MD
Cincinnati Eye Institute
Cincinnati, Ohio

SPENCER P.
THORNTON, MD, FACS
Founder, Thornton Eye Center
Nashville, Tennessee

MICHELLE VAN DER KARR
Consultant,
Center for Clinical Research
Evanston, Illinois

PREFACE

Others. Everything I do today is based on something I've learned from *others.* My hope is that I can give what I have learned to *others* – my patients and my collegues. We're simply transients here on earth, and we should be transients of information, whether it's the printed page or the electron. I think *"others"* is perhaps the most beautiful focus we can have in our lives – giving everything we can to *others* in vision, in information, in love, and in the concept of living with the Lord for eternity.

Our preoperative work-ups are very important, and they become more important as managed care and regulations become a greater part of our lives. We need to relate to our patients to the degree that their expectations are exactly what they receive. Topical anesthesia with intraocular lidocaine is a result of many people's works. We've been fortunate to be able to add the use of intraocular lidocaine to this progression of doing less invasive surgery in a way which eliminates injecting the eye with any medications. The patient can have a painless operation and have almost immediate visual rehabilitation without patches or even a red eye.

We have obtained the pharmacology of using intraocular solutions both for anti-inflammatory and antibiotics from the retinal people and the beautiful work of Drs. Peyman and Machamer. This application of the *"others"* to our field has greatly benefited our patients in the reduction of endophthalmitis and a quiet postoperative eye. There are fewer cases of CME and possibly fewer cases of all sorts of inflammation.

The advanced cataract incisions of the clear cornea, which have been developed by Drs. Fine, Fish, and Langerman, among others, all allow us to vary our corneal incisions to reduce astigmatism and to provide the safest incision with the least amount of irritation and inflammation for the patient. The SLiC incision, which blends the scleral, limbal and corneal incisions, allows a safer procedure with less irritation. The blade technology for both the diamond and metal blades has increased tremendously over the years. All of this we have contributed to each other and shared with each other so that all our patients may benefit.

Reduction of astigmatism is one of the most important aspects for the modern cataract surgeon to truly understand and implement. We applied the limbal relaxing incision, as first pointed out by Dr. Steve Hollis for corneal surgery, to cataract surgery. This incision has probably made the correction of astigmatism a much more applicable procedure for most surgeons and patients.

Dr. Gimbel, as he advanced the concepts of capsulotomy and phacoemulsification, thought of *others* – doctors and patients outside of his practice. When he shared his knowledge about the posterior capsulotomy and management of tears – he contributed to and gave to *others.* So his life has been multiplied by his writings, and his techniques incorporated into the practice of many doctors.

Dr. Kelman's original work on the phacoemulsifier has been utilized by many *others*, like Drs. Fine, Brown, Singer, Fukasaku, Nagahara and Maloney, to enhance different techniques which allow everyone to formulate different methods of phacoemulsification which work best for them.

The avoidance of complications is probably the true evidence of excellence in cataract surgery as Drs. Osher, Snyder, and Cionni have shown. And they help us and *others* by teaching us from their experience.

The manufacturers and many good clinicians have helped us study the new lens materials, and optic designs. Multifocal lenses have been delayed and possibly improved because of working with the FDA and the corporations. Drs. Brown, Gayton and myself all have used multiple implants for years and believe that they will be a wonderful addition to our armamentarium as ophthalmologists, allowing us to correct extreme hyperopia and myopia and help correct the pseudophakic refractive error. We've actually done multiple minus lens implantation for extremely high myopic patients with keratoconus. Dr. Holladay's scientific approach to the power calculations has saved many a doctor and patient much distress and lack of a satisfactory outcome.

Shared knowledge about the efficacy of additional viscoelastic has allowed us to safely use phacoemulsification even in Fuch's patients. New advances in technology introduced by Drs. Uram and Fyodorov, and clinical work by Drs. Gayton and Martin, are vastly improving the outcomes and minimizing the invasiveness of combined cataract and glaucoma surgery.

The ultimate *others* is when we carry our advanced techniques for cataract surgery to foreign countries and in their developing state try to help them give better care to their patients.

The purpose of this book, and the prayer of this book, is that we propose the most appropriate therapy for each individual case and that the patient receives the best rehabilitation possible.

James P. Gills, M.D.

PREOPERATIVE WORKUP

Maurice John, MD, Robert Fenzl, MD

CRITERIA FOR RECOMMENDING CATARACT SURGERY

There was a time when cataract surgery was always a difficult procedure, both operatively and with regard to postoperative course. The risk/benefit ratio was definitely high for immature, soft cataracts. Thus, it was better to wait until visual impairment was substantial, even severe, before operating. With the explosion of new IOL and surgical technologies, cataract surgery has become significantly less invasive with greater potential benefit.

With the risk side of the risk/benefit ratio significantly reduced for immature cataracts and the potential benefits increased, the added risks involved in operating on the cataract after it matures come into play. Losing the ability to perform the advanced microsurgical techniques in a difficult case can rob the patient of the benefits provided by capsulorhexis, phacoemulsification, and smaller incision surgery. In this regard, all cataracts are not equal. Other pre-existing conditions that could make the surgery more difficult may tip the balance in favor of earlier surgery to reduce the potential risks.

The presence of one or more of the following conditions may be enough to warrant recommending earlier cataract surgery. If a difficult surgery is anticipated, it is better to encourage the patient to have the cataract removed in an earlier stage.

1. Daily lifestyle complaints
2. Clinically significant glare and/or contrast sensitivity loss
3. Advanced cataract (mature, hypermature)
4. Poorly dilated pupil or impending addition of Pilocarpine
5. Bound down pupil with posterior synechiae.
6. Presence of a hard nucleus (LOCS System Grade III)
7. Presence of a posterior subcapsular opacity (PSC). The presence of a posterior residual plaque on the first eye should influence the decision of when to do the second eye with a similar impending PSC.
8. Symptomatic anisometropia—stereopsis
9. Narrow angle
10. Early, but significant, Fuch's dystrophy, or a low endothelial count with a normal appearing cornea on slit lamp examination
11. Multiple anterior subcapsular flecks, which can be very visually debilitating
12. Head tremor
13. Chronic obstructive pulmonary disease
14. Unusual head position or neck flexion
15. Senility or impending Alzheimer's
16. Prominent brow
17. Presence of a filtering bleb
18. Need for increased visibility of the retina for diagnosis or treatment
19. Obesity and/or a short, thick neck

One of the authors (MEJ) conducted a study of over 600 consecutive cases to determine the risk/benefit ratio of operating on immature cataracts versus mature cataracts. The Lens Opacity Grading System (LOCS II), developed by Dr. Leo Chylack, was used to classify opacification in three lenticular zones. In the nuclear region, color and opalescence were graded separately. The zones correspond to those regions defined by the Cooperative Cataract Research Group for in-vitro classification.

Figure 1-1 displays the distribution of LOCS II grades in this sample. Forty-two percent were graded 3 or 4, and 58% were graded as less than 3. Ninety-two percent of cataracts were immature, 7% were mature, and 1% were hypermature.

In the series in this study, significantly fewer mature cataracts could be removed by phacoemulsification. Only 59% of mature cataracts benefited from phacoemulsification,

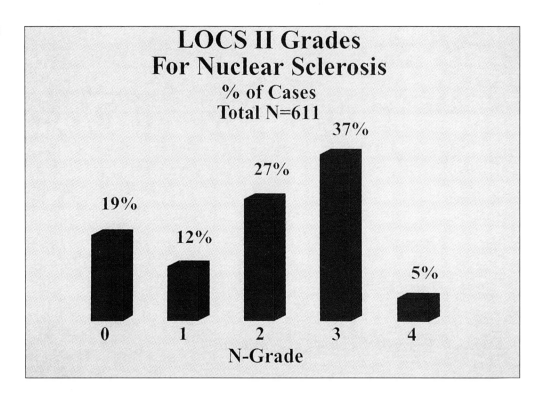

Figure 1-1. Distribution of LOCS II grades. Higher grades correspond with greater opacification. (John)

while 95% of immature cataracts were removed by phaco. Of mature cataracts that were phacoemulsified, 44% were graded as difficult compared to 21% of immature cataracts.

Hardness of nucleus as graded by the LOCS II system was positively correlated with ECCE, and overall difficulty of surgery and phaco, regardless of maturity of the cataract. Fifteen percent of cataracts graded 3 or more for nuclear hardness required an ECCE procedure compared with 1% of the less hard cases. Difficulty of phaco was greater in 30% of the harder nucleus cases compared with 15% of the softer cases.

We also found significantly more residual central plaque in cases with higher grades of posterior subcapsular opacities. The presence of residual plaque, which we refer to as dirty capsules, leads to increased risk of a ruptured capsule due to the extra manipulation required at surgery. There may be an increased probability for earlier Nd:YAG capsulotomy, causing the patient to lose the benefit of an intact capsule earlier.

Pupil size, of course, also impacts on surgical outcome. In our sample, only 30% of the small pupil cases (<6 mm) involved easy surgeries compared with 68% of normally sized pupils. The rate of vitrectomy was over three times higher (3.1% vs 0.8%), which was statistically significant. The small pupil, whether due to hereditary factors, miotic therapy, or synechiae, becomes a major risk factor for complications, because they offer significantly poorer visibility for the surgeon.

The decision of whether to perform cataract surgery obviously cannot be made on the basis of one factor alone. While Snellen acuity is a good guideline, the characteristics of the patient and the cataract must be taken into account. In addition to pupil size, the presence of other ocular disease or conditions, including problems such as Fuch's dystrophy, anisometropia, or a difficult first eye, can affect the ability to either perform complication-free surgery or the patient's ability to function. Some other indications for earlier surgery, such as head tremor, do not directly involve the eye but impact on the ability to perform optimal surgery. When combined with a harder nucleus or more mature cataract, these factors may add up to a technically more difficult surgery. However, earlier surgery in these cases may not only allow the patient the benefit of state-of-the-art cataract procedures depending on the level of surgical skill, but may also reduce the risk of complications or difficult surgery.

Finally surgeons must honestly assess their own skills. Surgeons in the early part of their learning curve or those with average skills should be operating sooner rather than later. While even the hardest of nuclei or the most difficult case can have a problem-free surgery by an excellent and experienced surgeon, not all surgeons can honestly claim that level of skill. An average skilled surgeon who timidly watches his or her patient develop a grade 4 nuclear sclerosis or a large posterior subcapsular plaque is not doing the patient any favors.

PATIENT EXPECTATIONS

As our ability to provide better quality cataract surgery improves, so do the expectations of our patients. It is now necessary for the cataract surgeon to deal with patients on the same level as the refractive surgeon. It must be determined whether the patient's impression of "good" vision means seeing clearly at distance or near. Many patients feel that clear vision means seeing detail on street signs ten blocks away, while others perceive clarity as reading a novel without glasses. If the expectations of these two types of patients are confused, the patient may perceive their outcome as a significant postoperative complication.

This problem is magnified when the wrong personality type is selected for monovision. As we all know, monovision offers an excellent visual compromise for many, but can present disappointment for the very discerning or critical patient. This author (RF) feels it can be disastrous for both patient and surgeon if a square peg is put in a round hole.

The necessity of surgeon-patient communication and accurate evaluation of the needs and wants of the patient will be even more critical with the advent of new IOL technology such as multifocal intraocular lenses. Significant dialogue with the patient will be necessary along with careful patient selection and education to ensure that the recipient of the multifocal lens will be excited by the advantages and not bothered significantly by the disadvantages. It is also important for the surgeon and staff to establish good rapport with the patient because data have shown that patients fare better with bilateral rather than monocular implantation of multifocal IOLs. Patients who have had monocular implantation and are awaiting surgery in the second eye will require significant support to carry them through this transition until they can be bilaterally implanted.

PREOPERATIVE WORKUP

Documentation

The chief complaint is the most vital piece of documentation for the cataract surgery workup. The specifics of the patient's complaints must be recorded precisely and should include exactly how the cataract is affecting the patient's vision and lifestyle. The importance of thorough documentation of the chief complaint for third party reviewers can not be underestimated and has become mandatory to properly document the need for surgery. Clear documentation also alerts the surgeon to the severity of the patient's visual problem, and provides clues as to the extent of visual loss related to the cataract. A well-recorded chief complaint makes the exam more efficient and less burdensome for the patient and also helps the surgeon provide appropriate counseling. As the debates continue around Snellen visual acuity, contrast sensitivity, and glare testing, the chief complaint has emerged as the backbone of the preoperative evaluation.

Visual Acuity

Despite the recent downplay of Snellen visual acuity, it remains an important part of the preoperative workup. Encouraging the patient to read the maximum amount of letters in order to record the best possible acuity can sometimes be a disservice to our patients. For example, if the individual fails to correctly read the majority of the 20/50 line, but can identify one or two letters on the 20/30 line, it is unreasonable to record the vision as 20/30. In a real-life scenario, we would not consider our vision *good* if straining and squinting were required to see a distant object.

Complaints consistent with glare disability or loss of contrast sensitivity should be documented objectively to determine whether the etiology of the complaint is truly cataract related. While there is no standard for these tests, their value lies in a relative indication of the problem rather than an absolute value. The surgeon may be more comfortable discussing surgery with a patient who complains of glare but has early nuclear sclerosis or moderate cortical spokes if there is objective documentation that the patient sees poorly under glare situations.

Obviously, a complete ophthalmological evaluation is required to rule out all other possible causes of the patient's symptomatology and to determine whether other ocular conditions such as keratitis sicca or glaucoma exist that could affect surgical outcome. When a complete evaluation has been performed, the patient must be made fully aware of the potential risks and benefits specific to his case so an informed decision can be made. The patient must understand how the cataract surgery will impact his lifestyle and solve the problems documented in the chief complaint.

Ultrasonography

After obtaining informed consent for cataract surgery, measurements for the intraocular lens are required. Since the advent of small, astigmatically neutral incisions, the accuracy of the postoperative refractive error is largely dependent on the ultrasound measurements. Accurate preoperative refraction, keratometry, and axial length are vital. Bilateral measurements of axial length are always performed, even if the patient is pseudophakic, because most patients' eyes measure within 0.2 mm of each other. Bilateral measurement improves accuracy and reduces measurement error. Factors such as staphyloma, nuclear sclerotic cataracts, amblyopia, and previous injury must all be considered when performing biometry.

Several years ago, on the recommendations of Ken Hoffer, MD and others, we (RF) changed to immersion ultrasound (Figure 1-2) rather than applanation. Immersion ultrasound provides the most reproducible results and eliminates the possibility of indenting the cornea, which is especially critical when measuring extremely high hyperopes where a small error is a greater percentage of the axial length. We use the Holladay IOL Consultant which requires additional measurements that include: corneal diameter (Figure 1-3), lens thickness and anterior chamber depth. By taking these measurements, it is possible to detect anterior segments disproportionate to axial lengths that may result in power surprises (see Chapter 15). It is also important to appoint technicians to specialize in ultrasonography. Redundancy improves skill, technique and therefore accuracy. This skill must be performed on a regular basis to obtain consistent, reproducible results, and the technician's skills should be re-evaluated periodically.

Figure 1-2. Measuring the axial length with immersion ultrasound (Fenzl).

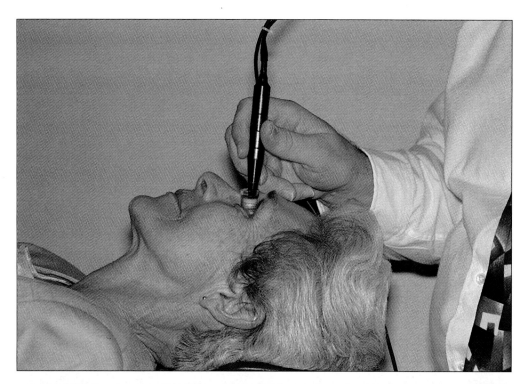

Figure 1-3. Measuring the corneal diameter (Fenzl).

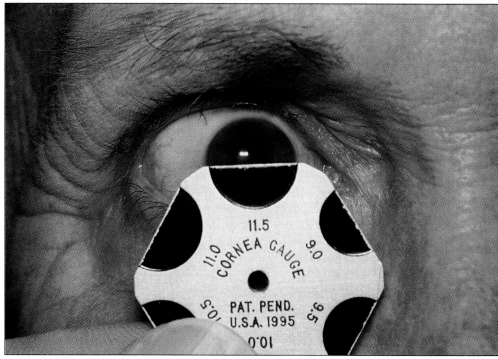

Although accurate biometry is critical, the formulas used to calculate IOL power are equally important. The advent of third-generation formulas such as the Hoffer Q, Holladay IOL Consultant, and the SRKT have greatly improved our outcomes.

Corneal Topography

Patients deserve the best postoperative refraction possible, including reduction of preoperative astigmatism. Astigmatically neutral incisions combined with limbal relaxing incisions can correct up to 3.5 diopters of astigmatism. Cases with greater than 3.5 diopters of astigmatism usually require additional corneal relaxing incisions. Accurate corneal topography is essential to formulate a surgical plan. While current technology is less operator dependent, new, state-of-the art maps and views of the cornea are available with units

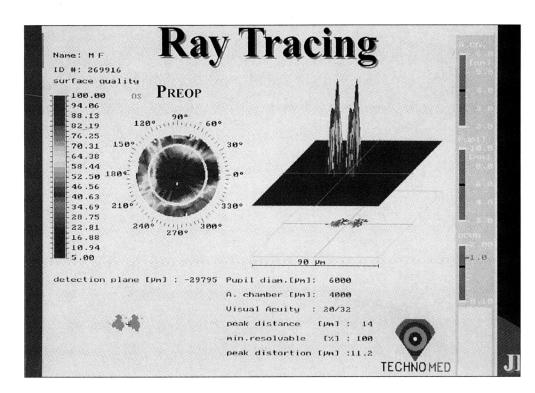

Figure 1-4. Technomed's ray tracing (Fenzl).

such as the Technomed C-Scan. Well-trained, computer-literate staff must provide the most relevant maps and information to the surgeon. If the patient has corneal astigmatism, topography should always be performed *before* immersion ultrasound or other tests that require corneal contact.

Corneal topography is also indicated to determine etiology of visual loss in the presence of minimal cataract and a normal fundus examination. The Technomed C-Scan offers Ray Tracing (Figure 1-4), a program that can predict potential corneal visual acuity. Variables such as pupil size, target size, and anterior chamber depth can be modified for the individual to determine potential acuity under different circumstances. From this program, we can learn the extent of peak distortion and resolution when the patient is presented two objects at a distant plane. With this data, we can understand how the patient performs in different lighting situations when presented with differently sized targets.

Calculating the Effective Corneal Power After Refractive Surgery

The aging baby boomer population created special refractive challenges to the cataract surgeon, since many have undergone corneal refractive surgery. The most significant problem lies in determining the corneal curvature accurately for IOL calculations (Figure 1-5). Routine keratometry readings do not accurately reflect the true corneal curvature in these cases and may result in power surprises if used for IOL calculations. Therefore, routine keratometry readings should *never* be used for IOL calculations in this population. There are three methods to determine the effective power of the cornea: historical method, contact lens method, and the topography method.

The simplest but least accurate method of determining corneal power is the historical method. The keratometry reading and refraction before refractive surgery must be known along with an accurate postoperative refraction. The corrected keratometry reading is determined by algebraically combining the original keratometry reading with the amount of refractive error corrected. The following formula would be used:

Corrected K = preoperative K - the change in refractive error

* Points to remember:
1. use an average of horizontal and vertical K-readings
2. factor in vertex distance of the glasses or refraction if the refractive error is greater than 4 diopters

For example, if a patient's preoperative cornea measured 44 diopters, the preoperative refraction was -4.0 and the postoperative refraction is plano, the corrected K reading would be calculated as follows:

Corrected K = 44 - 4

Corrected K = 40 diopters

The downfall of the history method is that cataracts frequently cause induced myopia. In many cases, calculation is complicated by the progressive flattening that occurs in about 25% of RK patients. It is nearly impossible to separate these two factors and determine each of their impact on the postoperative refraction.

The next most common method is to use the simulated keratometric measurements from corneal topography. These values may vary from one unit to another since each company's software has different methods of assessing the central corneal power. This information can be easily obtained by contacting the manufacturer.

Figure 1-5. Special care must be taken to determine the correct corneal curvature of the post-RK patient (Fenzl).

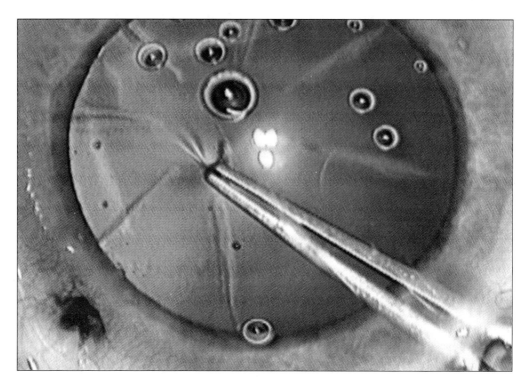

Probably the most accurate method of assessing the effective power of the cornea is the contact lens method. For this technique, a gas permeable contact lens with a known base curve is inserted and an over-refraction obtained. The contact lens must fit reasonably for an accurate over-refraction. This method is only accurate if the contact can ride centrally long enough to obtain a over-refraction. Air bubbles under the contact can also affect accuracy, which is why it is recommended to keep several base curves on hand. It may be more difficult to obtain a good fit in the post-RK patient that the post-PRK patient. The following formula is used to calculate the effective corneal power with the contact lens method:

Corrected K = Dioptric power of the contact + Base curve + (over refraction - refraction without the contact)

* Points to remember:

1. The base curve is recorded in diopters not millimeters.
2. Arithmetic is simplified by using plano contact lenses.

For example, if a patient's refraction is plano, and the over-refraction is -2.00 using a plano contact lens with a 40 D base curve, the K reading would be calculated as follows:

Corrected K = 0 + 40 + (-2.00 - 0)

Corrected K = 38

In other words, 2 diopters of tear film is between the cornea and contact. To work this formula backwards, the 40 diopter contact is 2 diopters steeper than the effective power of the cornea. Thus, the over-refraction of -2.00 is obtained.

Predicting Postoperative Acuity

Macular function tests, such as The Potential Acuity Meter, developed by David Guyton, MD, or the Super Pinhole, developed by David McIntyre, MD, have become essential in evaluating macular function preoperatively. These tests isolate visual loss due to media problems and help the clinician determine its impact on postoperative visual acuity consistently and reliably. Testing macular function is extremely important when gross examination of the cataract does not appear to be equal to visual loss or the patient's complaint. It is also useful to determine the significance of pigmentary abnormalities of the macula which may or may not represent macular dysfunction. This test should be part of the standard cataract evaluation of any patient who has any retinal pathology or where improvement of visual acuity is in question. Macular function tests along with predicted corneal acuity are useful in determining potential postoperative visual acuity. These tests are important to determine the potential visual benefit from cataract surgery and to help manage patient expectations.

If a dense cataract precludes examination of the posterior pole, B-Scan ultrasonography is indicated to rule out such problems as retinal detachment, dense macular scarring, or vitreous hemorrhage. In some cases, a skilled technician may be able to detect significant cupping of the optic nerve.

The Medical Workup

The main benefit of the medical workup in the preoperative evaluation of the cataract surgery patient is to provide the surgeon with any clues that could complicate or alter the approach to the surgery. It not only satisfies requirements by third party reviewers, but also gives the physician insight into systemic disorders and medications that may impact surgery. For example, it is important to know if the patient is using medications such as coumadin or aspirin when determining the type of cataract incision to be performed.

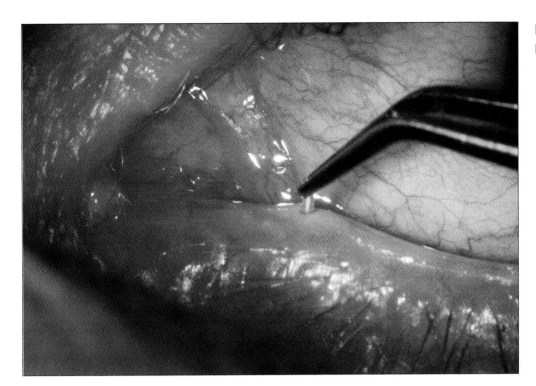

Figure 1-6. Insertion of punctal plug (Fenzl).

We have found preoperative medical testing to be of very little value for cataract surgery in an ambulatory surgery center. A patient who is medically unstable should be referred to the general physician to be stabilized before cataract surgery. We do not routinely order preoperative blood tests and only perform EKGs if the patient has significant history or symptoms that concern us.

Dry Eye

It is very important to assess the patient's tear film prior to surgery. Much postoperative discomfort is from keratitis sicca. If the patient is found to have an inadequate tear film, temporary or permanent punctal plugs (Figure 1-6) should be considered before surgery to prevent postoperative discomfort from the dryness. Many surgeons who perform punctal occlusion on nearly all their preoperative patients, while others are more selective. Before cataract surgery, we find at least 10-15% of patients require punctal occlusion. Patients who are symptomatic, stain with Rose Bengal, and are over 60 years old should receive permanent punctal plugs. Besides reducing irritation after surgery, punctal plugs actually extend the contact time of topical medications. For this reason, some doctors advocate temporary punctal plugs for all patients.

SUMMARY

Maximizing the outcome for the patient depends on proper patient selection, managing patient expectations, and accurate preoperative measurements and calculations. A thorough preoperative evaluation improves accuracy and surgical outcomes. Most importantly, the patient is well informed, feels well cared for, and is better prepared for the ultimate outcome.

TOPICAL ANESTHESIA AND INTRAOCULAR LIDOCAINE

James P. Gills, MD, Robert G. Martin, MD, Myra Cherchio, COMT

CATARACT SURGERY AND REGIONAL ANESTHESIA

Retrobulbar and peribulbar blocks have been used for years for ocular anesthesia. Retrobulbar anesthesia for ocular surgery was described as early as 1884 by Knapp.[1] Regional anesthesia definitely maintains its place in ocular surgery today, but is not without complications.[2,3] Although the complications are few, they can be quite serious. The more familiar among these include retrobulbar hemorrhage, respiratory depression, intramural or subarachnoid injection, optic nerve damage and globe perforation.

CATARACT SURGERY AND TOPICAL ANESTHESIA

In today's environment, akinesia is not the issue it once was and there is increasing concern to reduce the need for regional anesthesia and the morbidity associated with needle injections. Topical anesthesia was reintroduced by Dr. Richard Fichman[4] in October, 1991. The return to topical anesthesia effectively eliminates the risk of complications associated with regional blocks. Although it is not for every patient, topical anesthesia has gained wide acceptance as an effective, efficient, practical and safe form of ocular anesthesia for cataract surgery.[4-6]

Topical anesthesia has definite advantages over regional block over and above increased safety (see Table 2-1). Patients are less anxious knowing they will not be receiving an injection. They are physically more comfortable in the early postoperative period. Visual rehabilitation is greatly accelerated, leading to greater patient satisfaction. Topical anesthesia may obviate certain medical contraindications to surgery using regional block. For example, the patient on anticoagulant therapy may undergo clear-corneal cataract surgery with topical anesthesia without interruption of blood thinners.[4,5] There are also advantages for the surgeon. It is easier and more cost effective.

There are, however, disadvantages associated with topical anesthesia. Topical anesthesia can pose a problem for the surgeon when there is an anxious patient who cannot maintain fixation. Topical anesthesia alone is an effective method of anesthesia and is adequate for many patients. However it does not eliminate all sensation of pressure or discomfort in every patient. These sensations often arise from intraocular maneuvers that manipulate the iris root, such as occurs during phacoemulsification and lens insertion, which may cause undue anxiety and discomfort for the patient. These concerns have limited the use of topical anesthesia, especially for more complex procedures.

INTRAOCULAR ANESTHESIA

Anecdotal reports[7] of inadvertent intracameral injection of lidocaine indicated no complications and a normal postoperative course. These case reports led one of the authors (JPG) to hypothesize that intracameral injection of an appropriate solution of this drug could safely eliminate discomfort that patients may experience with topical anesthesia alone. In fact, R.A. Fichman, MD had already described the use of preservative-free tetracaine for intracameral injection to reduce intraoperative discomfort in selected patients undergoing surgery under topical anesthesia,[4] in instances where patient anxiety mounted during phacoemulsification.

The rationale for use of intraocular lidocaine is summarized in Table 2-2. We began using small doses of intracameral lidocaine for selected cases with limited visual potential and found no adverse effects. The solution used was 1% unpreserved and epinephrine-free. Lidocaine is potent and has a very fast onset. The duration, though relatively short, is

---

TABLE 2-1
ADVANTAGES OF TOPICAL ANESTHESIA

- Avoidance of unforeseen complications associated with retrobulbar block

    Retrobulbar hemorrhage
    Retinal vascular occlusion
    Prolonged diplopia
    Ptosis
    Systemic side effects

- Immediate return of vision - especially important for monocular patients
- "No needle" reduces anxiety
- Intact blink reflex - less risk of exposure keratitis, corneal abrasion
- Severity is reduced in the event of allergic reaction
- Time savings
- Cost savings

TABLE 2-2
USE OF INTRAOCULAR LIDOCAINE

- Documentation of Inadvertent Injection into A/C with No Adverse Effects
- Selected Clinical Use in Patients with Limited Vision Potential
- Gradual Dosage Increase
- Randomized Study
- Routine Use of 0.5 cc 1% Lidocaine

---

adequate. These features, combined with low toxicity, make it a good choice for intraocular anesthesia. Impressed with the efficacy observed in these cases and assured that there was no endothelial damage, we increased the dose to 0.1 cc.

Clinical Studies of Intraocular Lidocaine

Gills' Studies

We designed a masked, randomized, prospective, parallel group study to evaluate the safety and efficacy of intraocular lidocaine.[8] Patients were eligible for the randomized study if they were to undergo uncomplicated cataract extraction by phacoemulsification with insertion of a folded silicone IOL through an incision size of 3.2 mm or less and there were no contraindications for topical anesthesia. Contraindications included known allergic response to the topical anesthetics or lidocaine, any corneal or ocular conditions precluding the use of topical anesthesia. Patients scheduled for triple procedures (IOL + trabeculectomy) were also excluded. However patients with small pupils were not excluded as long as they were eligible for the phacoemulsification procedure. Patients scheduled for either corneal and/or limbal relaxing incisions to correct astigmatism were also eligible for the study.

All study patients received topical anesthesia under the following regimen: Proparacaine (0.5%), 1 drop administered twice; and Marcaine (0.75%), 1 drop instilled 4x. Patients who expressed anxiety were given Versed just prior to surgery regardless of study treatment.

The study treatments were as follows: 0.10 cc unpreserved, epinephrine-free Lidocaine at 1.0%, or 0.10 cc unpreserved BSS. Study medication for the day was dispensed by preloading the syringes ready for intracameral injection and was administered after entry into the anterior chamber. After intracameral injection, an interval of 1 minute passed before starting phacoemulsification. At specified intervals (1 minute, three minutes, and 5 minutes after administration) the patient's discomfort/pain level was measured using a predefined uniform scale administered by the nurse anesthetist. In addition the patient was asked if there was discomfort or pain midway during phacoemulsification and mid-way during lens insertion. The patient had also been instructed to utilize a predetermined hand motion to spontaneously signal any pain or discomfort if necessary, including both mild pressure and increased pressure. The goal was to evaluate all sensations the patient might feel, although mild pressure was not uncomfortable to the patient.

The surgeon would then determine, based on patient response, if an additional dose of lidocaine was needed. The level of pain or discomfort was quantified with a 5-point scale: 0= No sensation, 1+= Mild pressure (no discomfort), 2+= Increased pressure (uncomfortable), 3+= Moderate pain, 4+= Sharp pain, and 5+= Severe pain.

Efficacy of treatment was assessed by comparing pain or discomfort level as determined using the scale. The pain/discomfort scores were assessed during phacoemulsification, and during lens insertion. In addition, patients were classified according to the highest expressed pain/discomfort score occurring at any time during the procedure. The need for additional medication (added lidocaine for the lidocaine group or a first dose of lidocaine for the BSS group), and/or the need for sedation were also used to monitor efficacy. The safety of intraoperative lidocaine was assessed by IOP, visual acuity, anterior chamber cell and flare measurements, and endothelial cell counts.

Mean age, and the means of the pain scores for each group (range = 0 - 5) were compared using 2-tailed t-tests. The distributions of gender, pain/discomfort scores, visual acuities, and scores for aqueous flare and cells were compared between groups using a chi-square test with continuity correction. All statistical analyses were carried out using SAS[9] or Statmost.[10]

Results

Placebo-Controlled Study

A total of 303 procedures were performed under topical anesthesia: 183 received intraoperative lidocaine and 120

TABLE 2-3
DISTRIBUTION OF DISCOMFORT/PAIN SCALE SCORES BY TREATMENT GROUP AND INTRAOPERATIVE INTERVAL

Intraoperative Interval	Treatment	Discomfort/Pain Score N (%) of Patients				
		(0) No Sensation	(+1) Mild Pressure	(+2) Increased Pressure	(+3) Moderate Pain	TOTAL
Phacoemul-sification	lidocaine	152 (83%)	26 (14.3%)	4 (2.2%)	0 (0%)	182
	BSS	89 (74.2%)	19 (15.8%)	9 (7.5%)	3 (2.5%)	120
Lens Insertion	lidocaine	140 (76.9%)	31 (17.0%)	9 (4.9%)	2 (1.1%)	182
	BSS	78 (65%)	23 (19.2%)	14 (11.7%)	5 (4.2%)	120
Highest	lidocaine	123 (67.6%)	42 (23.1%)	15 (8.2%)	2 (1.1%)	182
Reported Level	BSS	58 (48.3%)	31 (25.8%)	23 (19.2%)	8 (6.7%)	120

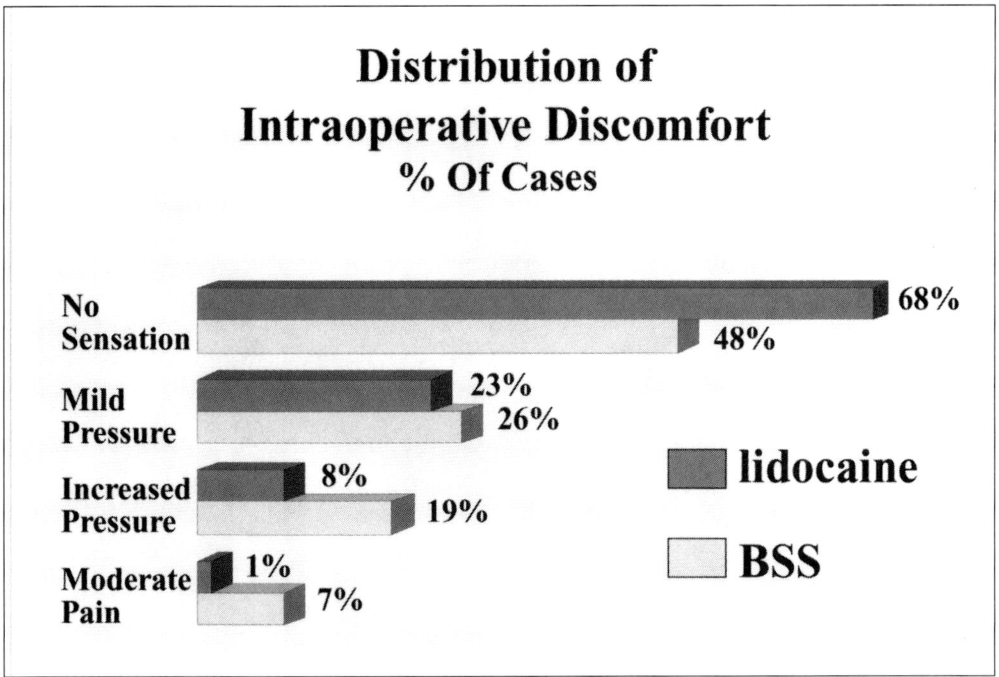

Distribution of Intraoperative Discomfort % Of Cases

No Sensation — lidocaine 68%, BSS 48%
Mild Pressure — lidocaine 23%, BSS 26%
Increased Pressure — lidocaine 8%, BSS 19%
Moderate Pain — lidocaine 1%, BSS 7%

lidocaine
BSS

Figure 2-1. Histogram illustrating the distribution of pain scores among patients treated with intraocular lidocaine (dark bars), and control patients treated with balanced saline solution (light bars) (Gills).

received BSS and constituted the control group. A pain/discomfort score was not obtainable from one of the lidocaine patients. The groups were comparable with respect to age and sex distribution, the use of Versed administered for anxiety, and the use of astigmatic keratotomy.

Discomfort or pain was assessed at several predetermined times during the operative procedure. The distribution of pain/discomfort scale scores is shown in Table 2-3 and in Figure 2-1 for each treatment group. First, we evaluated the highest score experienced at any point intraoperatively. The distribution of pain scale scores was shifted in the direction of increased discomfort among the BSS cases compared with lidocaine cases. Mild sensation, expressed as pressure, was reported by 26% of BSS patients and 23% of lidocaine patients. Increased pressure was reported in 19% of BSS pro-

cedures compared with 8% of procedures performed with lidocaine. Moderate pain (score 3+) was reported in 7% of BSS procedures versus 1% of lidocaine procedures. Thus 26% of patients with no lidocaine treatment experienced increased pressure or moderate pain versus 9% of lidocaine-treated cases. This finding was statistically significant (p<0.0001).

When the scores were examined according to when the discomfort occurred (during phacoemulsification or during lens insertion) it was found that pain/discomfort scores of 2 (increased pressure) or 3 (moderate pain) occurred more frequently during lens insertion than during phacoemulsification (Table 2-3, Figure 2-2). This result suggested that patients were describing, to some extent, sensation resulting from the wound manipulation as the IOL was introduced. During phacoemulsification only 4 lidocaine patients (2%) had reported

Figure 2-2. Histogram comparing the distribution of pain scores among patients treated with 0.5 cc of 1% unpreserved lidocaine (dark bars), with patients treated with 0.1 cc unpreserved lidocaine (light bars) (Gills).

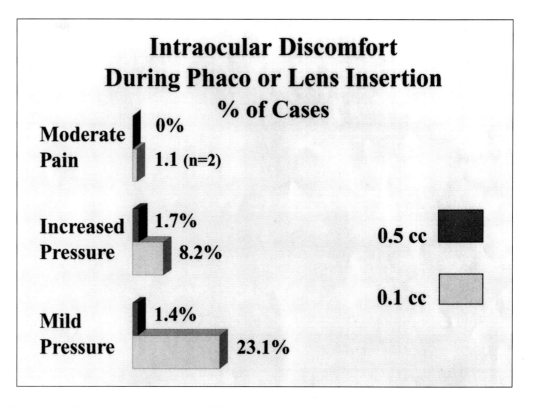

increased pressure (score = 2). None of the lidocaine patients reported pain (score >= 3) during phacoemulsification. Two of the 15 lidocaine patients expressing increased pressure during surgery did so before phaco began. In the BSS group, 9 (8%) reported increased pressure (score = 2) during phacoemulsification and 3 (2%) reported moderate pain (score = 3). No patient in the study reported sharp or severe pain (score = 4 or 5) at any time during surgery.

The two treatment groups were comparable with respect to the need for intraoperative Versed for anxiety. Nineteen percent of BSS patients and 18% of lidocaine patients required Versed to control anxiety.

There was no difference in pain score distribution between patients receiving astigmatic keratotomy and those with no relaxing incisions regardless of whether the patient was given lidocaine or BSS. However, patients receiving LRIs had more discomfort postoperatively.

There were no significant differences between the groups with respect to mean IOP at 1 day postoperatively, or in anterior chamber flare/cells measurements. Visual acuity (pinhole) at one day postoperatively was comparable between the groups, with 80% of BSS eyes and 83% of lidocaine eyes seeing 20/40 or better with pinhole.

Postoperative endothelial cell counts were collected for a 20% sub-sample of cases. No significant differences between treatment groups were found in cell counts or percent cell loss from baseline. Mean postoperative cell count for the sample was 1602 (s.d. = 279) for lidocaine patients and 1588 (s.d. = 285) for BSS patients. Mean central pachymetry measurements were also equivalent.

Blood pressures were compared between the groups just prior to surgery, intraoperatively and in the recovery room. If multiple measurements were charted at an interval, the highest was used for analysis. There were no group differences in the means of systolic or diastolic pressure at any time point. There were no adverse events among the study participants.

Secondary Studies

The statistically significant results of the controlled study documented the overall efficacy of intracameral lidocaine in optimizing patient comfort during surgery. After data analysis it was felt necessary to suspend the controlled study to avoid placebo treatment. Nevertheless there were remaining questions: 1) the optimal dose of lidocaine to eliminate any discomfort, and indeed, any sensation at all; and 2) whether a larger dose of lidocaine would impact on safety. To answer these questions a consecutive series of 300 patients were enrolled under the same general protocol but all patients were given 0.50 cc 1% unpreserved lidocaine. The pain scale was administered in the same way except that additional questions were asked to determine if the patient could distinguish between intraocular discomfort or pain and discomfort or pain felt extra-ocularly, that is, in the wound area or lids. This additional information was collected because of the finding that scores were much lower during phacoemulsification than for lens insertion which led the surgeon to believe that in some cases the source of discomfort to the patient came from manipulation of the wound during lens insertion and was not intraocular.

In this series, 286 of the 300 patients met study criteria and had complete data for analysis. Intraocular increased pressure

TABLE 2-4
EVALUATION OF CHANGES IN ENDOTHELIAL CELL COUNT (ECC) AND CORNEAL THICKNESS AT 2 WEEKS POSTOP AMONG 109 EYES RECEIVING 0.5 CC 1% LIDOCAINE

	Mean	Standard Deviation	Percentiles 10th	50th	90th
Preop ECC	1895	231	1500	1900	2200
Postop ECC	1884	244	1600	1900	2200
% Cell Loss	3.2%	1.86	11%(LOSS)	0%	10%(GAIN)*
Preop Pachymetry	0.57	0.028	0.54	0.58	0.60
Postop Pachymetry	0.56	0.096	0.54	0.58	0.60

*Recorded "gain" due to normal measurement error

(a score of 2+) was experienced by 0.7% of cases (2 patients) during phacoemulsification and by 1% (3 patients) during lens insertion. Two patients experienced external discomfort from wound manipulation which they rated as 2 or 3+. When the results of the 0.5 cc study were compared to the 0.1 cc lidocaine group from the randomized study (Figure 2-2), it was found that the rate of discomfort (any increased pressure or pain as defined by a score >= 2) was reduced to 1.7%. None of the 0.5 cc cases had 3+ scores. The presence of any intraocular sensation was reduced to 3.1%. At the 0.1 cc dose, 23.1% had felt mild pressure and 9.3% had increased pressure or moderate intraocular pain during either phaco or lens insertion.

Postoperative endothelial cell counts and pachymetry measurements were collected at two weeks from 109 patients who received 0.5 cc intraoperative lidocaine (Table 2-4). There were no differences in mean preoperative vs. postoperative endothelial cell count, and the mean percent change in cell count (preop to postop) was not significant. There were no adverse events among the 286 patients.

The results of the study documented a statistically significant decrease in pain or discomfort scores among patients receiving intraoperative lidocaine versus placebo. In the controlled study using a 0.1 cc dose, lidocaine patients mainly felt no sensation or mild pressure with no discomfort while placebo patients experienced increased pressure and moderate pain in many instances. In the subsequent study of 286 patients given 0.5 cc doses, no intraocular pain was experienced by lidocaine patients and increased pressure was felt by only 1.7 %. Furthermore, 97% felt no sensation at all, including mild pressure. Thus increasing the dose to 0.5 cc dramatically reduced even mild pressure.

There were no adverse events. Patients did not experience any untoward effects or significant endothelial cell loss at either the 0.1 cc dose or the 0.5 cc dose. The average 3% endothelial cell loss was less than that recently reported by Dick, et al. for clear-cornea cases.[7] Two-week endothelial cell count data is not generally considered stable. However, microscopy was done at this routine visit to check for any

acute toxicity effects. The decision not to alter the routine visit schedule was based on repeated observation of clear, healthy corneas. A long-term follow-up of these patients is underway to monitor endothelial health.

Currently all patients receive 0.5 cc unpreserved lidocaine intraoperatively. There is less need for supplemental anesthesia during phacoemulsification or lens insertion and fewer problems due to squeezing lids when lidocaine is administered. The effectiveness of lidocaine lasts for approximately 10 minutes and works best when administered prophylactically.

Since the study was performed, we have altered our regimen for topical anesthesia, because we observed that the repeated administration of proparacaine and marcaine tended to increase the rate of keratitis. Currently we use preservative-free tetracaine, administered just prior to the procedure (see Chapter 3).

Martin Study

We conducted a randomized prospective study of 100 patients undergoing phacoemulsification under topical anesthesia. Patients were randomly assigned to receive intracameral injection of either unpreserved lidocaine (0.5 cc of a 1% unpreserved solution) or BSS. Patients were administered a brief questionnaire in the recovery area to determine the comfort level of the procedure. However the main purpose of the study was to document the safety of intraoperative lidocaine as an adjunct to topical anesthesia.

The in-vitro study of Kim and colleagues had suggested that lidocaine instilled intracamerally could cause mild transient edema as evidenced by electron microscopy.[12] Their study had been performed on rabbit and human eyes using 15 minute perfusion intervals resulting in a total dose far in excess of that which would occur clinically. Even so, no pleomorphism or other cellular changes were noted.

The Kowa laser/flare cell meter was used to objectively quantify and compare the levels of anterior chamber reaction between the lidocaine and control groups at 1 and 10 days following surgery. Postoperative cell densities were obtained an

TABLE 2-5
DISTRIBUTION OF COMFORT SCORES ON DAY OF SURGERY: LIDOCAINE VERSUS PLACEBO

	No sensation	Mild pressure no discomfort	Increased pressure	Mild pain
Lidocaine	31 (78%)	8 (20%)	0 (0%)	1 (2%)
Placebo	30 (57%)	20 (38%)	3 (6%)	0 (0%)

P=0.048 (comparison of sensation vs no sensation: Fisher's exact

average of 115 (s.d.=27) days after surgery. The minimum number of days was 69 days. Cell densities were measured centrally using the Konan system which obtains an average cell density instantaneously within the specified area. The average cell size, the standard deviation of the average density, the coefficient of variation and the percent of cells hexagonal in shape (a measure of pleomorphism) were also obtained with the Konan system. Central pachymetry was also measured.

Results

Ninety-three patients (40 lidocaine, 53 control) completed the study and were evaluated. The two groups were comparable in age and sex distribution, surgery time, and type of cataract incision (mainly temporal clear corneal) and use of corneal relaxing incisions (6-8%).

There were no intraoperative complications. Only 8% of cases (one lidocaine and 3 control) reported any increased uncomfortable pressure or discomfort. However 78% of lidocaine patients versus 56% of controls reported no sensation at all (p=0.048, Table 2-5). The modest level of discomfort reported by any patient in the study was due in part to the methodology of the study in which patients were asked to grade intraoperative discomfort after surgery was over.

Cell density parameters are presented in Table 2-6. There were no significant differences between lidocaine cases and controls in the 2-3 month postoperative mean cell density or in the mean change in cell density from baseline. The mean coefficient of variation, standard deviation of density readings (within-patient), and mean percent hexagonal cells (within-patient) also did not differ significantly between the two groups. Kowa laser flare and cell measurements at ten days postop are presented in Table 2-7. The groups did not differ significantly in mean flare measurements or particle counts. Overall the study demonstrated that the use of intraoperative lidocaine is safe and efficacious.

Thus, we have found that intraocular lidocaine is safe, and when used as an adjunct to topical anesthesia, usually eliminates all discomfort. In most cases, patients have no sensation whatsoever. The patient is more relaxed and comfortable and is less likely to make any inadvertent movements. The sur-

TABLE 2-6
MEAN ENDOTHELIAL CELL DENSITY AT 2-3 MONTHS POSTOP

	Mean (standard deviation)		
	Lidocaine	Placebo	p-value*
Preop cell density	1694 (518)	1984 (613)	0.09
Postop cell density	2187 (473)	2169 (466)	0.90
Change at 5 weeks	317 (634)	256 (352)	0.77
Mean postop % hexagonal cells	48% (16.3%)	50% (10.3%)	0.65
Mean postop coeff. of variation	36 (10.3)	37 (7.5)	0.67
Mean postop pachymetry	0.56 (0.03)	0.55 (0.04)	0.22

* no significant differences, t-test of independent samples

geon and operating room staff are more at ease and can work more efficiently. Intraocular unpreserved lidocaine makes cataract surgery safer and allows a wider range of patients to enjoy the benefits of topical anesthesia. Because of intraocular lidocaine, the use of topical anesthesia can be extended to procedures such as glaucoma filtering procedures, iridectomies, and secondary implants.

Intraocular Anesthesia in Combined Surgery

Intracameral lidocaine may have a distinct advantage in patients with glaucoma, as it does not alter blood flow to the optic nerve, causing localized ischemia, as does retrobulbar and peribulbar anesthesia. Drs. Falck and Schenkman have conducted a prospective study of intracameral and peribulbar lidocaine in combined cataract and glaucoma filtration surgery (presented at the 1997 annual meeting of the American Society of Cataract and Refractive Surgery, Boston).

Lidocaine was detected in the aqueous after peribulbar injection. The concentration was significantly lower when compared with intracameral use. The lidocaine concentration at 10 seconds was not significantly different from that measured at 60 seconds. If one assumes that the 2 mg of lidocaine injected into the anterior chamber only distributes within the aqueous, the theoretic concentration is 10 ug/ul. If it distributes within the entire eye the concentration would be 0.3 ug/ul. The actual concentration was 3.8 ug/ul.

The data suggest that the lidocaine in the phakic eye is distributed mainly in the aqueous compartment with relatively slow clearance through the trabecular meshwork. There also is some diffusion of the un-ionized form (~50%) into the ocular tissues.

Anesthetic agents only bind to voltage sensitive sodium channels. Thus lidocaine within the vitreous cavity may cause a reversible inhibition of the ERG. The corneal endothelium does not contain voltage sensitive sodium channels, so that there is no danger of temporary loss of vision if the lidocaine is contained within the anterior segment.

Side Effects with Topical Anesthesia and Intraocular Lidocaine

In rare instances there could be a need to convert to regional anesthesia in the event of an intraocular complication requiring substantially more operating time.

One interesting effect we have observed is that lidocaine seems to have an effect on pupil size during surgery.[8] In the controlled study, almost three times as many lidocaine cases (24% vs. 9%) maintained pupil sizes of 9 mm or more. This effect was modest due to the overwhelming effect of the epinephrine we routinely use in our irrigating solution.

Our studies have indicated that intraocular lidocaine causes no endothelial cell damage; there is no cell loss and the corneas are clear and healthy. The rabbit eye study by Kim, et al. corroborated the safety of the procedure.[12]

We have found that in rare instances (4 cases among over 15,000 performed to date), intracameral irrigation with lidocaine can, in fact, result in a limited regional block with associated transient visual loss such as that which commonly occurs during retrobulbar block. In the 4 cases we have observed, the posterior capsule has not been intact. We have hypothesized that the preservative-free lidocaine migrated posteriorly into the vitreous where it bathed the ganglion cells. There was a complete visual recovery within hours, just as when retrobulbar blocks are used. The patients were given thorough retinal exams and no damage was found. In essence, these few patients, due to the non-intact posterior capsule simply received a regional block along with the concomitant transient visual loss. Nevertheless, it is important not to assume that any visual loss occurring under topical anesthesia is related to lidocaine use. The patient must have a thorough evaluation to rule out vascular occlusion and any other complications.

Effective Approaches to Cataract Surgery

Intraocular lidocaine has greatly broadened our inclusion criteria for topical anesthesia. However a select number of patients remain who still require regional anesthesia. Each patient is carefully evaluated to determine which anesthesia is best for them. Patients receive regional anesthesia for the following reasons: hearing problems, language barrier and no interpreter, extreme anxiety, senility, and nystagmus. Currently about 95% of our patients are given topical anesthesia with intraocular lidocaine.

The use of intraocular lidocaine has completely changed our approach to cataract surgery. Our patient preparation and care has become more personalized. Topical anesthesia, even

TABLE 2-7

MEAN KOWA FLARE AND CELLS AT 10 DAYS POSTOP

	Mean (standard deviation)		
	Lidocaine	Placebo	p-value*
1-day flare	11.38 (9.51)	14.35 (11.62)	0.19
1-day cells	7.18 (1.49)	7.14 (5.41)	0.99
3-5 wk flare	7.16 (4.39)	8.46 (8.59)	0.37
3-5 wk cells	1.23 (1.88)	1.43 (2.20)	0.65

* no significant differences

when supplemented by intraocular lidocaine, is most effective when there is a good rapport between surgeon and patient. Preoperative patient counseling and education are especially important. We make a point to establish communication preoperatively and earn the patient's trust. It is important that the patient view the doctor not only as his surgeon, but as his caregiver. This gives the patient the feeling that he is in a partnership with the surgeon and they are completely dependent on each other.

It is also important to give the patient a detailed explanation of what he will see and feel during surgery. The clinical and surgical staff join me (JPG) in reassuring the patients that they will feel no discomfort whatsoever. I do explain that there may possibly be some sensation of my fingers around the eye. Patients are encouraged to alert me if they feel any sensation other than the light pressure of my fingers. I also explain that if they are aware of any pressure whatsoever during the procedure, I can irrigate the eye with "special solutions" to eliminate it. In these occasional instances, the additional dose of lidocaine brings rapid relief from the increased pressure. I have found that most patients are very cooperative and less likely to move at inopportune moments when they are thoroughly educated. This allows the patient to enter the O.R. in a totally relaxed, cooperative state of mind.

The operating room staff is able to be more relaxed and focus their energy on the patient's needs, rather than worrying about the patient's next jump. I encourage the staff to focus all conversation on the patient. The nurse anesthetist holds their hand during the entire procedure.

Specific Preoperative and Surgical Procedures

Preservative-free tetracaine is used just prior to moving the patients into the O.R. As stated above, the switch to tetracaine was made to avoid excessive administration of drops prior to surgery. We had noted that excessive topical drops

Figure 2-3. Decision-tree diagram with suggested indications for I.V. and initiation of added anesthesia (Gills).

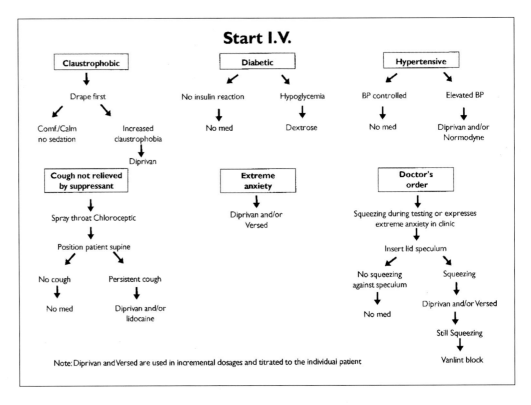

increases the rate of keratitis. The lidocaine is administered prophylactically during hydrodissection. Phacoemulsification is started after a 1-minute interval.

The duration of effect of the lidocaine is approximately 15-20 minutes. Rarely, irrigation with additional lidocaine is required later in the case if the patient has discomfort.

CHANGING SURGICAL PRACTICE PATTERNS

As ophthalmologists, we are always looking for ways to improve cataract surgery; to make it safer and more effective, while at the same time making it easier for our patients to experience. Topical anesthesia with intraocular lidocaine has an enormous impact on the roles played by patients, surgeons and surgical staff during surgery. The patient retains more control both during and after surgery and is better able to communicate and assist the surgeon and staff concerning his or her own comfort and well-being. The need for sedation is very low and can generally be predicted using good patient screening procedures. While routine intravenous access has traditionally been a standard part of cataract surgery, we have begun to re-assess its usefulness. The purpose of I.V. access is to allow for easy administration of medications which may be used during surgery such as those used in blood pressure control and sedation. It has been shown however, that receiving an I.V. creates almost as much apprehension as receiving a retrobulbar block.

We have found that there is less need for I.V. access during cataract surgery with the routine use of intracameral lido-caine and with thorough preoperative patient education. Avoiding the use of an I.V. line decreases patient anxiety and apprehension without the use of medications. This makes the procedure even easier for our patient to go through and increases the safety.

Dr. Kent Kirk has reported on the use of sublingual Versed as an alternative to I.V. sedation. This approach may be a viable alternative for many surgeons. However, we found the action of sublingual Versed to be too short to be practical in our practice.

Nevertheless, we have been able to eliminate the use of I.V.s in 90% of our cataract surgical cases. Some indications do remain for the use of I.V.s during cataract surgery. These include the very nervous patient, those with poorly controlled hypertension or diabetes, and the non-communicative patient. An I.V. is also valuable for patients with a cardiac condition who may become bradycardic with the use of sedatives. We may never totally eliminate the need for I.V. access during cataract surgery. However, limiting its use to only when it is indicated will make our patients more comfortable and ultimately more satisfied (see Figure 2-3)

Without the use of regional blocks, sedation and routine I.V. access, the role of the nurse anesthetist in cataract surgery at our facility has changed dramatically. At this time the need for the nurse anesthetist to be involved throughout the procedure is greatly changed. In this environment, the skills of the nurse anesthetist are better used for the infrequent complicated cases and for other intraocular procedures requiring blocks or general anesthesia.

SUMMARY

Since one of the authors (JPG) introduced the use of intra-cameral lidocaine as an adjunct to topical anesthesia, the use of this technique has increased rapidly. In the 1996 Leaming ASCRS survey, 52% of large-volume surgeons (>50 cases per month) were using intraocular lidocaine.[13] We believe that this technique is effective and safe and has had a great impact on postoperative outcome and patient satisfaction.

REFERENCES

1. Knapp H: On cocaine and its use in ophthalmic and general surgery. *Arch Ophthalmol* 1884; 13:402.

2. Hustead RF, Hamilton RC: Complications. In Gills JP, Hustead RF, Sanders DR, Eds, *Ophthalmic Anesthesia*, 1993; Thorofare, New Jersey, SLACK, Inc., pp 188-202.

3. Zahl K, Meltzer MA: The complications of regional anesthesia. *Ophthalmology Clinics of North America* March 1990; 111-123.

4. Fichman RA: Topical Anesthesia. In Fine IH, Fichman RA, Grabow HB, Eds, *Clear Corneal Cataract Surgery and Topical Anesthesia* 1993; Thorofare, New Jersey, SLACK, Inc., pp 97-162.

5. Blecher MH, ed: Four ways to approach topical anesthesia. *Review of Ophthalmology* 1996; 3(9):80-91.

6. Hustead RF, Hamilton RC: Technique. In Gills JP, Hustead RF, Sanders DR, Eds, *Ophthalmic Anesthesia*, Thorofare, New Jersey, SLACK, Inc., pp 166-183, 1993.

7. Gills JP, Hustead RF, Sanders DR, Eds, *Ophthalmic Anesthesia* 1993; Thorofare, New Jersey, SLACK Inc.

8. SAS® System for Windows, Release 6.11. SAS Institute Inc., Cary, NC.

9. StatMost™ Version 2.5 for Windows, DataMost Corporation. Salt Lake City, Utah.

10. Gills JP, Cherchio M, Raanan MG: The use of intraoperative unpreserved lidocaine to control discomfort during IOL surgery under topical anesthesia. *J Cataract Refract Surg* 1997; 23:527-535.

11. Dick HB, Kohnen T, Jacobi FK, Jacobi KW: Long-term endothelial cell loss following phacoemulsification through a temporal clear corneal incision. *J Cataract Refract Surg* 1996; 22(1):63-70.

12. Kim T, Lee J, Holley G, Broocker G, Edelhauser H: The effects of intraocular Xylocaine on the corneal endothelium. Poster presentation at the 1996 meeting of the American Academy of Ophthalmology, Chicago, IL.

13. Leaming DV: Practice styles and preferences of ASCRS members—1996 survey. *J Cataract Refract Surg* 1997; 23:527-535.

PHARMACODYNAMICS OF CATARACT SURGERY

James P. Gills, MD

The evolution of surgical practice has been to decrease the level of invasiveness to the body; that is, to achieve a highly specific, successful outcome with the least disruption to the patient's physical state. The goal is a minimal level of anesthesia, the absence of discomfort, minimal postoperative inflammation, and near-immediate visual recovery with no complications. As modern cataract surgical techniques have changed to achieve these goals, so has the composition of our pharmaceutical armamentarium. The goal is to use ocular pharmaceutics which are highly effective and very *specific* in their effects, thus producing minimal side effects. We also want to reduce as far as possible the length and complexity of the postoperative medication regimen. During the past few years, the main areas of change in the medication routines for cataract surgical patients have been in 1) anesthesia, 2) postoperative inflammation and early physical and visual recovery, and 3) prevention of infection.

ANESTHESIA

In the 1996 Leaming Survey of ASCRS members[1] the reported use of topical anesthesia almost doubled from 1995 to 1996. Fourteen percent of all respondents used topical anesthesia; 40% of surgeons performing more than 50 cases per month used topical anesthesia. The topical anesthetics are no longer chosen to prepare the eye for administration of regional blocks but to carry the patient throughout the procedure. Until recently we used proparacaine and bupivacaine hydrochloride (Marcaine®). The proparacaine was administered several times before the Marcaine to alleviate the stinging that the patient would feel upon instillation of the Marcaine. Usually the proparacaine had to be used at least twice (0.1%, 1 drop), 3 minutes apart. One drop of Marcaine was administered four times. It was also used repetitively throughout the procedure if the patient had any discomfort.

The use of intraocular lidocaine has been shown to be an effective adjunct to topical anesthesia.[2,3] Use of intraocular lidocaine provided a much higher level of comfort during the procedure reducing the need for repeated instillation of Marcaine (see Chapter 2). We found that the repeated instillation of topical anesthetics in the preop area led to an increase in keratitis and discomfort postoperatively.

Currently, we use preservative-free tetracaine (AK-T-CAINE™ PF, 0.5%, 1 gtt X 3) which is administered in the O.R. Instillations of drops are three minutes apart with the last dose given just before the procedure is started. This anesthetic has a very fast onset so we do not need to begin dosing the patient until just prior to the procedure. By not having to administer in the preop holding area, we have reduced the amount of topical anesthesia used, increased patient comfort, and reduced the prevalence of keratitis. The protocol for topical anesthesia is given in Table 3-1.

PROPHYLACTIC ANTIBIOTIC TREATMENT

Even with sterile surgical technique, infection can occur from many sources. In 1983, an epidemic of infectious endophthalmitis occurred which was traced back to commercially prepared balanced salt irrigating solution contaminated with *Candida parapsilosis*.[4] Prior to the manufacturer's recall, 110 of our patients were exposed.

However, none developed any sign of infection.[5] We believe our escaping this outbreak is directly due to our filtering of the irrigating solution. We had long been filtering our irrigating solution through a 0.2 micron millipore filter (Figure 3-1). Prior to our filtration, our incidence of endophthalmitis was 1-2 per 1000, which was the same as the national average. After filtration, our overall incidence dropped to 1 in 8000 to 10,000, but in a small series of 8 cases performed without filtration, we experienced a case of endophthalmitis.

TABLE 3-1

PREOPERATIVE, INTRAOPERATIVE, AND RECOVERY ROOM MEDICATIONS

Pre-Op

(exam area and again in pre-op holding area, 15 min. prior to transfer to O.R.)

Neosynephrine 10%	1 gtt x 1
Ocuflox .3%/Indocin	1 gtt x 1

Preparation: Reconstitute 1 mg of Indocin with Ocuflox. Reinject into Ocuflox bottle.

O.R.

AK-T-CAINE™PF (tetracaine)	.5% 1 gtt x 3 (3 min. apart with final gtt instilled just prior to beginning)
Betadine/BSS	1 gtt x 3 (2 gtts at the beginning of the case, 1 gtt at the end)

Preparation: Draw up 5 cc BSS followed by 5 cc of Betadine Solution 10%. Change needle to 18 g. filter needle and inject into sterile empty vial.

Ciloxan	1 gtt x 1 at case end

Intraocular Xylocaine 1%: (preservative free, without epinephrine, Astra Pharmaceuticals

0.5 ml is used prophylactically after the incision is made to minimize patient discomfort.

Irrigation Solution:

Epinephrine 1:1000
500 ml bottle BSS

Preparation:
To 500 ml bottle BSS add:
0.5 ml Epinephrine   (1:1000)

A 0.22 micron micropore filter is used to filter all irrigation solutions.
(# A5900) Surgin 1-(800) 753-7400 Tustin, CA

Post-op Anterior Chamber Injection of Indomethacin and Solucortef

Draw up 14.4 ml BSS injecting 12.4 ml into an empty sterile bottle.
Use the remaining 2 ml to reconstitute two 1 mg vials of Indomethacin.
Add both of the 1 ml vials of Indomethacin solution to the 14.4 ml bottle of BSS.
Add 8 gtts of Solucortef 125 mg/ml (8 minims using TB syringe), 0.06 Ceftazidime 50 mg/ml,
0.1 ml Vancomycin 500 mg/10 ml to the 14.4 ml bottle of Indomethacin solution.

Dosage per patient: 0.50 ml is injected into the A/C at the end of case.

Recovery Room:

Rev-Eyes	1 gtt x 1 (for topical patients)
Eserine	x 1 (for retrobulbar patients)
Polytracin ung	x 1

Ibuprofen 200 mg is given, 1 tab p.o. preoperatively and 1 tab postoperatively unless contraindicated.

Neumann et al. found particulate matter in all randomly chosen samples of BSS from seven different manufacturers with as many as 2,400 particles per millimeter.[4] Thus he has recommended filtration on all intraocular solutions, corroborating our practice.

Powe and colleagues,[6] have used a statistical pooling method to estimate the rate of endophthalmitis across a series of studies evaluating series of patients operated mainly during the eighties. They reported the pooled incidence to be 0.13% (95% confidence interval=0.09 to 0.17). Individual studies have reported rates between 0.05% and 0.5% during this time period.[7-15] The decrease in rates of endophthalmitis, when compared with levels earlier in the century (as high as 10%) and mid-century (up to 1.0%), has been attributed to better aseptic technique, smaller incisions, the switch to extracapsular surgery with an intact posterior capsule, decreased operative time, etc.[12] Nevertheless, the current average rate of 5 to 10 cases per 10,000 procedures (0.05 to 0.10%) results in perhaps one thousand to fifteen hundred cases of endophthalmitis per year in this country. While rare, this complication is associated with a high rate of ocular morbidity, often leaving the patient with severely compromised vision despite rigorous treatment. Over and above povidone iodine and other appropriate surgical prep, the value of prophylactic antibiotics administered both topically and by subconjunctival injection has been documented.[8,9,11,16] These studies show that the incidence of endophthalmitis was further reduced when both the topical and subconjunctival prophylactic measures were taken together. Clearly, the use of all available routes of prophylactic treatment should be considered.

In the mid 1980s, I initiated the use of antibiotics in the irrigating solution[5]. My protocol at that time was to use gentamicin sulfate (Garamycin®) solution (0.008 g/cc) filtered through a 0.2 micron millipore filter. During this period I modified the antibiotic protocol by adding Vancomycin® (0.1 cc at 100 mg/cc in each 500 cc bottle of BSS) to provide protection against gram positive bacteria which are the most prevalent organisms cultured in endophthalmitis cases (75% to 90% of positive cultures).[17,18] In a series of 27,000 cases of planned extra-caps with limbal-based flaps using filtered solution with antibiotic, we had no incidence of endophthalmitis[5]. Sterile hypopyons, which had been prevalent at a rate of one per 400 before the use of antibiotics, no longer occurred.[19] The positive effect of the antibiotic use combined with filtering of the infusate caused me to conclude that some transient hypopyons may be a form of mild infection. Currently our rate of endophthalmitis is less than one in every 10,000 cases. Thus we have reduced our rate to about a tenth of what it had been by use of the prophylactic treatment. We have had no safety problems with this procedure, and have seen no retinal toxicity.

In the 1996 Learning Survey of ASCRS members,[1] 41% of all respondents reported using antibiotics in the irrigating solution. Seventy-seven percent of respondents performing more than 50 cases per months reported using this method of prophylaxis.

Nevertheless, there is controversy as to whether the use of antibiotics in the infusion bottle or injected into the eye at the end of the case is appropriate.[20-22] Critics point out that there have been no prospective randomized clinical trials reported which show a statistically significant decrease in the rate of infection in the treated group. While that is certainly true, it is quite difficult to evaluate treatment or prophylactic modalities for very low-incidence complications.

However, there have been other reports of surgeons experiencing decreases in the rate of endophthalmitis after initiating prophylactic intraocular antibiotic treatment. Manus Kraff, MD began using antibiotics in the irrigation bottle in May of 1988 (presented at the summer ASCRS meeting, July 1993). He determined the respective rates of endophthalmitis among 2 series of patients (see Figure 3-2). The first series consisted of 3500 cases operated on between 1983 through April of 1988 and the second series consisted of 3600 cases operated on between May of 1988 (when he began intraocular antibiotics) and April of 1993. The rate of endophthalmitis before adding antibiotics to the irrigating fluid was 3.14 per thousand (9/3500). After adding antibiotics, no cases of endophthalmitis were seen among 3600 cases.

Masket reported the results of an endophthalmitis survey sponsored by the ASCRS.[23] Almost 19% of survey respondents

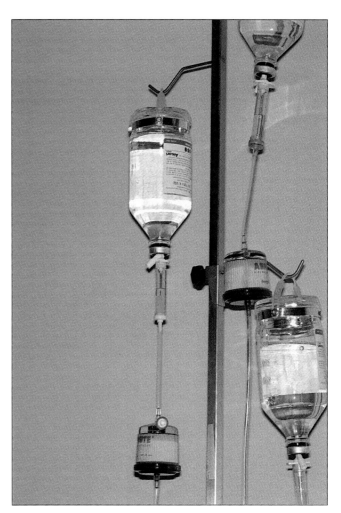

Figure 3-1. The use of a 0.22 micron micropore filter as a prophylactic measure against postoperative endophthalmitis.

reported having at least one case of culture-proven endophthalmitis during the previous year. The survey evaluation compared reported rates of endophthalmitis with various reported preventive practices and suggested a reduced likelihood of infection with the use of antibiotics in the irrigation fluid.

Another criticism of this method of endophthalmitis prevention is that widespread use of potent antibiotics (such as Vancomycin) could result in antibiotic-resistant bacterial strains unresponsive to treatment.[20-22] The Centers for Disease Control has discouraged general prophylactic use of Vancomycin[24]. Those recommendations were not specific to ophthalmic surgery, but were formulated based on the fact that resistant strains have developed in response to repeated systemic prophylactic use in hospital settings. Freeman and Freeman point out that in modern cataract surgery, this model of antibiotic resistance does not apply.[25] Very small total doses (3-4 mg) of Vancomycin are injected into a normally sterile compartment, which provides added protection against

Figure 3-2. Rates of endophthalmitis (per 10,000 cases) before and after changing surgical technique by adding antibiotics to the irrigation solution (courtesy of Manus C. Kraff, MD).

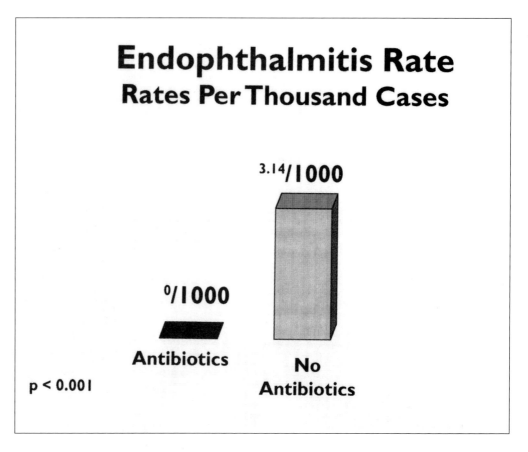

inoculation with a virulent organism. The antibiotic remains for a limited time, certainly not long enough to provide repeated selective pressure over many generations of bacterial replication.

A final criticism is that the use of Vancomycin prophylactically does not guarantee that there will be no cases of endophthalmitis.[21,22] This reasoning implies that the "benefit" must be *absolute* prevention to offset the "risk" of creating a resistant strain of bacteria. It has been shown in a randomized experiment that use of antibiotics in the irrigation solution decreased the likelihood of a positive postoperative aqueous culture.[26] In fact, the benefit of decreasing the rate of endophthalmitis far outweighs the very small risk of developing a resistant strain of bacteria through the use of intraocular antibiotics. The other risk critics point out is that of retinal toxicity.[21,22] Interestingly, the reason given is that clinical staff is likely to make mistakes when preparing the infusate, causing a toxic dose level. In fact, very low doses are used. The volume of irrigation fluid used may vary but the total dose load has a safe upper limit. As with all clinical/surgical practice, appropriate quality control of pharmaceutical preparation and dispensation is warranted.

My current preoperative, intraoperative and recovery room antibiotic regimens are presented in Table 3-1. Prior to transfer to the O.R., patients receive Ocuflox 0.3%/Indocin (1 gtt X1). During surgery the irrigation fluid is filtered through a 0.22 micrometer micropore filter (Figure 3-1). At this time,

rather than adding antibiotics to the irrigation solution, they are injected into the anterior chamber at the end of the procedure. I use Vancomycin and Cephtazidine prepared and administered as indicated in Table 3-1. I did use Amikacin, which also provides coverage for gram-negative bacteria. However, since Amikacin is an aminoglycoside, there is more risk of retinal damage should a dosing error occur. For this reason I changed to Cephtazidine, which also provides coverage for gram-negative bacteria while increasing safety. This regimen provides widespread coverage against endophthalmitis. Administering the antibiotics at the end of the case adds another measure of control over the total dose received by the patient. It should be noted here that in doses higher than those described in Table 3-1, Vancomycin and Cephtazidine would interact and precipitate out of solution. We have no problems with the minute concentrations used for intraocular injection.

At the beginning and the end of the case we also administer topical Betadine® drops, which is especially important during the early postoperative hours when the IOP is more likely to be low. Betadine eliminates flora in the cul-de-sac so they cannot enter the soft eyes that may occur within the first hour after surgery.[12,13] During this critical period it is important to make sure that the eye is clear and clean. We routinely instill polytracin ointment rather than antibiotic drops to increase the contact time of the medication to the cornea.

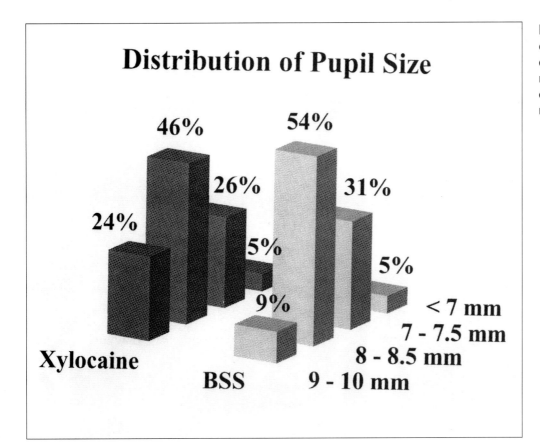

Figure 3-3. The distribution of intraoperative pupil diameters among patients receiving intraocular lidocaine and control patients receiving BSS.

INFLAMMATION CONTROL – THE ROLE OF NSAIDS

Over the last decade the use of non-steroidal anti-inflammatory agents has become highly effective in reducing inflammation and the incidence of postoperative cystoid macular edema (CME).[27-33] We do not need to rely on a heavy regimen of steroid treatment. We administer indocin prior to surgery (see Table 3-1 for dosage). Indocin has been specifically shown to be highly effective in preventing CME[27-30] and in controlling postoperative inflammation.[31] We had used NSAIDs additionally at the end of surgery to prevent the incidence of CME and because the administered dose will remain in the eye a long time. We discovered through KOWA cell/flare studies that although the NSAIDs administered preoperatively are only in the eye one minute before beginning phacoemulsification, the addition of postoperative NSAIDs is not needed.

The other indication for use of NSAIDs is to prevent miosis during surgery. Indomethacin, as well as a number of other NSAIDs have been shown to enhance mydriasis but not all are specifically indicated for this purpose.[34-36] Epinephrine has been shown to be safe and highly effective[34] for this indication. However, I have found that the use of intraocular lidocaine to eliminate intraoperative discomfort has the added benefit of enhancing mydriasis.[2] In a study comparing patients receiving intraocular lidocaine with a control group, 24% of lidocaine-treated patients maintained pupil sizes at 9-

10 mm versus 9% of BSS controls (see Figure 3-3). This mydriatic effect of a topical anesthetic was present in the early days when cocaine was the routinely used anesthetic. Enhancement of mydriais has also been demonstrated for chloroprocaine using animal models (personal communication, Donald Sanders, MD, PhD).

Postoperative regimen for inflammation control is shown in Table 3-1. At the end of the procedure in the intracameral antibiotic injection, the patient receives indomethacin and Solucortef. Voltaren® is administered for two weeks (1 gtt 4X). While I will also use Acular®, I prefer Voltaren for inflammation control and prevention of CME. I also prescribe Pred Forte gradually tapered over eight weeks.

POSTOPERATIVE COMFORT AND EARLY VISUAL RECOVERY

Small sutureless cataract surgery combined with topical anesthesia (facilitated by the use of intraocular lidocaine) results in a very fast visual recovery. Patients may be refracted the next day or even the same day and also usually achieve their optimal vision this early. Refractions and visions are always stable by two weeks postop. Crisp same-day visions are very important to the patient. Same-day refractions are especially important in cases requiring unusual powers (see Chapter 14) or in post-refractive surgery patients to ensure that appropriate power has been implanted.

Figure 3-4. The percentages of patients experiencing burning before and 2 hours after instillation of Voltaren drops, Acular drops, or commercial tears.

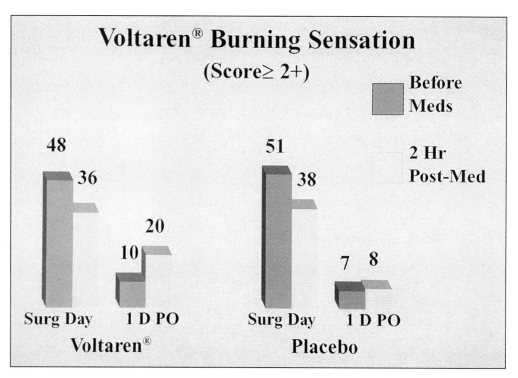

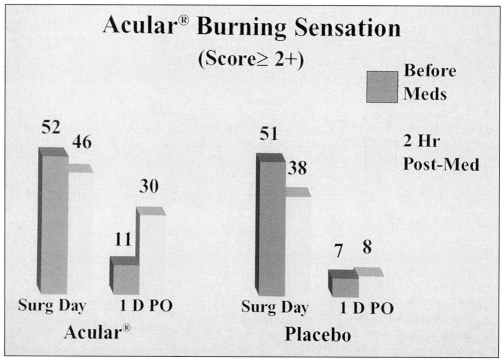

To provide good early postoperative vision, I occasionally administer Rev-Eyes® for most patients (1 gtt). For the few patients requiring regional anesthesia, Eserine is used (1 gtt). Formerly I used Carbochol to induce miosis after surgery. Over half of larger volume cataract surgeons (over 50 cases per month) use carbochol[1]. However, this drug is associated with early postoperative brow-ache, so I do not use it routinely.

Voltaren has been shown to be an effective corneal anesthetic.[37] NSAIDs are routinely used to control discomfort following photorefractive keratectomy.[38,39] To evaluate the possible role of NSAIDs in postoperative comfort among cataract patients we conducted a randomized 3-group study. In this study 274 patients scheduled for phacoemulsification procedures under topical anesthesia were randomized to receive Voltaren, Acular, or a BSS-based vehicle during the postoperative period. The dosages were equivalent (1 gtt QID for one week). Patients also received Pred Forte 1%, 8 X per day for 10 days then tapered over the next 2-week period. Patients completed day-of-surgery and one-day-postop diaries assessing several comfort attributes before and after dosing with the study medication.

About half of all patients experienced some level of burning, scratching, or aching upon arrival home. However, by the next morning 10% or less of all patients reported any symptoms before dosing with medications. We found that on the day of surgery both NSAIDs were equally effective in alleviating burning and scratchiness (in about 20%-25% of patients who had reported the symptoms). They were not as effective in alleviating achiness (probably brow ache associated with the administration of carbochol at the end of surgery during the time of the study).

However, on the next day after surgery, both NSAIDs actually increased burning sensations as long as two hours after instillation of the drops (Figure 3-4). Voltaren was associated with somewhat less burning upon instillation than was Acular, which is one reason I prefer Voltaren. Outright postoperative pain was reported only by about 1% of cases and among these the severity was mild. In general, postoperative discomfort is minimal for cataract patients and near-immediate visual and physical recovery are the norm.

SUMMARY

Modern micro-surgical techniques combined with topical anesthesia, intraocular lidocaine and efficient medication regimens provide the patient with a highly comfortable experience. We've reduced the length and complexity of the postoperative medication regimen. Rigorous prophylactic measures protect against endophthalmitis and optimize safety.

REFERENCES

1. Leaming DV: Practice styles and preferences of ASCRS members—1996 survey. *J Cataract Refract Surg* 1997; 23:527-535.

2. Gills JP, Cherchio M, Raanan MG: Unpreserved lidocaine to control discomfort during cataract surgery using topical anesthesia. *J Cataract Refract Surg* 1997; 23:545-550.

3. Koch PS: Anterior chamber irrigation with unpreserved lidocaine 1% for anesthesia during cataract surgery. *J Cataract Refract Surg* 1997; 23:551-554.

4. Neumann AC, Dzelzkalns JJ, Bessinger DJ: Endophthalmitis investigative protocol: A plan for source identification and patient protection. *J Cataract Refract Surg* 1991; 17:353-358.

5. Gills JP: Prevention of endophthalmitis by intraocular solution filtration and antibiotics. *J Am Intraocul Implant Soc* 1985;11(2):185-186.

6. Powe NR, Schein OD, Gieser SC, et al: Synthesis of the literature on visual acuity and complications following cataract extraction with intraocular lens implantation. *Arch Ophthalmol* 1994;112:239-252.

7. Stark WJ, Worthen DM, Holladay JT, et al: The FDA report on intraocular lenses. *Ophthalmology* 1983;90:311-317.

8. Christy NE, Lall P: A randomized controlled comparison of anterior and posterior periocular injection of antibiotic in the prevention of postoperative endophthalmitis. *Ophthalmic Surg* 1986;17:715-718.

9. Christy NE, Lall P: Postoperative endophthalmitis following cataract surgery: Effects of subconjunctival antibiotics and other factors. *Arch Ophthalmol* 1973;90:361-366.

10. Allen HF, Mangiaracine AB: Bacterial endophthalmitis after cataract extraction: A study of 22 infections in 20,000 operations. *Arch Ophthalmol* 1964;72:454-462.

11. Allen HF, Mangiaracine AB: Bacterial endophthalmitis after cataract extraction. II. Incidence in 36,000 consecutive operations with special reference to preoperative topical antibiotics. *Arch Ophthalmol* 1974;91:3-7.

12. Novak MA, Rice TA: The realities of endophthalmitis. In Weinstock FJ, ed, *Management and Care of the Cataract Patient* 1992; Blackwell Scientific Publications Inc., Cambridge, MA, pp 238-262.

13. Mamalis N: Postcataract inflammation and endophthalmitis: Diagnosis, prevention, and management. In: *Management and care of the cataract patient*. In Weinstock FJ, ed, *Management and Care of the Cataract Patient* 1992; Blackwell Scientific Publications Inc., Cambridge, MA, pp 222-237.

14. Kattan HM, Flynn HW, Pflugfelder SC, et al: Nosocomial endophthalmitis survey-current incidence of infection after intraocular surgery. *Ophthalmology* 1991;98:227-238.

15. Javitt JC, Vitale S, Canner JK: National outcomes of cataract extraction-endophthalmitis following inpatient surgery. *Arch Ophthalmol* 1991;109:1085-1089.

16. Christy NE, Sommer A: Antibiotic prophylaxis of postoperative endophthalmitis. *Ann Ophthalmol* 1979;11:1261-1265.

17. Gills JP: Antibiotics in irrigating solutions [letter]. *J Cataract and Refract Surg* 1987;13(3):344.

18. Gills JP: Filters and antibiotics in irrigating solution for cataract surgery [letter]. *J Cataract and Refract Surg* 1991;17(3):385.

19. Gills JP: Sterile hypopyon. *J Cataract Refract Surg* 1992;18(2):203.

20. Alfonso EC, Flynn HW: Controversies in endophthalmitis prevention. *Arch Ophthalmol*. 1995; 113 (11):1369-1370.

21. Donnenfeld E. Should we use antibiotics in the infusion bottle? No. They're ineffective and dangerous. In: *Point-Counterpoint. Review of Ophthalmology*. April 1997; Chilton Publications, Radner, PA.

22. Fiscella RG: Vancomycin use in ophthalmology [letter]. *Arch Ophthalmol* 1995;113(11):353-354.

23. Masket S: ASCRS endophthalmitis survey. Presented at the 1997 annual meeting of the ASCRS, Boston, MA.

24. Hospital Infection Control Practices Advisory Committee: Recommendations for preventing the spread of vancomycin resistance. *Infect Control Hosp Epidemiol*. 1995;16(2);105-113.

25. Freeman J, Freeman J: Should we use antibiotics in the infusion bottle? Yes. It is best to cover our bases. In: *Point-Counterpoint. Review of Ophthalmology*. April 1997; Chilton Publications, Radner, PA.

26. Ferro JF, de-Pablos M, Logrono MJ, et al.: Postoperative contamination after using Vancomycin and Gentamicin during phacoemulsification. *Arch Ophthalmol* 1997;115:165-170.

27. Kraff MC, Sanders DR, Jampol LM, et al.: Prophylaxis of

pseudophakic cystoid macular edema with topical indomethacin. *Ophthalmology* 1982;89:885-890.

28. Flach AJ, Stegman RC, Graham J, Kruger LP: Prophylaxis of aphakic cystoid macular edema without corticosteroids: A paired comparison. *Ophthalmology* 1990;97:1253-1258.

29. Miyake K, Sakamura S, Miura H: Longterm follow-up study on the prevention of aphakic cystoid macular oedema by topical indomethacin. *Br J Ophthalmol* 1980;64:324-328.

30. Yannuzi LA, Landau AN, Turtz AI: Incidence of aphakic cystoid macular edema with the use of topical indomethacin. *Ophthalmology* 1981;88:947-854.

31. Sanders DR, Kraff M: Steroidal and non-steroidal anti-inflammatory agents: Effect on post-surgical inflammation and blood aqueous humor barrier breakdown. *Arch Ophthalmol* 1984;102:1453-1456.

32. Kraff MC, Sanders DR, McGuigan L, Raanan MG: Inhibition of blood aqueous humor barrier breakdown with diclofenac: A fluorophotometric study. *Arch Ophthalmol* 1990;108:380-383.

33. Flach AJ, Kraff MC, Sanders DR, Tannenbaum L: The quantitative effect of 0.5% ketorolac tromethamine solution and 0.1% dexamethasone sodium phosphate solution on postsurgical blood-aqueous barrier. *Arch Ophthalmol* 1988;106:480-483.

34. Gimbel HV: The effect of treatment with topical nonsteroidal anti-inflammatory drugs with and without epinephrine on the maintenance of mydriasis during cataract surgery. *Ophthalmology* 1989;97:585-588.

35. Keates RH, McGowan KA: The effect of topical indomethacin ophthalmic solution in maintaining mydriasis during cataract surgery. *Ann Ophthalmol* 1984;16:1116-1121.

36. Keates RH, McGowan KA: Clinical trial of flurbiprofen to maintain pupillary dilation during cataract surgery. *Ann Ophthalmol* 1984;16:919-921.

37. Sun R, Gimbel HV: Effects of topical ketorolac and diclofenac on normal corneal sensation. *J Refract Surg* 1997;13:158-161.

38. Epstein RL, Laurence EP: Relative effectiveness of topical ketorolac and topical diclofenac on discomfort after radial keratotomy. *J Cataract Refract Surg* 1997;21:156-159.

39. Eiferman RA, Hoffman RS, Sher NA: Topical diclofenac reduces pain following photorefractive keratectomy. *Arch Ophthalmol* 1993;111:1022.

ADVANCED CATARACT INCISIONS

Harry B. Grabow, MD, James P. Gills, MD,
John R. Fish, MD, Michelle Van Der Karr

Only ten years ago the majority of cataract surgeries were by extracapsular extraction through 12 to 14-mm wounds. The advent of foldable lens technology and the increasing popularity of phacoemulsification spurred an interest in reducing the often visually disabling iatrogenic astigmatism caused by cataract incisions. In just a decade, we have seen the evolution of cataract surgery to today's sutureless, minimally invasive, micro incisions with little or no clinically relevant induced astigmatism.

THE SUTURELESS REVOLUTION

In an attempt to further reduce induced astigmatism of small (3-4 mm) incisions, Dr. Sam Masket introduced the scleral tunnel pocket incision.[1] Dr. Mike McFarland noticed that the architecture of this wound created a valve and actually allowed it to seal itself.[2] By eliminating stitches, the tissues have better apposition as they are not distorted by tension from the sutures. The resulting incision is stronger with less irregular induced astigmatism. In 1992, Fine[3] introduced the clear-corneal incision, which was originally described as a stab incision temporally located in avascular tissue. Since then, many modifications and variations have been developed, encompassing a wide variety of sutureless incisions.

INCISION TECHNOLOGY

The design of modern sutureless, self-sealing cataract incisions involves the consideration of three design parameters: site, size and shape.

Incision Site

The location of cataract incisions may be categorized according to two geometric classifications. The first classification relates to location on the imaginary circle that we commonly use to describe the corneal circumference, which would locate an incision at a certain "axis". The second relates to the distance along a radius of that circle, which would locate a corneal incision at a certain "optical zone" and a scleral incision at a certain millimeter distance from the limbus.

In the first classification, the incision is usually described as located at one of four possible sites on the corneal circle: superiorly, obliquely, temporally, or on steep axis. The superior location is still the most common site used, being the most familiar to the majority of the current generation of cataract surgeons. Superiorly located incisions, when not under the influence of sutures, are known to have an against-the-rule astigmatic effect, greater with longer incisions, due to the effects of gravity and/or lid closure on wound gape.

The oblique location, whether nasal or temporal, is espoused by some who prefer this site not only for ergonomic advantage, but also for greater wound stability when compared to superior incisions. These wounds are believed by some to be the only ones not affected by transmitted tractional forces of a rectus muscle, a theory yet to be documented.

The temporal location has been shown to be the most astigmatically stable of these three locations,[4] achieving stability almost immediately and maintaining stability for life or until further astigmatic intervention. First, the temporal location is farthest from the visual axis, and so there will be less impact on the corneal curvature at the visual axis. Second, the wound is parallel to the effects of both lid blink and gravity. The temporal location has an added advantage in that it provides the easiest anatomic access to the surgical site, being unimpeded by the bony orbital rim.

On-axis surgery is the most recent option available in our pre-surgical planning armamentarium. On-axis cataract incisions for correcting pre-existing astigmatism will be discussed in Chapter 5.

The second classification of location involves the radial distance from the optic axis. These locations for cataract incisions

Figure 4-1. Schematic of SLiC incision (Gills).

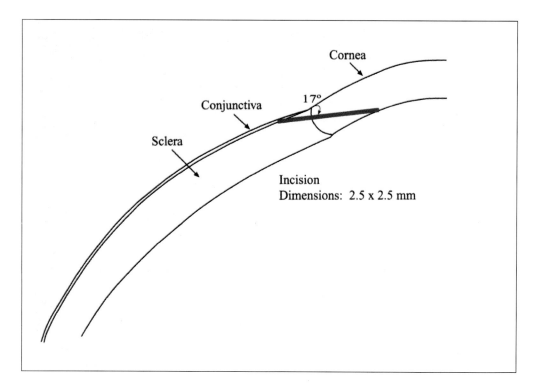

have traditionally been designated by their anatomic location: the sclera, the cornea, and the junction of these two—the limbus. Scleral incisions, being farthest from the optic axis, when compared to corneal and limbal incisions of equal dimension, have less effect on both corneal astigmatism and the corneal endothelium, and the same is true for peripheral corneal incisions compared to more central corneal incisions.

The external entry incision for small, self-sealing sclerocorneal incisions as originally described was made 3.0 to 4.0 mm posterior to the limbus. The distance from the limbus has become progressively less as surgeons have mastered creating the self-sealing internal corneal lip. Most now are comfortable about 1.5 mm posterior to the limbus, giving a total sclerocorneal tunnel length of approximately 2.5 to 3.0 mm.

The clear-corneal incision is made just anterior to the limbus. More recently, the "near-clear" incision has been introduced, which is moved back from clear cornea to the limbus.

Gills Scleral/Limbal/Corneal (SLiC) Incision

The SLiC (scleral/limbal/corneal), or scleral-corneal stab, incision was designed to provide the advantages of the scleral incision with the advantages of the corneal incisions, with the disadvantages of neither. The advantages of this technique are:

1. It can be safely enlarged to accommodate PMMA lenses, such as the Array Multifocal IOL
2. The conjunctiva covers the incision, providing added safety and comfort for the patient. The chance of late infection appears rare, which is a particularly important advantage of clear-corneal incisions
3. The incision is nearly invisible on the first postoperative day

4. It does not cause corneal edema and/or compromise corneal integrity
5. The location of the incision adds to its self-sealing nature, and it seals better than other incisions
6. The entrance is posterior enough so that the cornea is not affected, but anterior enough to avoid iris prolapse.

This incision may be an excellent transitional technique for the beginning surgeon who is still learning phacoemulsification. Conversely, it is also excellent for the experienced surgeon who simply requires a larger incision for the new multifocal IOL technology, but is not willing to give up the advantages of the clear-corneal incision.

The scleral-corneal stab cannot be combined with a limbal relaxing incision. Therefore, patients having against-the-rule astigmatism receive a modified Langerman Hinge (described below) combined with an LRI. With-the-rule cases may have a scleral-corneal stab since the incision is not in the same meridian as the LRI. The SLiC is also used for patients who do not require astigmatic keratotomy.

The design of the incision is very important. The incision is basically a corneal incision that is partly scleral (Figure 4-1). The most important part of any wound architecture is the inner aspect which forms the seal. The outer aspect is not as important. There should be a straight line across the cornea where the keratome enters, which can be tested by checking to make sure that the IOP remains stable, not intraoperatively, but twenty minutes after surgery. We have found that there may be hypotony in the early postoperative period, and then a return to normal IOP within several hours.

The incision may be made with the Rhein diamond 3D blade (Figure 4-2) or a similar disposable model (Figure 4-3).

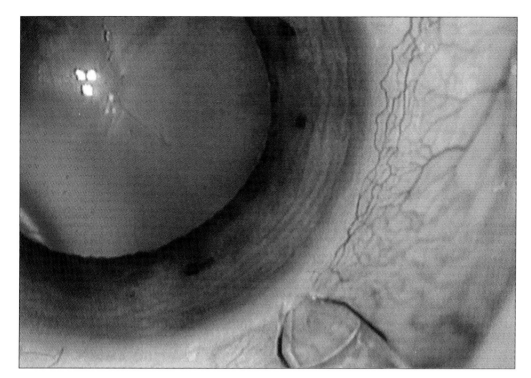

Figure 4-2a. Creating the SLiC incision with the Rhein 3-D diamond blade (Gills). (A) The incision begins about 0.5 mm posterior to the limbus, catching some conjunctiva. (B) The blade is kept flat as it enters. (C) Keep a 17° angle of incidence between the keratome and the endothelium. (D&E) Advancing the keratome into the anterior chamber. (F) The SLiC incision is covered by conjunctiva and is usually invisible by the first postoperative day.

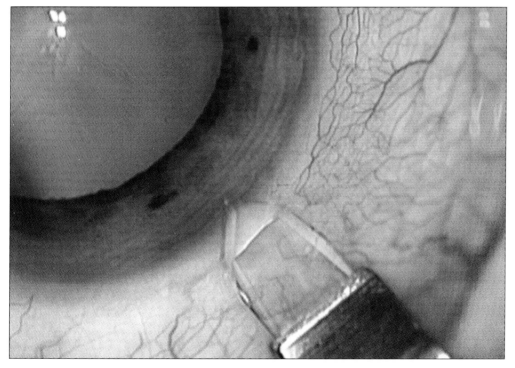

Figure 4-2b.

This incision is difficult to make with the previous diamond keratomes because they can cut the edges of the incision. The incision begins 0.5 to 1 mm posterior to the limbus, catching the conjunctiva, going into the limbus, then through clear cornea. It is important to avoid Tenon's capsule, which is located approximately 2 mm posterior to the limbus. If Tenon's capsule is cut, swelling of the conjunctiva will result (Figure 4-4). Keep the knife flat so the sides enter in the same plane.

Point the blade toward the dome of the cornea as soon as the arms of the keratome are in. As you begin to enter the anterior chamber, pull back slightly and then enter. A 17° angle of incidence is desired between the keratome and the endothelium to produce a firm inner seal. This technique produces a perfectly square incision as described by Dr. Paul Ernest.[5]

As mentioned above, conjunctival swelling may occasionally occur if the incision is made too posterior to the limbus.

Figure 4-2c.

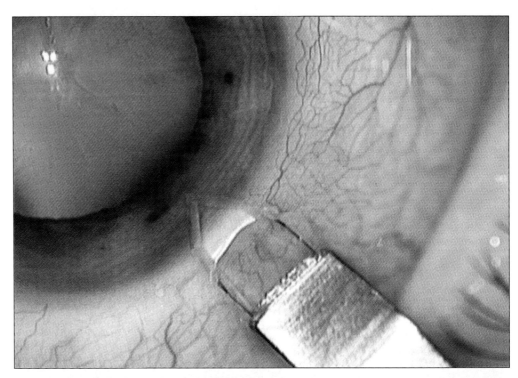

Figure 4-2d.

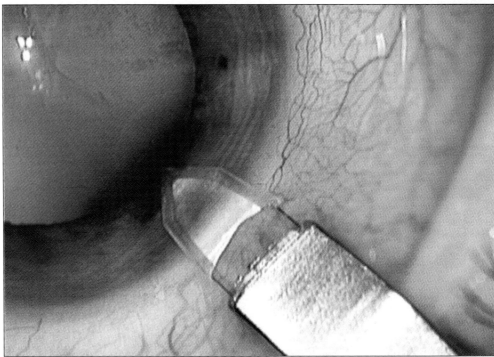

It usually disappears within a few minutes and rarely causes problems for the surgeon. If using a phaco tip with a tight seal, it is more controllable and does not usually become as significant. Rarely is there swelling to the point of "kissing conjunctiva", which greatly reduces the red reflex. A small cut in the conjunctiva and Tenon's allows the fluid to dissipate and keeps the swelling from worsening. Another technique to reduce the conjunctival swelling is to "rock" the eye back and forth until the visualization improves.

Paul Koch, M.D. points out that the bleb produced from the swelling may actually prove beneficial. He found that he never had a case of endophthalmitis when he had swelling of the conjunctiva during surgery (personal communication). The bleb may reduce the risk of infection in two ways:

1) by physically protecting the incision from opening, and
2) by filling with steroids and antibiotics.

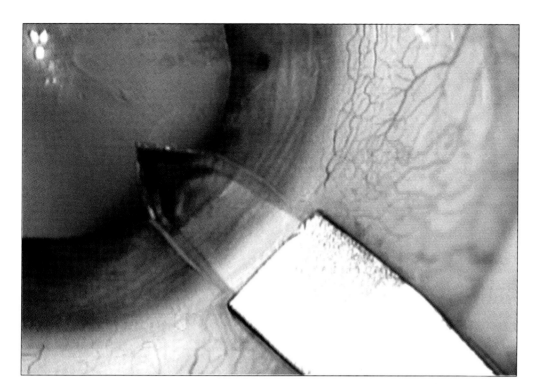

Figure 4-2e.

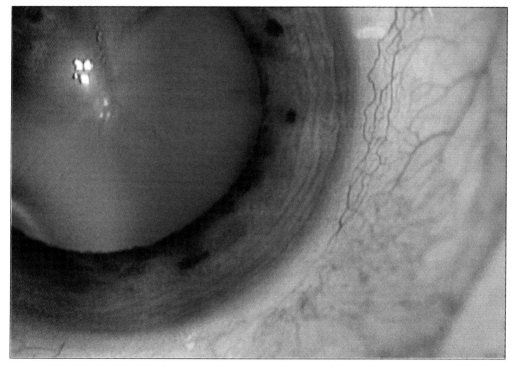

Figure 4-2f.

Fish Mini-Flap Limbal Corneal Incision

The mini-flap limbal-corneal incision is started 0.5 mm posterior to the clear cornea. It is made 2.8 mm wide and the limbal-corneal tunnel enters the anterior chamber 2.3 mm after entering clear cornea, creating a square 2.8 x 2.8 mm wound (Figure 4-5). Since the wound is more posterior, beginning in vascularized limbal tissue, the wound heals more rapidly and is stronger than a corneal wound.[6] At the end of the case, the external wound margin is covered by a mini conjunctival flap which protects the wound postoperatively.

Creation of the mini-flap corneal wound is begun by fabricating a two-snip conjunctival mini-flap at the temporal limbus. This flap is actually a 3 mm wide peritomy. No undermining of the tissue is done, and a bipolar cautery is used to achieve a bloodless field. A ceramic blade is used to score the limbus 0.5 mm behind clear cornea 2.8 mm wide. A 2.8-mm

Figure 4-3a. The same technique can be applied when making the SLiC incision with a disposable blade (Gills).

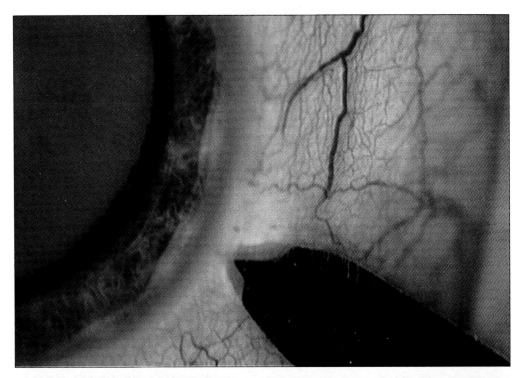

Figure 4-3b.

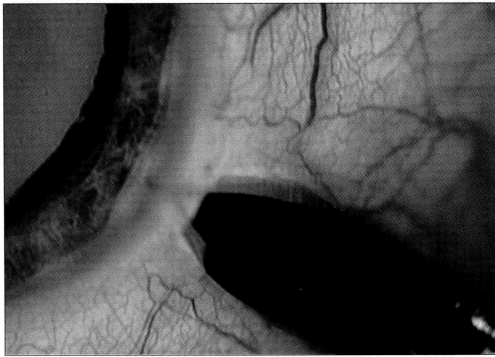

keratome is then used to fashion a mini-scleral tunnel 0.5 mm in length, the full width of the scored area, to prevent tearing the sides of the wound during creation of the tunnel.

The keratome is then advanced into clear cornea 2.3 mm before entering the anterior chamber through Descemet's. After the implantation of the IOL, the wound is self sealing and can be left unsutured. However, if the surgeon suspects a leak on wound manipulation or simply wants to close the wound, a 10-0 Vicryl suture can be placed horizontally starting the suture through the floor of the wound on the right, coming through the surface on the left side, and entering back through the roof on the right to bury the knot. The conjunctival flap is then cauterized into place over the wound margin.

Incision Size

The size of incisions, referring to their length along an arc

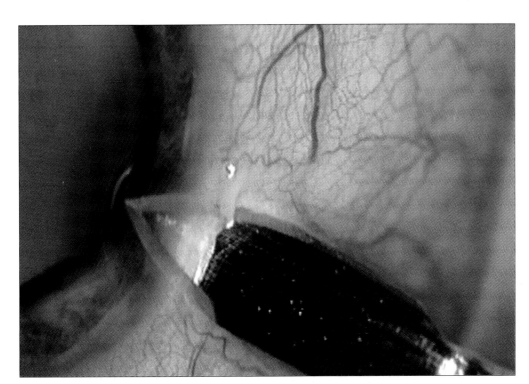

Figure 4-3c.

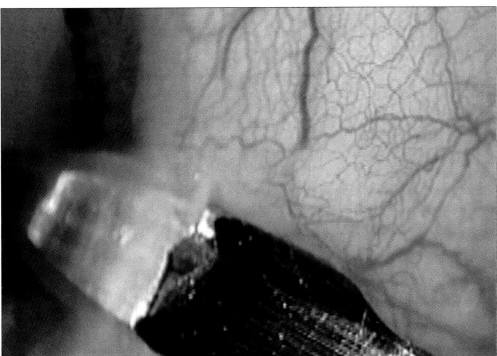

Figure 4-3d.

of the imaginary corneal-limbal circle, is another critical factor determining the astigmatic outcome. Self-sealing sclerocorneal incisions have been safely made up to 8 mm in length without sutures, and clear-corneal incisions up to 5 mm in length, for insertion of PMMA IOLs, but not without significant astigmatic effect. Early attempts at unsutured temporal clear-corneal incisions up to 6 mm in length resulted in as much as 5 D of induced astigmatism. Moreover, unsutured superiorly placed clear-corneal incisions greater than 5 mm in length demonstrated a decrease in wound integrity resulting in a transient increase in the incidence of early postoperative infectious endophthalmitis.

Paul Ernest subsequently demonstrated in cadaver eye studies that a short clear-corneal incision whose limbal length more closely approximated its intracorneal tunnel length, tending toward a square incisional configuration, was signif-

Figure 4-3e.

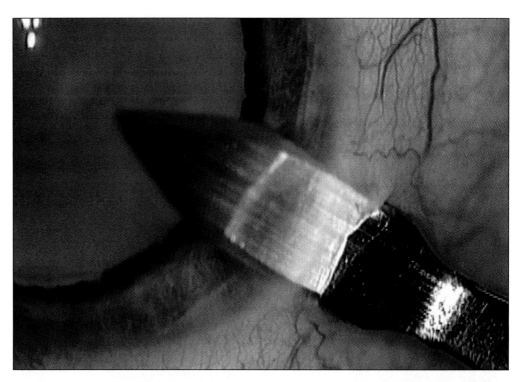

Figure 4-4. Note conjunctival swelling with SLiC incision (Gills).

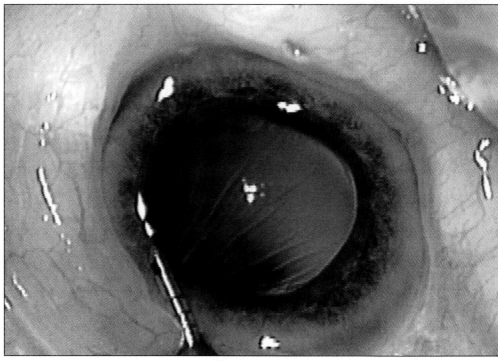

icantly more resistant to external pressure than incisions with limbal lengths greater than their intracorneal lengths.[5] Sclerocorneal incisions have both a scleral tunnel portion and a corneal tunnel portion, the combination of which produces a tunnel that is almost always longer and stronger than pure corneal incisions. For sclerocorneal incisions with limbal lengths of 4 mm or less, the intracorneal tunnel should be no less than 1 mm, regardless of the intrascleral tunnel length.

Clear-corneal incisions, on the other hand, can be considered to be only the intracorneal portion of a sclerocorneal tunnel incision. For safety, therefore, clear-corneal tunnels should be no less than 1.5 mm in length. Using tunnels less than 1.5 mm may risk wound leak. Tunnels greater than 2 mm are not only unnecessary for self-sealability, but also create unwanted corneal striae during wound instrumentation, distorting the surgeon's clear view and causing instrument

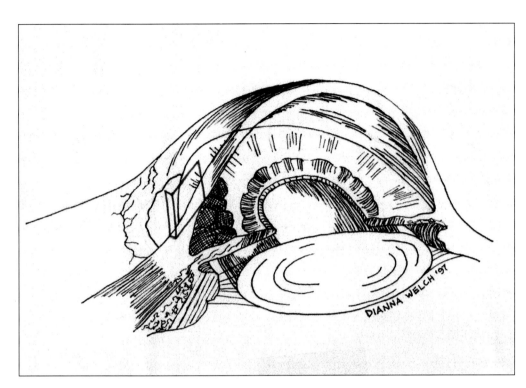

Figure 4-5. Mini-flap limbal-corneal incision. (Fish)

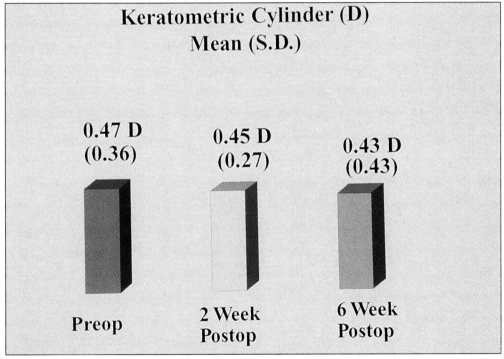

Keratometric Cylinder (D)
Mean (S.D.)

0.47 D
(0.36)

0.45 D
(0.27)

0.43 D
(0.43)

Preop

2 Week
Postop

6 Week
Postop

Figure 4-6. Mean keratometric cylinder power preoperatively and at 2 and 6 weeks postoperatively in a series of 78 cases receiving 2.4-2.5 mm clear-corneal incisions in the horizontal axis. Standard deviations are given in parentheses. (Gills)

"oarlock", reducing intraocular maneuverability. In addition, the more central the internal opening in the anterior chamber, the closer to the cornea is the tip of the phacoemulsifier, increasing the potential for greater endothelial cell loss. The ideal intracorneal tunnel length, therefore, may be 1.75 mm, and for purposes of phacoemulsification and foldable lens implantation by today's technology, the limbal length dimension need not be any longer than 2.8 mm. It is the current practice of this author (HBG) to perform an incision measuring 2.7 mm by 1.5 mm for routine cases and to suture corneal incisions with limbal lengths greater than 4 mm.

Micro Incisions

One of the advantages of the clear-corneal incision technique is the ability to insert the foldable IOL through a smaller wound than is possible with scleral-tunnel incisions. When

Figure 4-7. Mean refractive cylinder power preoperatively and at 2 and 6 weeks postoperatively in a series of 78 cases receiving 2.4-2.5 mm clearcorneal incisions in the horizontal axis. Standard deviations are given in parentheses. (Gills)

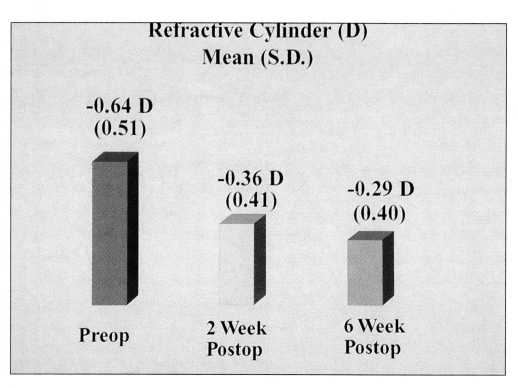

Figure 4-8. Histogram showing the distribution of keratometric cylinder power 6 weeks postoperatively in a series of 78 cases receiving 2.4-2.5 mm clear-corneal incisions in the horizontal axis. (Gills)

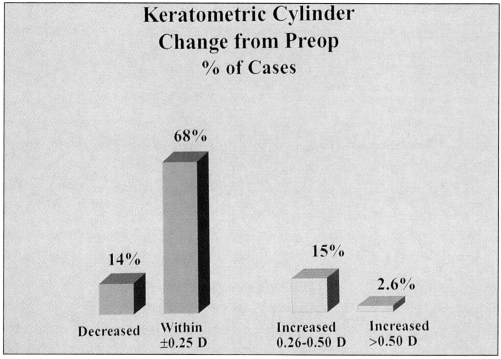

clear-corneal incisions were in their infancy, Chuck Williamson, MD, and many others were saying that the incision should be larger on the outside than the inside, which would allow the injector to fit more easily in the incision without stretching the sclera. The ultimate goal is to have no tissue stretch. The trapezoid incisions that Dr. Williamson describes are about 0.5 mm wider on the outside than the inside. If the difference between the inner and outer aspects of the incision is kept minimal, the injector can be only partially inserted.

The concept of decreasing tissue stretch has been taken one step further by modifying the injector cartridge. Inserting the injector partially into the incision allows for an even smaller incision. By adapting technique and hand position, and assistance, a 2.2-2.6 mm incision can be obtained. Implantation should be done with gentle pressure on the

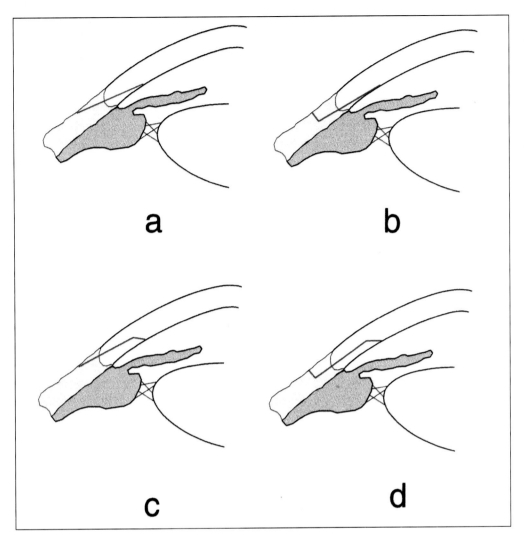

Figure 4-9. Sagittal views of sclerocorneal incision shapes (Grabow). (A) Single-plane one-step "stab" incision. (B) Biplane two-step grooved incision. (C) Biplane with internal incision bevel. (D) Tri-plane three-step incision with scleral groove and internal bevel.

a

b

c

d

inserter. The upper lip should be kept against the endothelium as the lower lip is pressed against the sclera. Gentle pressure on the sclera during lens insertion provides good control of the IOL as it emerges, and keeps it from bulging out and pushing itself out of the eye. When half of the IOL has cleared the inner mouth of the incision, the injector can be withdrawn.

Results of Micro Incisions

One of the authors (JPG) evaluated a consecutive series of 78 cases in which an incision size of 2.4 or 2.5 mm was used. In all of these cases the Gills-modified Langerman Hinge incision (described below) was made just anterior to the limbus in the horizontal axis.

Preoperatively, mean keratometric cylinder was 0.47 D (standard deviation=0.36). Ninety-two percent of the cases had no more than 0.75 D of keratometric cylinder and 60% had less than 0.50 D of keratometric cylinder. None of these cases received any corneal or limbal relaxing incisions.

Mean postoperative keratometric cylinder power was 0.45 D at 2 weeks and 0.43 D at 6 weeks, which was equivalent to the preoperative level (Figure 4-6). Refractive cylinder power

is summarized in Figure 4-7. The data demonstrate a mild reduction of refractive cylinder power. Figure 4-8 shows a summary of individual change in keratometric cylinder following surgery. Sixty-eight percent of cases were within 0.25 D of the preoperative keratometric cylinder level while 15% had an increase in cylinder between 0.26 and 0.50 D. Only 2.6% had a cylinder increase greater than 0.5 D. Fourteen percent of the cases had decreases in cylinder power. Mean absolute change in keratometric cylinder power was 0.21 D (standard deviation = 0.26). Vector analysis was used to determine the amount of surgically induced keratometric cylinder power taking into account any shift in the steep axis. Mean surgically induced cylinder power was 0.35 D (standard deviation = 0.32). Ninety percent of cases had 0.75 D or less of surgically induced cylinder, and about 75% had 0.5 D or less.

Incision Shape

After site and size, shape is the remaining anatomic parameter in the geometric consideration of cataract incision construction. There are two aspect views of these incisions: **sagittal** and **anteroposterior**; and three components: the *external*

Figure 4-10. Sagittal views of the external component of clear-corneal incisions (Grabow). (A) Single-plane one-step stab incision. (B) Bi-plane two-step shallow-groove incision (C) Deep-groove "hinged" incision.

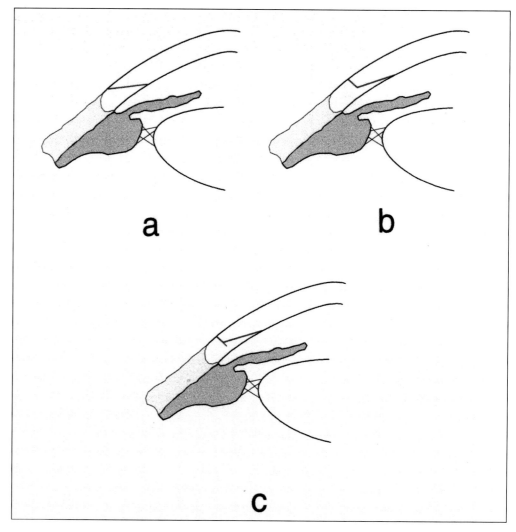

incision, the intratissue *tunnel*, and the *internal* incision. From the **sagittal** aspect, sclerocorneal incisions may be made in one of four possible configurations (Figure 4-9), varying between single-plane, grooved, beveled, and triplane with a groove and a bevel. The *external* component of clear-corneal incisions also may be in one of three theoretical configurations (Figure 4-10): the single-step "stab" incision as initially introduced by I. Howard Fine, M.D.; the two-step grooved incision with a shallow 300-μ or 400-μ groove introduced by Charles Williamson, M.D.; and the "hinged" incision with a deep 600-μ groove introduced by David Langerman, M.D. Grooved incisions provide a superficial corneal flap that has a thicker edge, which helps to avoid avulsion when grasping with forceps or when suturing. The deep groove of Langerman in believed to physically separate the sclera from the internal corneal flap sufficiently to allow scleral indentation (patient rubbing) without internal wound separation, thereby reducing the potential for wound leak. The Langerman hinge incision will be discussed in more detail below.

The sagittal shape and direction of the *tunnel* may also vary. Most tunnels are made flat or planar by flat blades

advanced in a single plane. Some surgeons believe there may be superior sealability with a convex sagittal curve to the corneal tunnel (Figure 4-11), although it is technically difficult to create and to reproduce.

The third component of these incisions, the *internal* opening, may have one of two sagittal shapes: single-plane "stabs" in the same plane as the corneal tunnel, or bi-planar "stepped" (Figure 4-12). In addition, Singer proposes that the most accurate anatomic angle of entry into the anterior chamber through the endothelial surface is 17.5°, that which duplicates the average angle of perforation of scleral veins.

The **anteroposterior** aspect of cataract incisions may begin first with analysis of the *external* component of the sclerocorneal incision, which assumes the shape of a line. The line may be straight, angled, or curved (Figure 4-13). The limbus-parallel incision is the oldest external incision shape, historically, and has the greatest astigmatic effect. The "frown" incision, popularized by Singer and Fukasaku, and the "chevron" incision, popularized by Gills and others, are the more recent shapes for scleral external incisions and have less effect on astigmatism. The radial incision of Steve

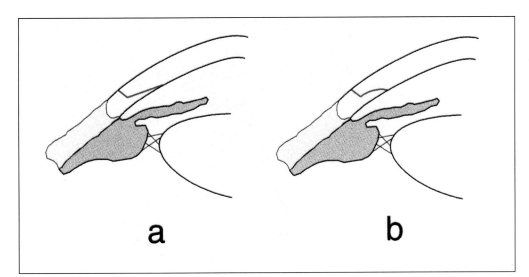

Figure 4-11. Sagittal views of corneal-tunnel incisions (Grabow). (A) Planar. (B) Convex-anterior.

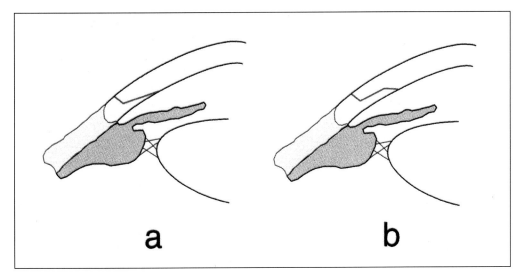

Figure 4-12. Sagittal views of the internal opening of corneal incisions (Grabow). (A) Planar entry in the same plane as the corneal tunnel. (B) Beveled.

Seipser, M.D. has a limbal length of "zero" because its external scleral component is a line in a radial direction. Theoretically, this incisional configuration is the most astigmatically "neutral" of all sclerocorneal shapes. The anteroposterior aspect of the external component of clear-corneal and limbal incisions has, to date, been of only one configuration: limbus parallel (Figure 4-14).

The anteroposterior aspect of the second component of clear-corneal incisions, the tissue *tunnel*, is summarized in Figure 4-15. The original configuration was a parallelogram introduced by Fine. The second configuration, discussed in more detail below, was a convergent trapezoid, introduced by Williamson. In this design, the external incision is longer than the internal incision, to improve instrument maneuverability while preserving the smallest internal opening for self-sealability. The third configuration, the divergent trapezoid of Hoffer, has its external opening smaller than its internal opening, to reduce the astigmatic effect, while allowing maneuverability internally.

Langerman Hinge and Gills Modification

Although clear-corneal incisions appear to be watertight at the end of surgery, Langerman[7] and Ernest[5] have shown that both straight-in and two-plane clear corneals can leak. This ability to leak indicates a less than perfect seal. John[8] has shown a higher incidence of sterile endophthalmitis in clear corneals compared to scleral tunnels. This increased incidence is probably due to reflux of flora into the anterior chamber through the incision. The lack of culture positive infection can be attributed to John's aggressive prophylactic antibiotic regimen, after the Gill's method (see Chapter 3).

Langerman has developed a hinge technique which involves making the initial vertical groove deeper than the point at which the horizontal shelf is started. The deep groove then functions as a hinge, with the inner aspect of the incision flexible and malleable, allowing it to adhere to the outer portion of the incision.

The Gills' modification of the Langerman hinge involves a vertical incision that is 85% deep. The next step is to create a deep longitudinal bevel in the stroma in either a single- or

Figure 4-13. Various shapes of the external groove of sclerocorneal incisions (Grabow). (A) Limbus-parallel. (B) Straight-linear or tangential. (C) Limbus-antiparallel or "frown". (D) Angled limbus-antiparallel or "chevron". (E) Radial. (F) Tangential-radial.

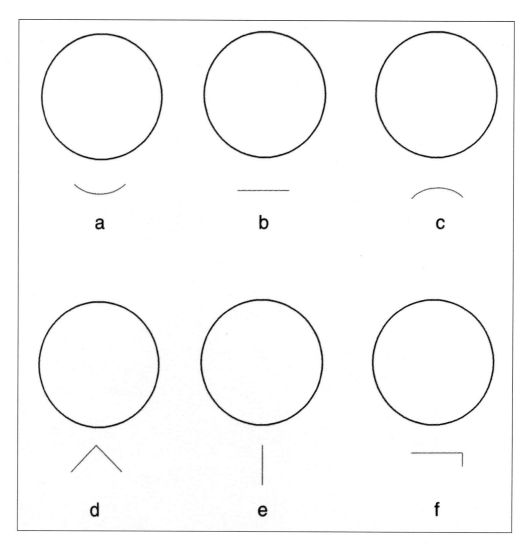

two-plane fashion. This portion is deeper and longer than Langerman describes. Because the inner flap is very thin, it allows for greater flexibility and better contact when pressure is applied to any portion of the wound (Figure 4-16).

The key to creating a very deep, thin incision is to pick up the distal aspect of the corneal wound with forceps. This step is essential for two reasons: 1) it allows the surgeon to have control over fixation of the eye when using topical anesthesia, and 2) it allows the surgeon to make a deep incision with greater ease. The flap is created by directing the keratome (diamond or metal) toward the dome of the eye. After tunneling through the posterior stroma for a distance of approximately two-thirds the keratome width, the incision is beveled posteriorly through Descemet's membrane and into the anterior chamber. Using a 2.3-mm to 2.5-mm trapezoidal keratome and beveling it into the anterior chamber approximately 2 mm will create a 2.3-mm to 2.5-mm by 2.0-mm incision. The incision performs similarly to navigational valves, when pressure against the rubber forces the aperture closed.

The anteroposterior aspect of the third incisional component, the *internal* opening, has only recently come under

investigation. Three directional possibilities exist for this incision (Figure 4-17): limbus-parallel, tangential, and limbus-antiparallel ("corneal frown"). Limbus-parallel *internal* incisions, unlike limbus-parallel *external* incisions, have been demonstrated to be the most stable and most resistant to deformation and leakage. Conversely, corneal frown internal incisions are the weakest. Therefore, cutting strokes to enlarge an internal incision should move either in a central direction, by advancing the blade, or in a lateral direction, so as to preserve a limbus-parallel configuration, rather than in a peripheral direction, as when withdrawing the blade.

INCISION PHYSIOLOGY

Beveled cataract corneal incisions, by creating overlying superficial and deep lamellae on each side of a tunnel, possess an intrinsic anatomic structural integrity not architecturally available to vertical corneal incisions, such as those used in incisional refractive keratotomy. Superficial lamellar hydration at the conclusion of surgery, by injection of balanced salt solution (Figure 4-18), as described by Fine, tem-

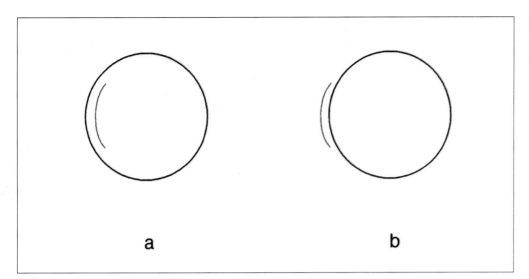

Figure 4-14. (A) External component of clear-corneal incision (Grabow). (B) Limbal-corneal incision (Grabow).

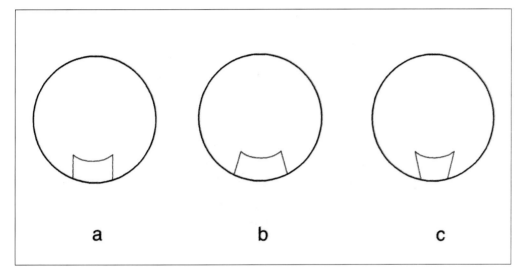

Figure 4-15. Antero-posterior aspect of corneal tunnels (Grabow). (A) Convergent trapezoid. (B) Parallelogram. (C) Divergent trapezoid.

porarily iatrogenically closes the corneal tunnel by superficial lamellar expansion and compression. The space is physiologically closed internally by aqueous pressure against the endothelial surface of the deep lamella, the so-called internal corneal "flap", "lip", or "valve". Closure is not only dependent on the rates of aqueous production and drainage, but also on the surface area of the flap.

An additional physiologic closure mechanism is offered by Fine: the endothelial pump. Theoretically, the endothelial pump may dehydrate the deep lamellae, which may in turn draw fluid from the edematous superficial lamellae across the tunnel, thereby creating a negative closing pressure in the tunnel.

The clinical concerns regarding early postoperative wound integrity are truly bi-directional; that is, there is concern regarding egress of aqueous out of the eye, and greater concern regarding ingress of conjunctival contaminants into the eye. The experiences of endophthalmitis with early clear-corneal incisions certainly did nothing to alleviate this apprehension, and the subsequent cadaver demonstrations by

Ernest only elevated the level of skepticism regarding the clinical integrity of unsutured clear-corneal incisions. However, the self-sealing clear-corneal incision has proven to be *clinically* competent in thousands of cases, creating confidence and many new converts in recent years. The anticipated rise in the rate of endophthalmitis, after the initial spike, did not occur. In addition, the clear-corneal incision has also proven to be a new and very powerful tool in the management of astigmatism in the cataract patient.

BLADE TECHNOLOGY

When clear-corneal incisions were first introduced, surgeons attempted their traditional three-step approach in the cornea with their favorite metal scleral blades (Figure 4-19). If the blades were new—that is, if they had not been dulled from previous use—they worked. However, it rapidly became apparent that metal blades could not be used as repeatedly with clear-corneal incisions as they had been used with scleral incisions.

Figure 4-16. Gills-modified Langerman Hinge incision (Gills).

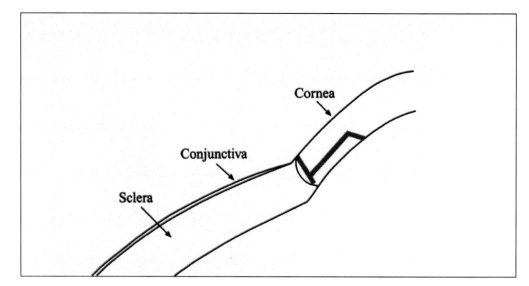

Figure 4-17. Antero-posterior aspect of internal corneal openings (Grabow). (A) limbus parallel. (B) Tangential. (C) Limbus-antiparallel or "corneal frown".

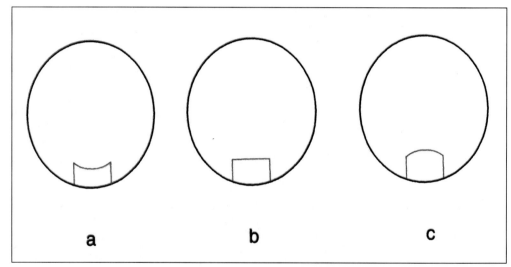

What made the difference? Bowman's membrane. Bowman's membrane is the firm internal cuticular skeleton imparting rigidity, curvature, and elasticity to the cornea. Unlike the softer texture of the sclera and the stroma, the hardness of Bowman's membrane requires a sharper blade for incision.

Gem blade technology evolved first, as surgeons found it easier to enter the cornea with the sharper edge of a diamond, compared to that of stainless steel. The anatomy of the blade became a new focus of study. Topics of interest included bevels on the tip; bevels on the sides; the angle of the point; the diameter, thickness, and shape of the blade; the shape of the handle; the material and cost of the blade; and the care and handling of the blade.

Early diamond blades had beveled tips with acutely angled points. The non-beveled sides, it was soon learned, made it difficult to move these blades through the tissue, and would occasionally cause radial tears in the superficial corneal flap. Beveling the sides alleviated these problems. However, as

always, a solution can also create a new problem. The sharp beveled sides now also allowed for inadvertent lateral wound extension due to uncontrolled ocular movement during topical anesthesia, another factor to be mastered in the surgeon's learning curve.

The acute angle on the point, it was soon learned, allowed inadvertent, premature entry, and did not provide the surgeon with a geometric guide to tunnel length. Therefore, tunnel length was an approximation with great variability. Blades were then designed with 90° angled points and 3-mm widths, which also had an axial point-to-shoulder dimension of 1.5 mm (Figure 4-20). The surgeon desiring to perform phaco and foldable implantation through a corneal tunnel of 3.0 x 1.75 mm now had an intracorneal "ruler for reproducibility". If the point was kept in the corneal stroma until the angles of the shoulder exactly reached the external incision (Figure 4-21), the surgeon knew the tunnel was now 1.5-mm long. Advancing then through Descemet's membrane into the anterior chamber would result reproducibly in a tunnel length of

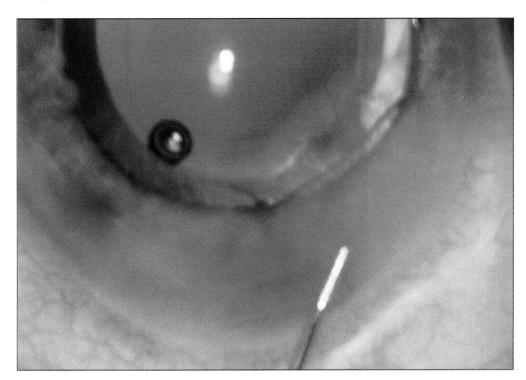

Figure 4-18. Stromal hydration with balanced salt solution of the superficial corneal lamellae of clear-corneal incision at the conclusion of surgery (Grabow).

approximately 1.75 mm. These incisions demonstrated safety, reproducibility, predictability, self-sealability, and have become somewhat blade dependent.

For surgeons preferring disposables, the same blade design became available in stainless steel. Bob Kellan, M.D. designed a metal blade with marks on the surface to let the surgeon know exactly how far the blade has entered the stroma.

Special diamonds have been designed for specific incision sizes and shapes. Charles Williamson, M.D. designed a two-blade system. The 1-mm "step blade" (Figure 4-22) is for making both the sideport paracentesis (Figure 4-23) and the vertical groove (Figure 4-24) for a two-step phaco incision (Figure 4-25). The "trap blade" has non-parallel sides (Figure 4-26) to automatically create a convergent trapezoid incision. These trapezoid diamonds are manufactured in several sizes to accommodate different sizes of phaco tips (Figure 4-27).

David Brown, M.D. has designed the "buck knife", which is a 1-mm wide diamond that has sharp beveled sides. With this one blade, he can make all of his incisions: the sideport, the groove, and the phaco incision. To make the phaco incision, he simply enters the anterior chamber, making an initial 1-mm opening and then, keeping the blade in the incision, slides the blade to the side to create a 3-mm opening.

A similar blade has been developed by Doug Mastel (Rapid City, SD) with a square tip designed to be used with a corneal incision marker. This marker first makes an imprint on the cornea of the entire incisional area. The blade is then introduced into the stroma and is moved forward and laterally until the surgeon has "drawn" the incision with the blade in the stroma under the imprinted template. The blade, remaining in the

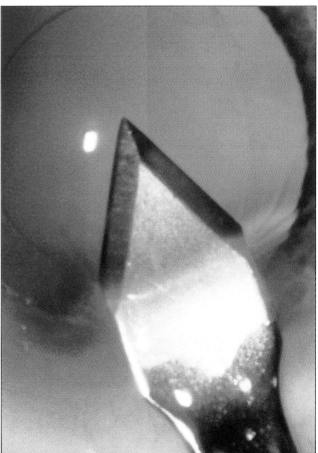

Figure 4-19. Bi-beveled, acute-angled, metal keratome clear-corneal incision (Grabow).

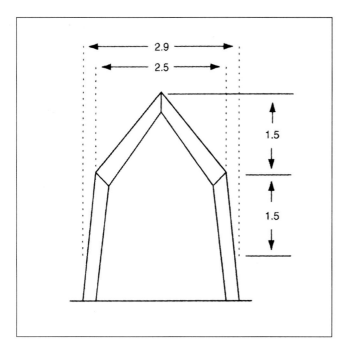

Figure 4-20. Diamond clear-corneal blade design for creating a trapezoid incision measuring 2.5 mm x 2.9 mm x 1.5 mm (Grabow).

planar tunnel created, is then advanced into the anterior chamber and moved laterally to complete the internal opening.

The 3-mm wide diamonds are also available in step handles so that both the guarded groove and the phaco incision can be made with one blade (Figure 4-28). Fine has developed a blade called the "3-D" or "three-dimensional blade" (Figure 4-29). This blade has different bevels on the point, designed to create perfectly linear entry incisions into both Bowman's and Descemet's membranes.

The original diamond blades manufactured in the 1980s for refractive surgery, and later for cataract surgery, were relatively thick, measuring 200 μ. Most of the current generation blades are thinner, measuring from 80 μ to 130 μ. In addition, blades have become available in less expensive materials, such as cubic zirconium, ruby, and sapphire (HUCO/Switzerland). These materials make blades that are sharper than metal blades, almost as sharp as diamond blades. They retain their sharpness much longer than metal blades, but still not as long as diamonds.

THE FUTURE

It appears that cataract incisional technology may have reached its ultimate level of design. Although phacoemulsification has been performed through smaller than 1-mm incisions, with present phaco technology that is not practically feasible, nor is it necessary. As phaco and foldable lens technology has downsized incisions to under 2.5 mm, surgically induced astigmatism and wound integrity are no longer issues. The only remaining reason to perform 1-mm cataract surgery would be for the purpose of injecting a liquid cataract replacement material into an intact capsular bag which had its contents removed through a 1-mm capsulotomy. Although this technology is available now, the problems of lens power determination and lens epithelial cell proliferation still remain. In addition, if the desired result is to attempt to restore accommodation to a senile eye with a cataract (or a pre-senile eye with presbyopia), it seems unlikely that simple lens replacement would reverse this complex, progressive physiologic process.

REFERENCES

1. Masket S: Astigmatic analysis of the scleral pocket incision and closure technique for cataract surgery. *CLAO Journal* 1985, 11:206-209.
2. McFarland, MS: The Clinical history of sutureless surgery. in Gills JP, Martin RG, Sanders DR, eds, Sutureless Cataract Surgery, 1992; Thorofare, NJ
3. Fine H: Clear corneal incision. *J Am Soc Cat and Refract Surg*, 1991.
4. Fine IH, Fichman RA, Grabow HB, eds, *Clear-Corneal Cataract Surgery and Topical Anesthesia*. Slack, Thorofare, NJ, 1993.
5. Ernest PH, Fenzl R, Lavery KT, Sensoli A: Relative stability of clear corneal incisions in a cadaver eye model. *J Cataract Refract Surg* 1995, 21:39-42.
6. Ernest PH: The healing process as a function of incision construction—evaluation in an animal model. *Fifth Annual Ocular Surgery News Symposium*.
7. Langerman DW: Architectural design of a self-sealing corneal tunnel, single-hinge incision. *J Cataract Refract Surg* 1994; 20:84-88.
8. John, ME: Incidence of sterile endophthalmitis in scleral-tunnel vs clear-corneal incisions. Presented at 1997 annual meeting of American Society of Cataract and Refractive Surgery.

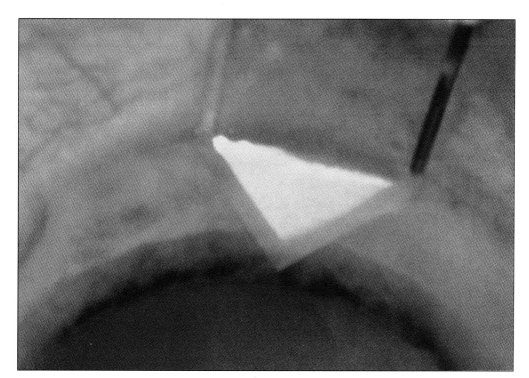

Figure 4-21. Diamond blade in cornea 1.5 mm, ready to enter anterior chamber (Grabow).

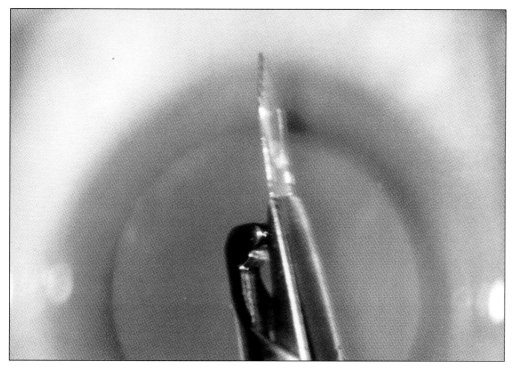

Figure 4-22. Williamson 1 mm "step" blade fully extended for sideport paracentesis (Diamatrix).

Figure 4-23. Sideport paracentesis with Williamson 1 mm "step" blade (Diamatrix).

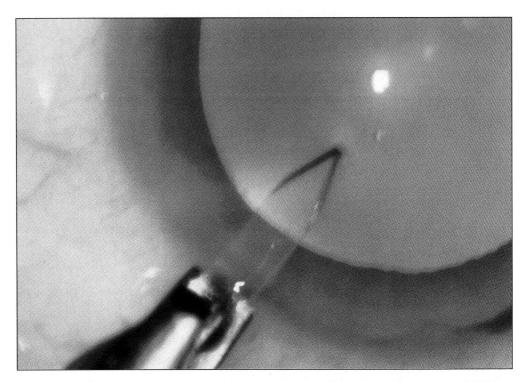

Figure 4-24. Williamson 1 mm "step" blade with guard for grooved incision (Diamatrix).

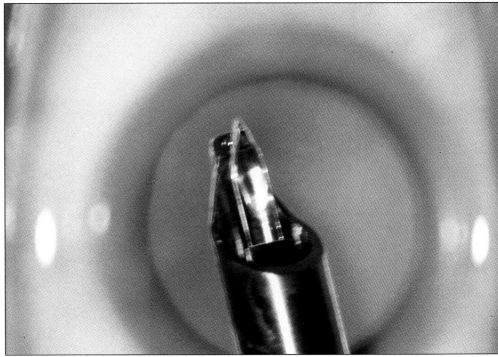

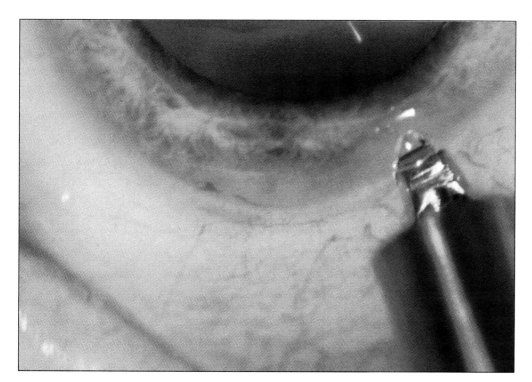

Figure 4-25. Clear-corneal groove with Williamson "step" blade (Diamatrix).

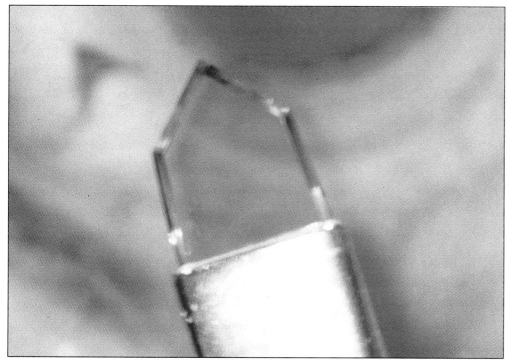

Figure 4-26. Williamson trapezoid diamond blade (Diamatrix).

Figure 4-27. Various sizes of clear-corneal trapezoid blades (Mastel).

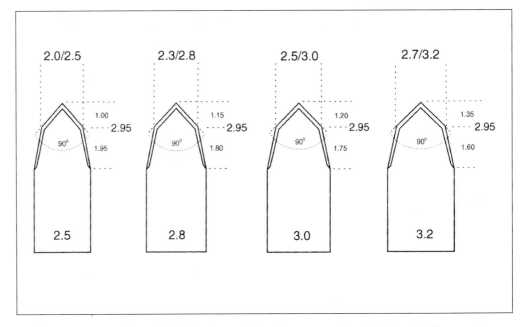

Figure 4-28. Trapezoid diamond blade for guarded groove and clear-corneal entry (Rhein).

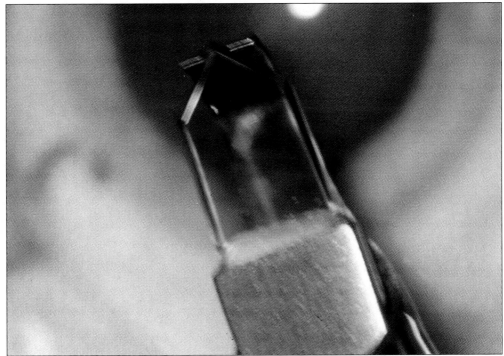

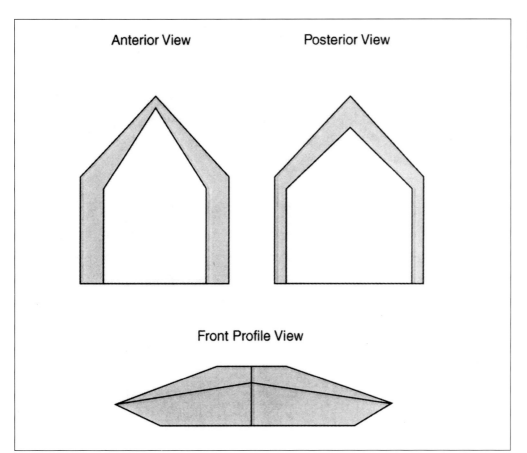

Anterior View   Posterior View

Front Profile View

Figure 4-29. 3-D diamond blade design (Rhein).

REDUCING PRE-EXISTING ASTIGMATISM

James P. Gills, MD, Johnny L. Gayton, MD

Optimizing vision is the ultimate goal for the cataract patient. In today's state-of-the-art cataract environment, optimal vision includes not just excellent best-corrected vision, but uncorrected vision as well. In order to achieve these excellent visual results, the effect of astigmatism on postoperative vision must be minimized. Control of surgically induced astigmatism along with reduction of pre-existing astigmatism has become a clinical efficacy benchmark when evaluating cataract surgical outcomes. Minimizing postoperative astigmatism is achieved through appropriate cataract incision management, proper use of relaxing incisions, and the customization of surgical strategies utilizing corneal topography.

There have been a number of major advances in the past 10 years that have dramatically impacted astigmatism management. These advances include:

1. foldable lens technology with a concurrent rise in phacoemulsification use that spurred the development of small-incision surgery
2. sutureless incision architecture, which eliminated distortion caused by sutures
3. side incision surgery, which can control or reduce against-the-rule astigmatism
4. corneal cataract incisions, which represent the ultimate in minimally invasive cataract surgery, and include the clear and "near-clear" corneal incisions made just at or anterior to the limbus
5. improvement in relaxing incision techniques, that can reduce or eliminate pre-existing astigmatism with fewer overcorrections

These advances address two issues involved with astigmatism management. First, today's cataract incisions provide better control of surgically induced astigmatism, either by producing "astigmatism neutral" surgery or by using induced astigmatism at the steep axis to counteract low levels of pre-existing astigmatism. Second, improved techniques for correcting astigmatism allow many patients with moderate to high levels of pre-existing astigmatism to have better vision postoperatively than they have ever had.

For the patient with pre-existing astigmatism, especially those with the more visually disabling against-the-rule astigmatism, there are a number of strategies for reducing or eliminating astigmatism at the time of cataract surgery. Surgeons have their own techniques and nomograms for dealing with pre-existing astigmatism, but these nomograms generally all deal with some modification to the cataract incision and/or some form of relaxing incision.

GILLS TECHNIQUE—LIMBAL RELAXING INCISIONS

Previous experience has shown us that corneal relaxing incisions (CRIs) have limited predictability and often result in overcorrections, especially in lower-level astigmats. We no longer employ CRIs as a "first-line" correcting technique. They are used only in high astigmats.

We have moved our relaxing incisions off the cornea, and now create 4- to 12-mm relaxing incisions 0.5 to 0.6 mm in depth at the limbus (limbal relaxing incisions, or LRIs) in the steep meridian. The LRIs can be used with any type of cataract incision. We initially developed this technique in conjunction with a modification of the Langerman 3-plane hinge self-sealing clear corneal incision (CCI, see Chapter 4). By modifying the Langerman hinge, we were able to incorporate the LRI into the cataract incision. Currently we employ scleral-limbal-corneal (SLiC) cataract incisions for most of our spherical and lower astigmatism cases (see Chapter 4).

Limbal relaxing incisions have definite advantages compared with CRIs. Use of LRIs results in better corneal

Figure 5-1. Limbal relaxing incision created with the Lab Instruments L320 micrometer knife. The incision is placed in the steep axis at the limbus, just anterior to the Palisades of Vogt (Gills).

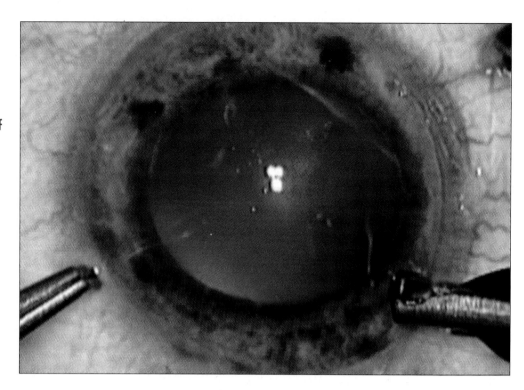

Figure 5-1. Limbal relaxing incision created with the Lab Instruments L320 micrometer knife. The incision is placed in the steep axis at the limbus, just anterior to the Palisades of Vogt (Gills).

topographies with less corneal distortion or irregularity and is quite effective in low and moderate astigmats (<=3D). They are easier to perform and more comfortable for the patient. LRIs are more "forgiving" due to the placement and length of the incision. Precise placement "on-axis" is not as critical because the length is 4 to 12 mm. They are also more forgiving of variation in depth than CRIs. There is less variability of refraction, and overcorrections are rare.

We have found that extending the length of LRIs to 10-12 mm can produce significant added effect for cases with astigmatism >3 D. However, customization of the surgical plan based on topography is essential. LRIs combined with CRIs placed near the limbus can correct even higher levels of astigmatism (up to 8 D).

Incision Technique

The amount, axis, and symmetry of the corneal cylinder are determined by keratometry and topography. The refractive cylinder is not considered in phakic patients, because any lenticular astigmatism would be removed by the cataract surgery and thus cannot be figured into the surgical plan. Topography is extremely important to tailor surgery to the patient. We currently use the Technomed C-Scan topography system. This system provides high-resolution mapping in the center zone with no smoothing or interpolation, and error-free focusing. We find that for our astigmatism cases, the Technomed astigmatism evaluation feature with vector analysis is very helpful. The ray tracing feature allows us to determine the optical quality of the cornea within the entire pupil area. The steep axis of astigmatism is marked with a cautery based on the keratometry and topography measurements.

The LRIs are made using a Lab Instruments L320 micrometer knife (Figure 5-1), and are placed in the steep axis at the limbus just anterior to the Palisades of Vogt. The number and length are determined according to the nomogram described below. The surgical keratometer is used to confirm the result.

The Gills' nomogram for correcting astigmatism with LRIs is shown in Table 5-1 and Figure 5-2. This is a "starting point" nomogram, which titrates surgery by length and number of LRIs. However, the length and placement can vary based on topography and other factors. The goal is to reduce cylinder power and absolutely avoid overcorrecting with-the-rule cases, because we want to minimize against-the-rule astigmatism. In cases with 0.5 D of cylinder or less, only an astigmatically neutral cataract incision is used.

Patients with low (<1.5 D) against-the-rule (ATR) astigmatism (180 degrees) receive only a single LRI in the steep meridian, placed opposite to the SliC incision (See Chapter 4). However, if astigmatism is greater than 1.5 D, a pair of LRIs must be used. In ATR cases, one of the pair of LRIs is incorporated into a modified Langerman hinge incision by elongating the first plane of the hinge (Figure 5-3). The length of the LRI is not affected by the presence of the cataract incision.

In low with-the-rule cases, a single 6.0 mm LRI is made at 90°, 0.6 mm in depth. The LRI is always independent of the cataract incision in WTR cases (Figure 5-3).

A 6-mm relaxing incision generally relieves about 1 D of astigmatism for the 73-year-old patient. For more astigmatism, paired limbal relaxing incisions are used. If the patient has 2 to 3 D, the pair of LRIs can be extended up to 8 mm. Four diopters can often be corrected or substantially reduced with a pair of 10- to 12-mm LRIs.

TABLE 5-1

LIMBAL RELAXING INCISIONS FOR PATIENTS > 73

	1 D	1-2 D	2-3 D	3-4 D	>4 D
No. of LRIs	1	2	2	2	2 + CRIs
Length	6 mm	6 mm	8 mm	10 mm	10-12 mm

PARAMETERS FOR ASTIGMATISM >4 D

Incisions	Blade Setting	Length	Optical Zone	No. of Incisions
LRI	600 microns	10-12 mm	at limbus	2
CRI	99% depth (pachymetry)	2 mm for every D over 4 D	8 mm	based on correction desired over 4 D

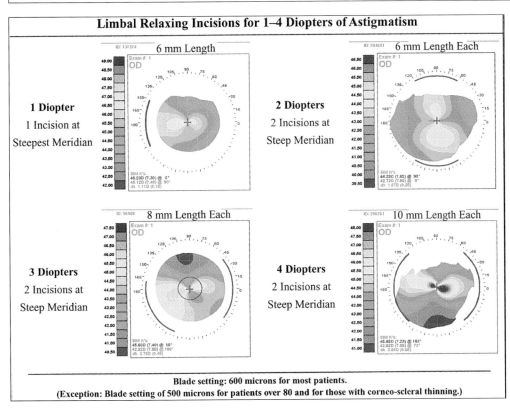

Limbal Relaxing Incisions for 1–4 Diopters of Astigmatism

6 mm Length

1 Diopter
1 Incision at
Steepest Meridian

6 mm Length Each

2 Diopters
2 Incisions at
Steep Meridian

8 mm Length Each

3 Diopters
2 Incisions at
Steep Meridian

10 mm Length Each

4 Diopters
2 Incisions at
Steep Meridian

Blade setting: 600 microns for most patients.
(Exception: Blade setting of 500 microns for patients over 80 and for those with corneo-scleral thinning.)

Figure 5-2. Gills' nomogram for the use of LRIs to correct mild to moderate levels (up to 4 D) of astigmatism. This nomogram applies to patients older than 73. Younger patients require somewhat longer incisions to achieve the same effect. The number and length of the LRIs determine the level of correction achieved. The blade setting is 600 microns for most patients. However, for patients over 80 years of age and for patients with corneo-scleral thinning, the knife is set at 500 microns (Gills).

Recently we have found that LRIs can be quite effective in substantially reducing astigmatism even in high astigmatism cases. Two LRIs are placed and lengthened to 12 mm to correct the first four diopters. Corneal relaxing incisions may then be added to provide additional correction. If CRIs are used, they are at 99% depth at the 8- or 9-mm optical zone, 2 mm in length for every diopter over four. Added corneal relaxing incisions are reserved only for cases with higher levels of pre-existing astigmatism keeping in mind that we are careful to avoid overcorrecting WTR cases. (see Table 5-1).

We do take a conservative approach to astigmatism. It is better to make a long incision at the limbus than to use a small relaxing incision on the cornea. In the case of high astigmats,

there is often contributing pathology, such as corneal scarring or keratoconus. In these cases, the surgical effect is less predictable, so we often are conservative in planning surgery, preferring undercorrection. We can improve the quality of vision substantially in these high astigmatism cases, even if there is residual cylinder.

Results of the Gills Program

Low to Moderate Astigmatism

Case studies of 2 patients with moderate astigmatism are illustrated topographically in Figures 5-4 and 5-5. The first patient (Figure 5-4) had 1.12 D of preoperative keratometric cylinder at axis 154. The refraction was +1.75 –1.5 X 150 =

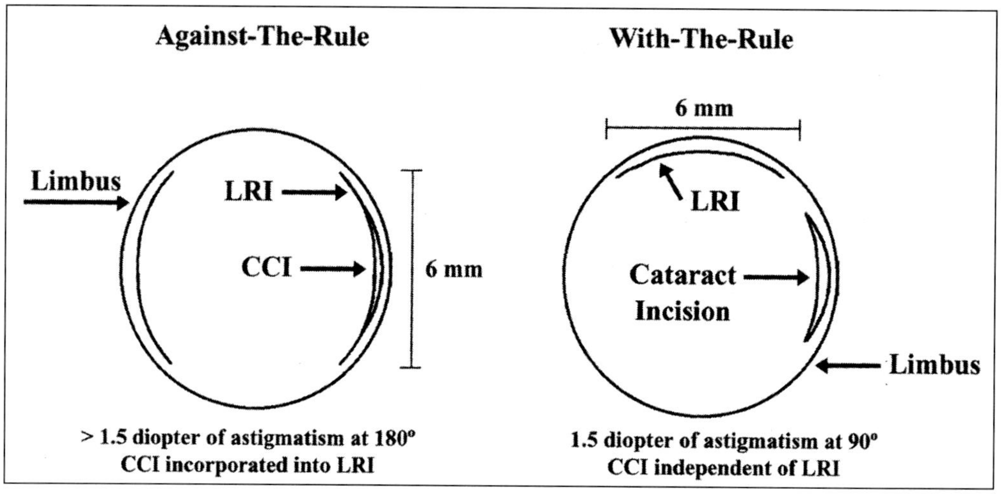

Figure 5-3. Schematic diagram of the relationship between the cataract incision and the LRI. In WTR cases and for lower levels of ATR astigmatism (requiring only a single LRI), the incisions are independent. However in ATR cases requiring a pair of LRIs, one LRI is incorporated into the top plane of the 3-plane hinge incision (Gills).

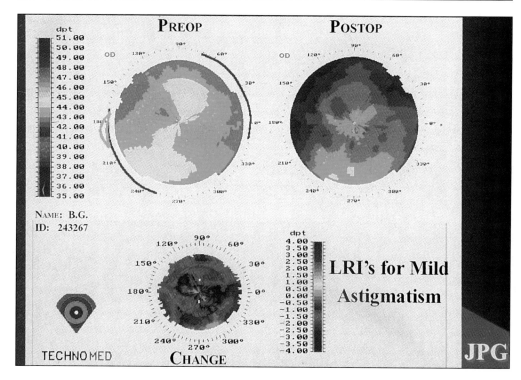

Figure 5-4. Preoperative, postoperative and change map topographies of a patient receiving a pair of LRIs for low to moderate astigmatism. The incisions are indicated on the preoperative map. The change map shows flattening in the desired meridian (Gills).

20/30. A 2.4 mm modified Langerman Hinge incision was made temporally and a pair of 6.0-mm LRIs were placed in the steep meridian (2:00 and 8:00). As discussed above, the LRI centered at 8:00 was incorporated into the first plane of the hinge incision. The blade was set at 0.5 mm. The postoperative refraction at 2 weeks was plano-sphere. Both corrected and uncorrected vision was 20/20. Postoperative topography indicated a near-spherical corneal surface.

The next case (Figure 5-5) had 1.65 D of preoperative keratometric cylinder at axis 84. Refraction was +3.0 –2.75 X 85 = 20/25. A 2.4-mm modified Langerman hinge CCI was made at 2:00 and a pair of 6.0-mm LRIs were placed in the horizontal meridian. Final refraction was plano –0.5 D = 20/20. Uncorrected vision was also 20/20.

We analyzed a series of mild to moderate astigmatic cases to evaluate the efficacy of this surgical approach. Sixty-two eyes with refractive cylinder powers ranging up to 3 D received single or paired LRIs. Mean preoperative refractive cylinder was 1.16 D, which was reduced postoperatively to a mean of 0.47 D. Figure 5-6 displays the postoperative versus preoperative cylinder for every case. All but one patient was improved by the LRI procedure.

Figure 5-7 shows the distribution of refractive cylinder pre- and postoperatively. Preoperatively 86% had over a half diopter, and 46% had over a diopter of cylinder. After receiving LRIs, 68% had 0.5 D and 36% had no more than a quarter diopter. Only 3% had more than a diopter of cylinder postoperatively.

The overall effectiveness of the LRI approach can be illustrated quite dramatically by the use of vector plots (Figures 5-

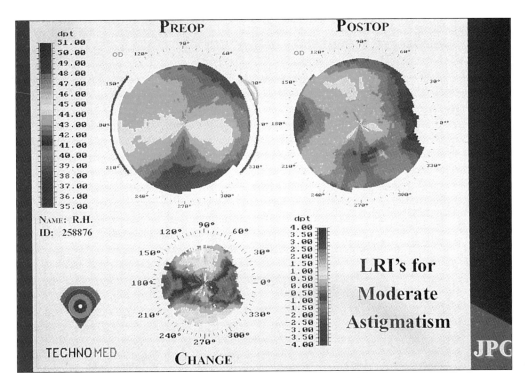

Figure 5-5. Preoperative, postoperative and change map topographies of a patient receiving a pair of LRIs for moderate astigmatism. The incisions are indicated on the preoperative map. The change map shows flattening in the desired meridian (Gills).

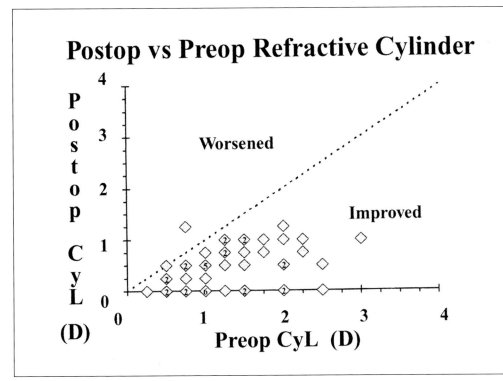

Figure 5-6. Scatterplot of preoperative versus postoperative refractive cylinder for individual cases receiving LRIs for the correction of mild to moderate astigmatism. Note that all but one of 62 patients was improved by the procedure (Gills).

8A&B, and Figures 5-9A&B). The length of each vector arrow represents the amount of cylinder for each patient. The orientation of the vector depicts the axis of the cylinder. Each concentric ring represents 0.5 D of cylinder power. The preoperative and postoperative cylinder vectors for ATR cases are shown in Figures 5-8A&B. The surgical approach is aggressive for ATR cases; ATR cylinder is eliminated or substantially reduced. Minor overcorrection to the WTR direction is tolerated. In contrast, we are more conservative with WTR astigmatism. The preoperative WTR cylinder vectors (Figure 5-9A) are lessened (Figure 5-9B) but no cases are converted to ATR astigmatism through overcorrection.

Figure 5-7. Bar chart showing the distribution of refractive cylinder pre- and postoperatively for 62 cases receiving LRIs to correct mild to moderate levels of astigmatism (Gills).

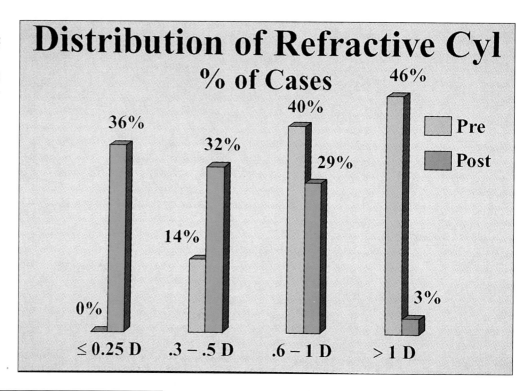

TABLE 5-2
GAYTON LRI WITH CATARACT INCISION NOMOGRAM

Cylinder (D)	Arc Pairs
1.25	30°
1.50	40°
1.75	50°
2.00-2.25	60°
2.50-2.75	65°
3.00-3.25	70°
3.50-3.75	75°
4.00	80°

- Use foldable AcrySof lens through temporal incision and 0.65 depth limbal arcs.
- For asymmetrical astigmatism, arc lengths should not be symmetrical. Use topography as a guide.
- Care must be taken with arc lengths above 60°, as they can cause wound gape.

High Astigmatism

Twenty-two cases with preoperative keratometric cylinder over 3 D received either LRIs or a combination of LRIs and CRIs. Surgery was planned conservatively in most cases. One case received an enhancement. Most cases had clear corneal incisions, but a few had scleral incisions.

The mean preoperative keratometric cylinder of 3.72 D was reduced to a mean of 1.91 D postoperatively. Mean per-cent reduction of keratometric cylinder was 49%. All cases were reasonably improved, most without the use of corneal relaxing incisions. Seventy-two percent of the cases could see 20/40 or better uncorrected.

An example of the use of LRIs for high astigmatism is illustrated topographically in Figure 5-10A&B. This case shows that we can provide substantial correction with LRIs, then enhance the surgery if a more spherical final refraction is desired. This patient had 4.37 D of keratometric cylinder. Refraction was +3.25 –4.0 X 005 = 20/50. A temporal Langerman hinge CCI was used, and a pair of LRIs was placed in the vertical meridian. The superior LRI was 8 mm and the inferior LRI was 9 mm. As shown in Figure 5-10A, the result was not optimal. Therefore, another pair of 6-mm LRIs was placed in the same meridian just anterior to the first pair. Final refraction was +0.75 –0.50 X 180 = 20/30. Postoperative keratometric cylinder was reduced to 1.18 D. The overall surgical change is shown in Figure 5-10B.

A pseudophakic patient with high astigmatism received secondary 7-mm LRIs followed by enhancement with a CRI to correct 3.53 D of keratometric cylinder at axis 106 (Figures 5-11 A&B). Preoperative refraction was plano –3.0 X 95 = 20/40. Following enhancement, the final refraction was plano –0.75 X 25 = 20/16. Uncorrected vision was 20/25.

GAYTON TECHNIQUE—LRIs

Surgical Technique

After removing the cataract and inserting the IOL, the globe is pressurized with balanced salt solution. The limbal arcuate

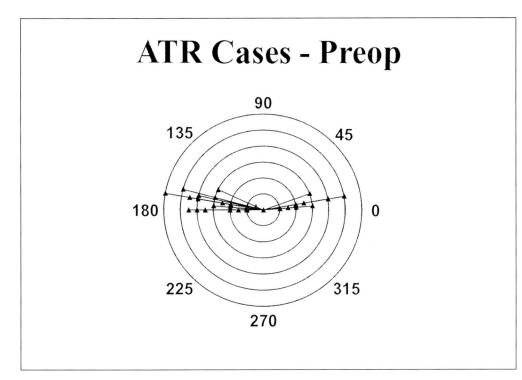

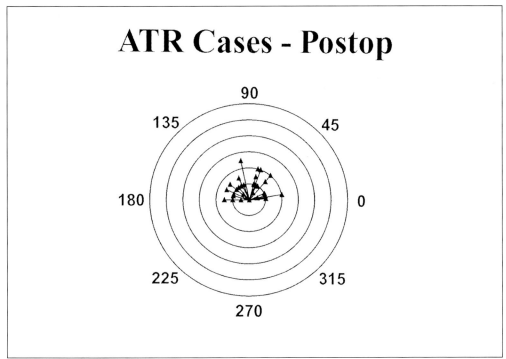

Figure 5-8. Plot of individual cylinder vectors for patients receiving LRIs to correct ATR cylinder (Gills). (A) Preoperatively. (B) Postoperatively.

relaxing incision is then made. Table 5-2 outlines the Gayton nomogram. The Gayton Limbal Degree Marker (Storz) is inked with a Visitec pad and applied to the limbus. A triple edge arcuate blade is then used to cut the predetermined number of degrees at the appropriate axis. I strive for 90% to 95% depth as determined by limbal pachymetry. TobraDex (Alcon) drops are used postoperatively for 5 to 7 weeks.

Results of Gayton Program

A consecutive series of 20 cases with limbal relaxing incisions were collected. At the time of the study, cases received a 6- to 7-mm cataract incision. The current procedure is to use a foldable AcrySof lens through a small temporal incision. Eighty percent of the cohort had more than 6 month follow-up.

Figures 5-12A&B show the preoperative vs postoperative

Figure 5-9. Plot of individual cylinder vectors for patients receiving LRIs to correct WTR cylinder. Note that there were no conversions to ATR cylinder (Gills). (A) Preoperatively. (B) Postoperatively.

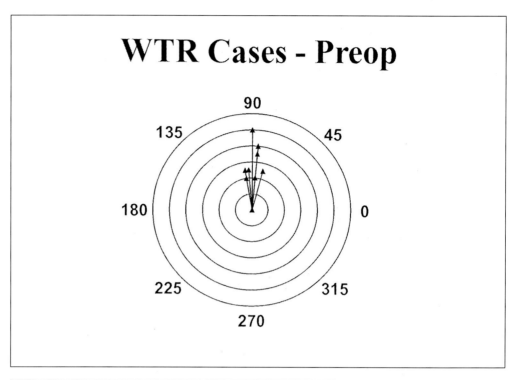

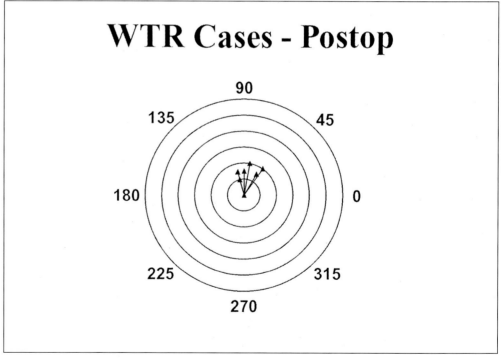

keratometric cylinder at 2-4 weeks and >6 months. Cases below the equivalency line had reduced cylinder postoperatively. Cases between the dashed lines were within 1 D of their preoperative level. Sixty-five percent of cases at 2-4 weeks and 62.5% at >6 months were reduced by more than 1 D. At >6 months, mean reduction in cylinder was 1.32 D (s.d. 0.90) with a mean percent correction of 46%.

Figures 5-13A&B show the amount of induced cylinder in the correcting axis at 2-4 weeks and >6 months, respectively. The correcting axis is the axis in which cylinder should be induced to correct pre-existing astigmatism, which is 90 away from the steep preoperative cylinder axis. Cases above the equivalency line are overcorrected, below the line are under-corrected, and within the dashed lines are within 1 D of a per-

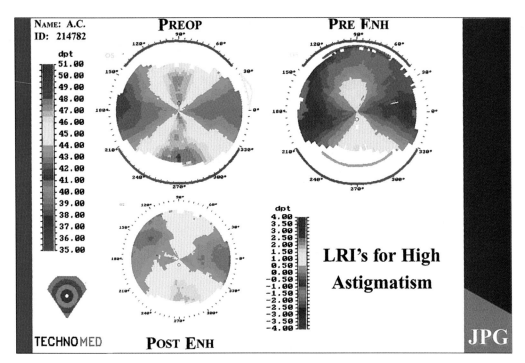

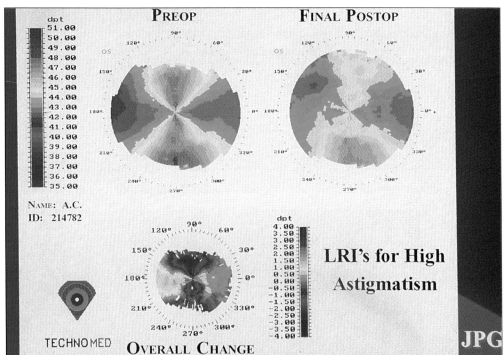

Figure 5-10. Topography maps of a patient who received LRIs to correct higher astigmatism (Gills). (A) The preoperative, pre-enhancement, and final postoperative topography maps show the first pair of LRIs and the second pair of LRIs used to enhance the result. (B) The overall change map shows that a significant reduction of cylinder was achieved.

fect correction. Mildly overcorrected cases may have a shift in axis but still experience a substantial reduction in cylinder. At 2 to 4 weeks, some cases are mildly overcorrected, but by >6 months, the effect has regressed slightly such that no case is overcorrected. Forty percent of cases were within 1 D of a perfect correction.

Figure 5-14 further illustrates that no case was overcorrected, by demonstrating preoperative versus postoperative

cylinder axis. All cases are close to the equivalency line, indicating no major axis shifts, as would be seen with an overcorrection.

Figure 5-15 shows the mean keratometric cylinder over time. Preoperatively, the mean keratometric cylinder was 3.54 D (s.d. 1.67), ranging from 1.50 D to 8.75 D. One day postoperatively, the mean cylinder was reduced to 2.66 D (s.d. 1.90), and at the final postoperative visit (>6 months) was

Figure 5-11. Topography maps of a pseudophakic patient who received LRIs followed by enhancing CRIs to correct higher astigmatism (Gills). (A) The preoperative, pre-enhancement, and final postoperative topography maps show the first pair of LRIs and the CRI which was used to enhance the result. (B) The overall change map shows that a significant reduction of cylinder was achieved.

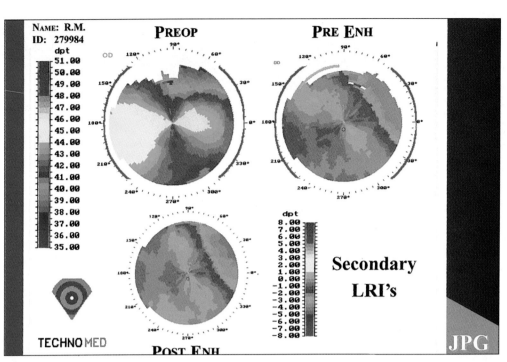

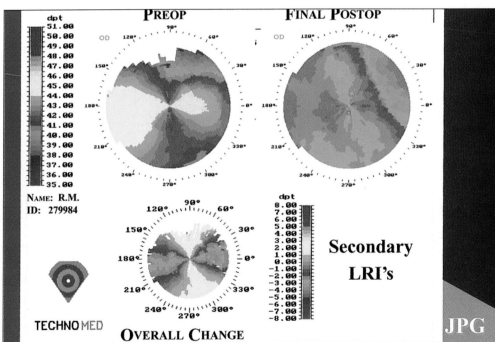

1.71 D (s.d. 1.24), ranging from 0.13 D to 4.37 D.

Figure 5-16 shows the mean surgically induced keratometric cylinder over time. At 1 day postoperatively, about 4 D on average are induced by the combined cataract/astigmatic keratotomy surgery, but the effect regresses to about 2 D at the final visit (>6 months).

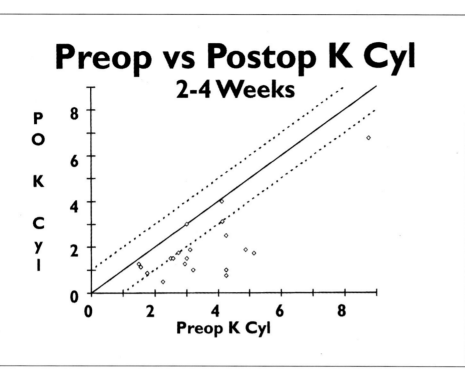

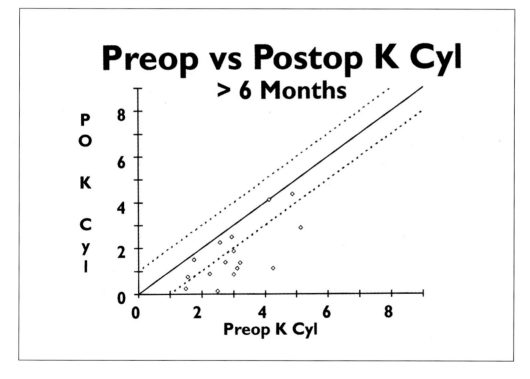

Figure 5-12. Preoperative versus postoperative keratometric cylinder. Cases within the dashed lines are within 0.5 D of their preoperative level (Gayton). (A) Results at the 2-4 week postoperative visit. (B) Results at >6 months.

Figure 5-13. Induced cylinder in the correcting axis. The correcting axis is defined as 90 away from the steep preoperative axis. Cases above the equivalency line are overcorrected, below the equivalency line are undercorrected, and within the dashed lines are within 0.5 D of a perfect correction. An overcorrected case may still have a reduction in cylinder level, but the cylinder may be in an opposing axis (Gayton). (A) Results at the 2-4 week postoperative visit. (B) Results at >6 months.

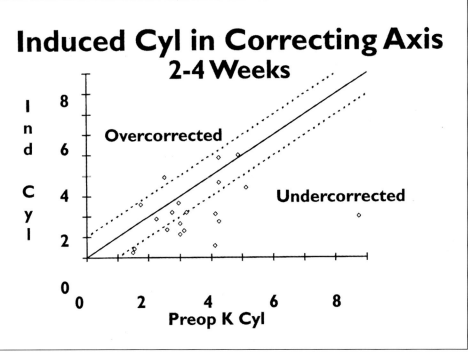

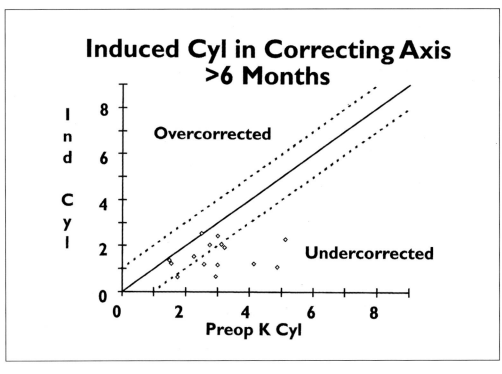

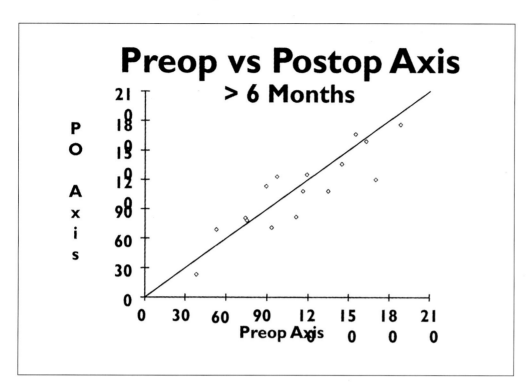

Figure 5-14. Preoperative versus postoperative cylinder axis for cases with >6 months (Gayton).

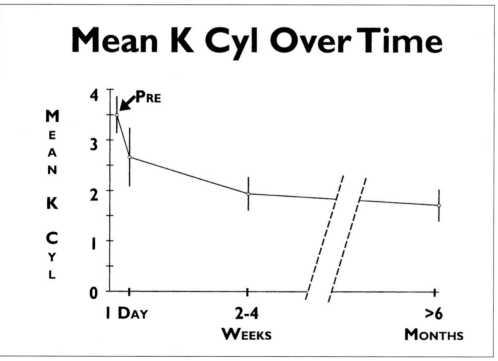

Figure 5-15. Mean keratometric cylinder over time (Gayton).

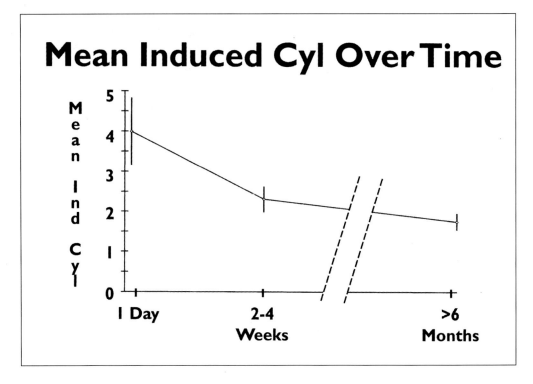

SUMMARY

Cataract surgery provides the opportunity for improving the patient's vision, not just by removing the cataract, but also by correcting preoperative refractive error. While the appropriate lens power can provide a level of refraction not present preoperatively, LRIs can improve the refraction further by correcting astigmatism. Astigmatism need not be eliminated for the patient to benefit. A conservative approach that minimizes any residual against-the-rule cylinder can vastly improve the patient's uncorrected vision.

CHAPTER 6

ADVANCED CAPSULOTOMY

Howard V. Gimbel, MD, FACS

HISTORY OF CAPSULORHEXIS

Capsulorhexis is a direct outgrowth of the capsulotomy techniques of the early 1980s. Capsulotomies, incisions into the capsule, were developed to provide access to the nucleus for phacoemulsification as well as for capsule-fixated irido-capsular intraocular lenses and then posterior-chamber intraocular lens (PC-IOL) implantation. An early technique, the can-opener capsulotomy developed by James Little, involved V-shaped incisions around 360°, resembling a lid that had been removed from a can. This technique tended to produce numerous radial tears emanating from the incisions.

Continuous Curvilinear Capsulorhexis, CCC or capsulorhexis for short, was developed to address the tendency of currently-used capsulotomy techniques to form radial tears, thus compromising the integrity of the capsule. Developed simultaneously and independently by Gimbel and Neuhann,[1-3] the capsulorhexis is formed by a continuous curvilinear tear (capsulorhexis meaning "to tear the capsule"). Due to uniform stress distribution across a relatively elastic rim, the resultant continuous curved border of the capsular opening is resistant to radial tears, even when the rim is stretched during lens implantation.

The development of the capsulorhexis, which consistently and reliably delivers a capsular opening that leaves the bag intact, has made possible many of the advanced cataract techniques in use today. Small incision surgery with soft IOLs, hydrodissection, in situ nucleofractis phacoemulsification, and pediatric posterior chamber in-the-bag implantation are all techniques that require or are facilitated by an intact capsule.

Many methods of performing capsulorhexis have been developed. In addition to the more traditional methods using cystotomes, bent needles, or forceps, capsulorhexis has been described using a vacuum method,[4] radio-frequency endodiathermy,[5] and mechanized anterior capsulectomy.[6]

Vacuum capsulorhexis uses a modified 25-gauge cannula attached to a manually controlled hydraulic line. After a tear is punctured in the capsule, the system creates a suction which attaches the capsular flap to the cannula. In creating the capsulorhexis, the vacuum cannula functions similarly to a forceps.

Capsulorhexis using radiofrequency endodiathermy was originally described by Klöti in 1984.[7,8] The technique uses a probe with a platinum alloy tip, heated to approximately 160°C by a modulated high-frequency current of 500 kHz, to coagulate and cut the capsule. The technique is most useful in pediatric cases, in which the capsule is so elastic as to be difficult to direct the rhexis inward, with the risk of extending the tear to the zonules. A diathermy capsulorhexis is easier to perform, and thus may provide some advantages in difficult cases. However, the diathermy capsulorhexis does not have the elasticity of a manually torn capsulorhexis, and hence lacks the integrity and resistance to radial tears of the more traditional manual technique.

Similarly, mechanized anterior capsulectomy, made by cutting the capsule with a vitrector, is suggested only for pediatric cases. The slightly scalloped edge created by the vitrector is not well tolerated by the less elastic capsule of the adult eye, which can lead to radial tears during phacoemulsification.

FORCEPS-PUNCTURE CONTINUOUS CURVILINEAR CAPSULORHEXIS

Initially we used an irrigating cystotome to start the capsulorhexis and Kraff-Utrata forceps (Storz Instrument Co.) to complete it. Later, we used a nonirrigating cystotome to start the CCC and viscoelastic to maintain the anterior chamber. Our technique gradually evolved into a single-instrument method using Gimbel-modified Kraff-Utrata forceps (E2002G, Storz) for the entire process. This forceps has a

Figure 6-1. The Kraff-Utrata forceps exerts controlled tension on the anterior lens capsule.

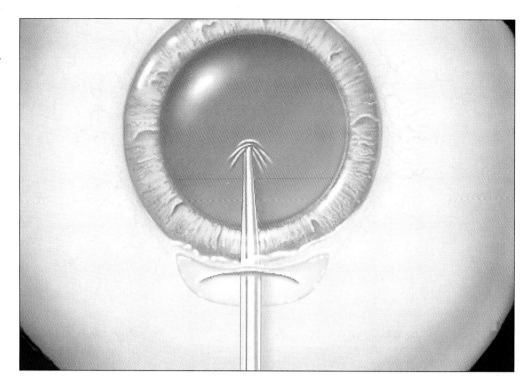

slightly longer shaft and sharper, longer tips than similar forceps. Using less instrumentation during the procedure decreases the chance of inadvertent damage to ocular structures and reduces surgical time.[9]

A single puncture is placed centrally and brought inferiorly to raise a capsular flap. While the pointed capsulorhexis forceps are used to accomplish this task, a cystotome or bent needle may be necessary in young, elastic capsules. A central location for the initial puncture is used because it decreases the tendency for the first tear to extend toward the periphery, facilitates a central circular capsulorhexis, and reduces zonular stress.

The forceps is held with the tips together and slightly tilted to create the start of the capsulotomy by applying pressure and forward movement toward the forceps tips while in contact with the center of the lens capsule (Figures 6-1, 6-2). The tip of the forceps is used to grasp the capsular flap close to the torn edge for better control. In addition, the forceps are positioned slightly ahead of the advancing tear to allow for the use of shearing forces.

The resulting tear is guided radially with the forceps toward the 3 o'clock position. The tear is then turned, using the forceps to grasp the edge of the flap, and is continued counterclockwise to complete the capsulotomy (Figure 6-3).

The shearing technique of tearing the capsule creates the CCC. The torn edge of the flap is grasped with the forceps and lifted off the plane of the capsule.[10] The force applied to the capsule is in the direction of least resistance of the tear. Thus, minimal force is required to tear it, which is particularly useful in eyes with weakened or damaged zonules. The tear is led in the desired direction using the forceps to grasp and

regrasp the flap as the tear progresses. The capsular flap is regrasped as often as necessary to control the tear.

The CCC is completed when the tear has progressed through a full circle and meets the edge of the torn capsule from the outside inward (Figure 6-4), once the required capsulorhexis diameter is achieved. The free capsular flap is removed from the eye at the start of phacoemulsification.

MATURE CATARACTS

Continuous curvilinear capsulorhexis is more challenging in intumescent cataracts.[11] Because a red reflex is absent in intumescent cataracts and milky cortex exudes through the capsulotomy, visualizing the edge of the capsulorhexis is difficult. Visualization can be improved by dimming the operating room lights and increasing the operating microscope's magnification and coaxial lighting's illumination. A 26- to 30-gauge needle can also be used to aspirate lens milk.

Dr. James Gills has suggested using a light pipe to follow at the edge of the tear with the microscope light off. The pipe illuminates the edges of the capsule that would normally not be visible (see Chapter 18). Another technique to increase visualization of the capsule has been reported by Dr. Robert Fenzl. He begins by eliminating the fluid from the anterior chamber and fills it with air. He then "paints" the capsule with fluorescein, removes the air, and fills the anterior chamber with viscoelastic.

Two-staged Capsulorhexis

In cases with intumescent or brunescent cataracts with diminished red reflexes, or cases with small pupils with lim-

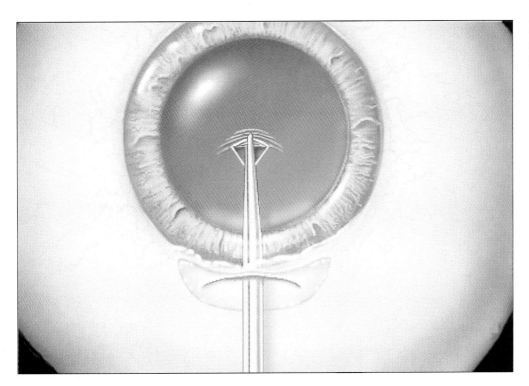

Figure 6-2. The initial capsule puncture is made with the Kraff-Utrata forceps.

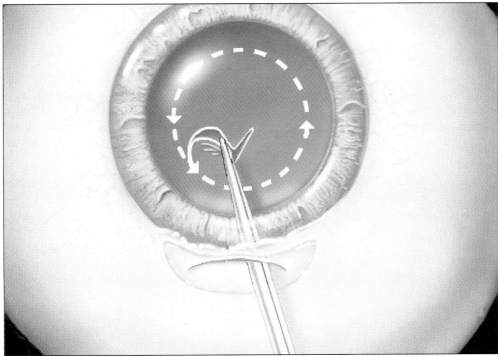

Figure 6-3. The capsulotomy is guided past the 3 o'clock position with forceps.

ited visualization, a small capsulectomy may be desirable. The small opening should be large enough to accommodate the phacoemulsification probe and a second instrument for lens manipulation. This smaller capsulectomy can then be enlarged for cortical removal as well as lens implantation using a two-staged CCC technique.[12]

After removal of the nuclear material, additional viscoelastic is used to reinflate the capsular bag. Capsule scissors are then used to make a tangential snip on one side of the opening. Care should be taken to prevent the side of the capsule opening from folding at the scissors tip, which would result in a V-cut, destroying the integrity of the continuous tear. Complete closure of the scissors should also be avoided because the point of the scissors may cause an irregularity in the line of the cut. Capsule forceps are then used to complete the larger curvilinear tear by removing a strip, or ribbon, of additional capsule.

Figure 6-4. A completed CCC.

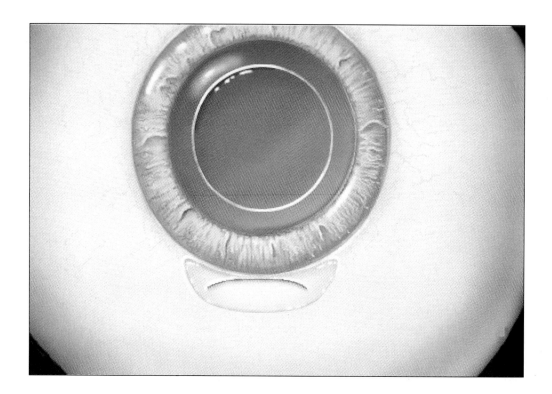

The 2-CCC technique may also be useful for corneal endothelial protection in intercapsular and endocapsular cataract extraction, when the original capsulorhexis is inadvertently too small, or for conversion of a small, traumatic opening in the anterior capsule.

MINICAPSULORHEXIS

Solomon[13,14] and Michelson[15] have both described a "minicapsulorhexis" which is large enough to permit phacoemulsification, but maintains the anterior chamber to serve as a barrier between the phacoemulsifier and the corneal endothelium. A puncture is made near the superior iris border and converted to a capsulorhexis between 0.5 to 4 mm in size. Following phacoemulsification, the "minicap" is enlarged using the 2-CCC technique for IOL insertion. The technique may significantly reduce endothelial cell loss.[16-19]

Nishi has described a buttonhole capsulotomy.[20,21] A horizontal capsulotomy is made in the superior portion of the capsule and the ends are then rounded off using forceps or a microcapsulopunch. This configuration may reduce stress concentrations so that the capsulotomy does not tear easily.

Pop[22] has developed a minicapsulorhexis technique that accommodates a two-handed phaco technique. A very small minicap is made at 2 o'clock for entry of a spatula, while a second minicap of about 3 mm in diameter is made at 11 o'clock for the phaco tip. Following phacoemulsification, the bridge between the two CCCs is incised, and the IOL implanted. A small snip is then made in the margin of the 3-mm CCC and a complete capsulorhexis is then performed.

The disadvantage of the minicapsulorhexis technique for endocapsular phaco is an increased risk of posterior capsule tears. If a posterior capsule tear occurs during phacoemulsification, loss of nuclear material into the vitreous is more likely if the anterior rim is present. Anterior capsule tears may occur during manipulation of the instruments through the small CCC. The range of movement of the phaco tip is more limited, challenging the dexterity of the surgeon, which can lead to the possibility of extending an anterior capsular tear into or through the zonules.

POSTERIOR CAPSULORHEXIS

If a small linear or triangular tear occurs in the posterior capsule, it can be converted to a continuous curvilinear tear, thus preventing the tear from extending and preserving the integrity of the bag.[23,24] The posterior continuous curvilinear capsulorhexis (PCCC) technique is accomplished by grasping one of the advancing tear flaps with forceps and completing a curvilinear tear that encompasses the extent of the original tear. To control the progressing tear, use capsule forceps to grasp the capsule flap near one point of the tear and turn the tear in the desired direction so as to blend the tear from the periphery. The opening should be kept as small as possible to preserve maximum support for the IOL.

The PCCC technique may also be used for making primary posterior capsulectomies or in removing posterior plaques. The PCCC technique is not applicable to tears that extend to or are near the equator.

OPTIC CAPTURE

In the case of a posterior capsule tear that cannot be converted, or when capsular support is otherwise compromised, the IOL can be implanted in the sulcus while "capturing" the optic within the anterior capsular rim.[25] An intact rim, as provided by CCC, is required. A spatula is used to push the optic edges underneath the anterior capsule while the haptics remain sulcus-fixated.

Optic capture can also be used in conjunction with PCCC in pediatric cases to prevent secondary cataract formation. The optic is manipulated through the posterior opening with a spatula or blunt cannula, while the haptics remain in the capsular bag. The size of the PCCC must be large enough to allow the optic through, yet small enough to capture it. The PCCC is performed before IOL implantation into the bag, with viscoelastic in place. After the procedure, the viscoelastic in the anterior chamber is removed, while the viscoelastic behind the IOL remains.

MANAGING ANTERIOR CAPSULAR TEARS

If a short anterior capsule tear occurs, it can be blunted or turned back toward the CCC using forceps[26] or by tearing a small strip or ribbon of capsule which encompasses the short tear. Although the opening will be eccentric, a radial extension of the tear will be avoided. If a longer anterior capsule occurs that cannot be blunted or turned back, care must be taken during nuclear prolapse or tipping for in-the-bag phacoemulsification, and nuclear cracking must be avoided or performed with extreme care so that no undue pressure will extend the tear into the posterior capsule.

Careful selection of IOL design is important in the presence of an anterior capsule tear. Three-piece IOLs with C-loop designs or one-piece IOLs no longer than 11 mm cause the least capsule stress. One-piece plate-haptic silicone lenses should not be implanted in the presence of a tear, as they may subluxate out of the bag when the capsule contracts.

During IOL insertion in the presence of an anterior capsule tear, viscoelastic agents can help in avoiding an extension around to the posterior capsule. The IOL haptics should be oriented perpendicular to the tear, and the tear matched 180° away to create symmetric tension on the anterior capsular rim as the capsule contracts postoperatively.

SUMMARY

Continuous curvilinear capsulorhexis is the safest means of opening the anterior capsule during cataract surgery because it preserves the elastic rim of the capsule and lessens the chance for radial tears. The principles of CCC can be used to manage anterior or posterior capsule tears that do occur, because a curved edge blunts a tear and provides resistance to further tearing. The CCC technique ensures capsular bag fixation and good centration of the IOL, and has greatly facili-tated the development of modern small-incision cataract surgery techniques.

REFERENCES

1. Gimbel HV, Neuhann T. Development, advantages and methods of the continuous circular capsulorhexis technique. *J Cataract Refract Surg* 1990; 16:31-37.

2. Gimbel HV, Neuhann T. Continuous curvilinear capsulorhexis [letter]. *J Cataract Refract Surg* 1991; 17:110.

3. Neuhann T. Theorie und Operationtechnik der Kapsulorhexis. *Klin Monatsble Augentreilkd* 1985; 16:372-376.

4. Brierley L. Vacuum capsulorhexis. *J Cataract Refract Surg* 1995; 21:13-15.

5. Luck J, Brahma AK, Noble BA. A comparative study of the elastic properties of continuous tear curvilinear capsulorhexis versus capsulorhexis produced by radiofrequency endodiathermy. *Br J Ophthalmol* 1994; 78:392-396.

6. Wilson ME, Bluestein EC, Wang X-H, Apple DJ. Comparison of mechanized anterior capsulectomy and manual continuous capsulorhexis in pediatric eyes. *J Cataract Refract Surg* 1994; 20:602-606.

7. Klöti R. Bipolar-Nassfeld-Diathermie in der Mikrochirugie. *Klin Monatsbl Augenheilkd* 1984; 442:184.

8. Gassmann F, Schimmelpfennig B, Klöti R. Anterior capsulotomy by means of bipolar radio-frequency endodiathermy. *J Cataract Refract Surg* 1988; 14:673.

9. Gimbel HV, Kaye GB. Forceps-puncture continuous curvilinear capsulorhexis. *J Cataract Refract Surg* 1997; 23:473-475.

10. Arshinoff S. Mechanics of capsulorhexis. *J Cataract Refract Surg* 1992; 18:623-628.

11. Gimbel HV, Willerscheidt AB. What to do with limited view: The intumescent cataract. *J Cataract Refract Surg* 1993; 19:657-661.

12. Gimbel HV. Two-stage capsulorhexis for endocapsular phacoemulsification. *J Cataract Refract Surg* 1990; 16:246-249.

13. Solomon LD. Endocapsular phacoemulsification. In Solomon LD (ed): *Practical Phacoemulsification: Proceedings of the 2nd Annual Workshop* [Supplement to *Ophthalmic Practice*]. 1990, pp 10-13.

14. Solomon LD. Endocapsular (intercapsular) phacoemulsification. In Solomon LD (ed): *Practical Phacoemulsification: Proceedings of the 3rd Annual Workshop* [Supplement to *Ophthalmic Practice*]. 1991, pp 29-39.

15. Michelson MA. Endocapsular phacoemulsification with mini-capsulorhexis. In Koch P, Davison J (eds): *Phacoemulsification Techniques*. Thorofare, NJ, Slack, Inc, 1991, pp 275-309.

16. Patel J, Apple D. Protective effect of the anterior lens capsule during extracapsular cataract extraction. *Ophthalmology* 1989; 96:598-602.

17. Hara T, Hara T. Subcapsular phacoemulsification and aspiration. *Am Intraocular Implant Soc J* 1984; 10:333-337.

18. Wan WL, Gindi JJ, Schanzlin DJ. Endocapsular cataract surgery—II. Effects on the corneal endothelium. *Cataract* 1985; 2:11-14.

19. Solomon KD, Gwin TD, O'Morchoe DJC, et al. Protective effect of the anterior lens capsule during extracapsular cataract extraction. Part I: Experimental animal study. *Ophthalmology* 1987; 96:591-597.

20. Nishi O, Nishi K. Endocapsular phacoemulsification follow-

ing buttonhole anterior capsulotomy: A preliminary report. *J Cataract Refract Surg* 1990; 16:757-762.

21. Nishi O. Endo-Intercapsular cataract surgery following buttonhole anterior capsulotomy. In Yalon M (ed): *Techniques of Phacoemulsification Surgery and IOL Implantation.* Thorofare, NJ, Slack, Inc, 1992, pp 249-266.

22. Pop M. Two-port endocap phaco: Safe and quick. *Ocular Surgery News* 1991; 9:1,40.

23. Gimbel HV. Posterior capsule tears using phacoemulsification: Causes, prevention and management. *Eur J Implant Ref Surg* 1990; 2:63-69.

24. Gimbel HV. The prevention and management of capsule complications. *Asia-Pacific J of Ophthalmol* 1995; 7(3)5-8.

25. Gimbel HV, DeBroff BM. Posterior capsulorhexis with optic capture: A new method to maintain a clear visual axis after pediatric surgery. *J Cataract Refract Surg* 1994; 20:658-664.

26. Gimbel HV. Continuous curvilinear capsulorhexis and nucleus fracturing: Evolution, technique, and complications. *Ophthalmology Clinics of North America* 1991; 4(2):235-249.

COMPLICATIONS RELATING TO CAPSULORHEXIS

John R. Shepherd, MD, FACS, Maurice John, MD

Capsulorhexis has become the cornerstone of modern phacoemulsification surgery. It alone preserves the capsular bag, a space spoken about for years but which did not actually exist with earlier methods of capsulotomy. The structurally sound capsular bag allows better centration with the earlier open-loop haptic implants and is absolutely required with plate haptic designs.[1]

In addition, capsulorhexis makes possible more complete removal of cortex, allows stable fixation of the implant in the face of severe zonular dehiscence, and prevents anterior capsular tears from extending to the posterior capsule in the presence of chamber collapse or positive vitreous pressure. Clear-corneal cataract surgery with topical anesthesia would be highly dangerous without the employment of capsulorhexis.

But all of these advantages come at a price. That is, the retention of large numbers of anterior lens epithelial cells (LEC) and the resulting complications.

According to Apple, residual lens epithelial cells are responsible for:
1. Posterior capsular opacification.
2. Optic decentration or excessive distortion of loops.
3. Phacotoxis or phacoanaphyactic inflammatory reaction.
4. Soemmering's ring
5. Difficulty in achieving long-term success with IOL implantation in children.
6. Decentration of foldable implants.[2]

Of course all of the above complications have been seen for years prior to capsulorhexis. Most are due to peripheral lens epithelial cell proliferation either alone or in conjunction with anterior lens epithelial cells and retained cortical fibers. However, with the widespread use of capsulorhexis, we are now seeing two new complications: capsular phimosis, and anterior inflammatory membranes.[3]

What is the mechanism by which these problems occur? In the past, the more destructive, can-opener capsulotomy left only a tattered fringe of anterior capsular flaps which retracted and quickly adhered to the posterior capsule in the periphery. Few of these remained over the optic of the implant. This technique not only left little anterior capsule upon which the epithelial cells were attached, but the early adherence of the capsule prevented the retained epithelial cells from proliferating. The earliest mention of the anterior proliferative membrane was reported by surgeons using an envelope capsulotomy which retained a large sheet of anterior capsule.[4-7]

With capsulorhexis, one retains a large section of anterior capsule densely populated with epithelial cells and separated from the posterior capsule by the optic in conventional open-looped haptic implants and both the optic and the haptic in the newer plate-haptic IOL.

Nishi has proposed that the juxtaposition of LEC with a solid foreign object has some stimulative effect on proliferation of these cells,[10] which probably explains their more exuberant proliferation with plate-haptic implants following capsulorhexis and open-looped implants following envelope capsulotomies. Certainly, any breakdown in the blood-aqueous barrier such as in iritis patients or glaucoma patients with miotic pupils can act as a catalyst in the reaction.

Proliferation of LEC takes place primarily at the inner edge of the rhexis. In the early postoperative period, small gray digital projections can be observed extending from the torn edge of the capsule toward the center of the implant (Figure 7-1). The routine use of steroids for two weeks seems to inhibit their growth and they usually disappear by week two to three.

More commonly, this proliferation takes the form of encircling the inside edge of the rhexis. These proliferating cells undergo metaplastic change to become a white, fibrotic membrane demarcating the inner border of the tear. With wide dilation of the pupil, this ring can be seen on many if not most patients. It is usually benign (Figure 7-2).

Figure 7-1. Small gray digital projections can be observed extending from the torn edge of the capsule toward the center of the implant caused by proliferating lens epithelial cells (LECs) (Shepherd).

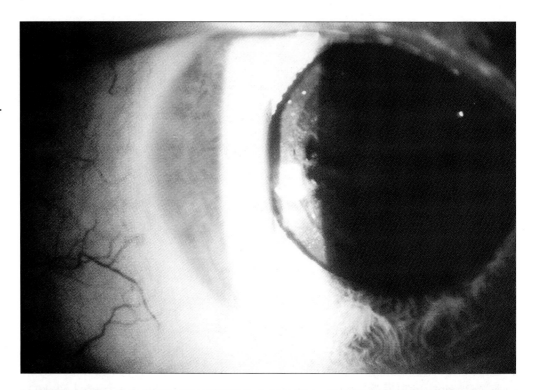

Figure 7-2. Proliferation of LECs encircling the inside edge of the rhexis. These proliferating cells undergo metaplastic change to become a white, fibrotic membrane demarcating the inner border of the tear (Shepherd).

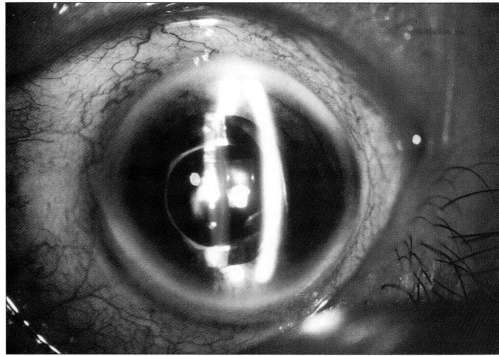

However, if this membrane is substantial enough, it can contract, gradually shrinking the opening as if by drawstring until only a pinpoint opening remains (capsular phimosis) (Figure 7-3). If the capsular bag is unnaturally large, the capsulorhexis opening may be asymmetrical and subsequent contraction may cause the implant to become decentered.

The most dramatic form of proliferation is the inflamma-tory membrane that covers the entire anterior surface of the implant.[4-9] Although most prevalent in Asian literature, it has been described in the U.S., and one of the authors (JRS) has experienced five cases out of 1500 cataract surgery patients in 1994. The following case history is typical.

A 72 year-old women of Japanese ancestry had an uncom-plicated phacoemulsification with implant of a solid-haptic

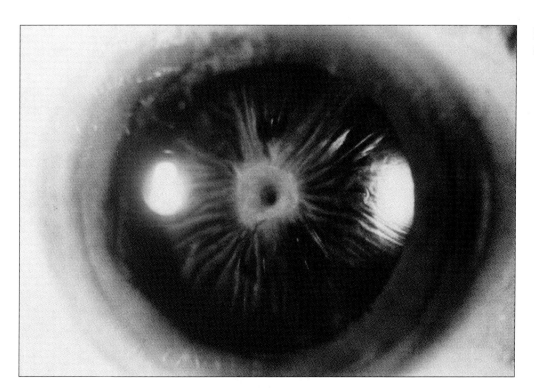

Figure 7-3. Capsular phimosis (Shepherd).

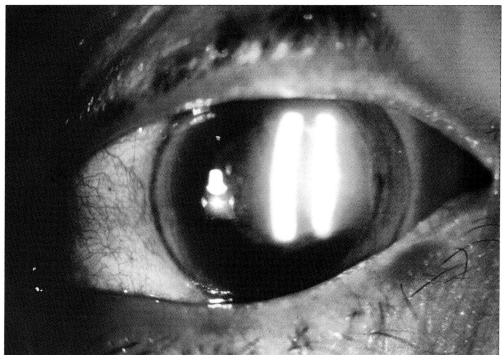

Figure 7-4. Proliferation of LECs which created an inflammatory gray membrane that covers the entire anterior surface of the implant attached to the anterior capsulorhexis (Shepherd).

silicone implant. She had a normal postoperative course and was discharged on no medications at two weeks. Six weeks later she returned with acute iritis and was treated with topical steroids and mydriatics. Four days later she presented with a gray membrane covering the anterior surface of the

implant attached to the anterior capsulorhexis edge (Figure 7-4). This patient was taken to surgery and the entire membrane stripped and sent to ophthalmic pathology at the University of Utah. The slides revealed metaplastic LEC and fibrous tissue (Figures 7-5).

Figure 7-5. Pathology slides from same eye shown in Figure 7-4 revealed metaplastic LEC and fibrous tissue (Shepherd).

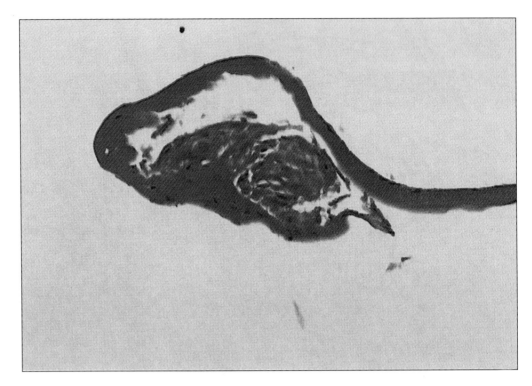

PREVENTION OF COMPLICATIONS

If the underlying cause of these complications is the retention of lens epithelial cells, then the solution is apparent. Most of these cells need to be removed at surgery.[9,13]

Removal of LECs—Shepherd Technique

Removal of LECs is accomplished in two steps.

1. Make a large capsulorhexis—The most effective method of removing the LECs is by making a large capsulorhexis. Since the anterior zonules insert at about the 6-mm ring, the ideal size that would not tear into the zonules would be about 5.5 to 6 mm. This size would allow overlap at the edge of the optic and would remove a large section of anterior capsule with epithelial cells attached.

A capsulorhexis of this size is not always possible to do at the beginning of the procedure. Not infrequently, it is safer to make a smaller rhexis. Sometimes the size seems larger before the cataract is removed and the IOL inserted than after. In both of these situations, it is advisable to enlarge the capsulorhexis after the implant is inserted (see also Chapter 6).

To enlarge the rhexis opening after the implant is inserted, the following points may make the procedure easier.

- Control the anterior chamber by inflating with viscoelastic, which prevents a chamber collapse and subsequent radial tears in the anterior and even posterior capsule.
- Make a small nick in the capsule with Vannas scissors.
- Tear a larger opening by pulling this flap in a circular motion with the Utratta forceps (Figure 7-6).

2. Clean the LEC off the remaining anterior capsule—The remaining anterior capsular flap should have the bulk of the epithelial cells removed by scraping the posterior surface of the anterior capsule with some type of instrument. I prefer a modification of the chalazion curette in which both sides of the curette are sharp. This instrument allows us to scrape the posterior capsule as well as the anterior capsule. Because of the large area of the curette, it will not cut and can be used quite safely without fear of rupturing the capsule. I use the following technique:

- Following removal of all cortex, I inflate the anterior chamber with BSS (unless there is a large amount of vitreous pressure, in which case I use a viscoelastin).
- A right Shepherd-Rentsch curette (Morning STAAR Surgical Instruments) is placed in the anterior chamber and the central posterior capsule is cleaned. Then the curette is placed between the right anterior and right posterior capsules and both surfaces are scraped. The anterior is the more important of the two, so it commands the most attention. We clean from 6 to 12 o'clock and then remove the curette (Figure 7-7).
- The anterior chamber is re-inflated with BSS or viscoelastin and the same procedure is performed on the left anterior and posterior capsule using the left curette.
- Lastly, the patient is placed on a steroid eye drop four times daily for two weeks.

Preventing Decentration

An asymmetric capsulorhexis may lead to a significant decentration of the IOL as the fibrotic forces from the irregu-

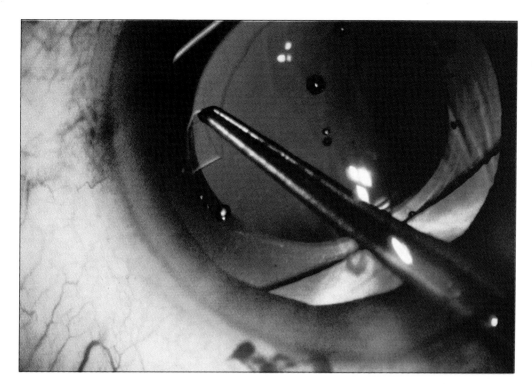

Figure 7-6. Enlarging capsulorhexis with Utrata forceps (Shepherd).

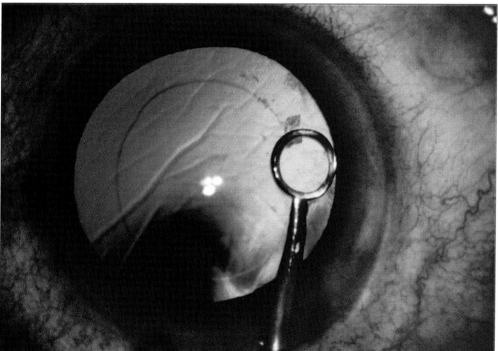

Figure 7-7. Cleaning the capsule (Shepherd).

larly shaped capsule push the lens (Figure 7-8). If the haptics are aligned parallel with the irregularity in the rhexis, the haptic will provide a counter force against the fibrotic forces from the capsule, resisting lens decentration. As the fibrotic forces are balanced, the capsule will reorient itself so that the capsulorhexis becomes more symmetrical.

TREATMENT OF COMPLICATIONS

Posterior capsule opacification

Posterior capsule opacification is the most common complication of cataract surgery and economically by far the most important. Its prevention by diligent cleaning of the capsular

Figure 7-8. An asymmetric capsulorhexis may lead to a significant decentration of the IOL as the fibrotic forces from the irregularly shaped capsule push the lens (Shepherd).

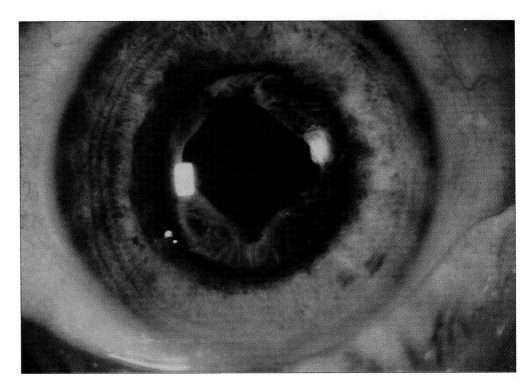

bag and choice of IOL should be the goal of all cataract surgeons. However, some capsules will opacify despite all precautions. It is ironic that the solid plate silicone lens, which has the lowest incidence of capsular opacification, is the lens that can cause the most problems if YAGed too early or too strenuously.[11-13]

The technique of removing lens epithelial cells described above makes early opacification (within one year of surgery) very rare. In addition, if YAG capsulotomy becomes necessary in later years, the capsule will be very thin and easily opened. The tough fibrotic capsule or the capsule thickened by enormous pearl proliferation will almost never be seen.

In our experience of inserting several thousand of these plate lens over the last ten years, rarely is a capsulotomy required within the first three to six months following surgery. If it is necessary, however, wait a minimum of three months and preferably six to perform it.

We have observed for some time that the capsular bag undergoes shrinkage in the early postoperative period. Previous opinion held that the anterior and posterior capsule fused in a sequential manner from the periphery to the center of the capsule. This fusion would frequently decenter the haptics of J loop implants, in some occasions bending the haptics completely over their optics, requiring amputation.

After opening several capsules while performing lens exchanges or repositioning, we have not found strong adhesions between the peripheral anterior and posterior capsules. The progressive contraction of the capsular bag appears to be generated by the annular fibrosis around the rhexis opening, drawing the anterior capsule tighter and tighter. This process occurs for an undetermined period following cataract surgery.

If YAG capsulotomy is performed during this period of active contraction, the posterior capsule can split, dumping the plate haptic implant into the vitreous.

There have been reports of this complication occurring as late as two years following surgery. The prudent surgeon will then avoid capsulotomy as long as possible.

John YAG Capsulotomy Method

The typical cruciate technique used for PMMA lenses with prolene or PMMA loops should be abandoned for plate haptic lenses (Figure 7-9). These plate haptic lenses are relatively inert and are relatively small, when compared to an expanded loop-style lens. If too large a posterior capsule opening is made, the plate haptic lens may dislocate into the vitreous. I have seen cases where I placed two vertical shots in the posterior capsule, and the opening enlarged vertically 4 mm due to severe posterior pressure from the anterior capsule.

To avoid this complication, start by evaluating the anterior capsule. If there is a fibrotic anterior capsular rim, involving 140° or more of the anterior capsule, the laser surgeon should first create small V-shaped breaks in this anterior capsular ring. While creating each V-opening, in the anterior capsule, usually 2-10 laser shots will be required.

Once the actual ring is broken through, usually the interruption will extend about 0.5 mm to 1 mm peripherally on its own, because of the release of tension in the circular band which the surgeon has created (Figure 7-10 A,B). This extension certainly verifies that there is indeed some very significant forces at work, which need to be abated before addressing the cloudy posterior capsule.

There is no need to treat near the transparent areas of the

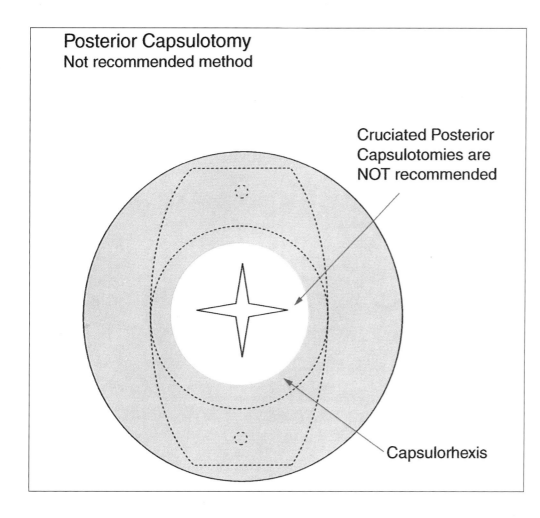

Posterior Capsulotomy
Not recommended method

Cruciated Posterior
Capsulotomies are
NOT recommended

Capsulorhexis

Figure 7-9. The typical cruciate YAG capsulotomy technique used for PMMA lenses with prolene or PMMA loops should be abandoned for plate haptic lenses (John).

anterior capsule. Only the whitish, fibrotic purse string-like bands need to be "fractured". This constrictive anterior capsule, whether partial or complete, creates a great deal of posterior pressure on the IOL. If the anterior capsule is not treated first, then the posterior opening may be too large, and the anterior capsule will push the lens posteriorly.

After creating about 1-4 of these V-shaped fractures in the anterior capsule, then address the posterior capsule. Starting centrally, in a spiral fashion according to the Shepherd technique, the posterior capsule is carefully opened (Figure 7-10C). The posterior capsule should be enlarged to a diameter of about 2.5 mm. Ultimately, we want a circular opening which is hopefully nearly as strong as the original anterior capsulorhexis at the time of the initial surgery (Figure 7-10D). Using this technique, I've never had a plate-haptic IOL dislocate either posteriorly or anteriorly.

Shepherd YAG Capsulotomy Method

When capsulotomy is necessary, I use the following technique:

1. Dilate the pupil widely
2. Place an Abraham YAG capsulotomy contact lens in the patients eye.

3. Use 2.0 milli-joules of power, and retro-aim the HeNe beam as follows: Focus the beam on the posterior capsule. Push the joy stick forward until the two HeNe spots are separated by a distance of two spot sizes. This procedure will place the explosion about 200 microns posterior to the capsule and implant.
4. Fire once in the visual axis. Then make a second shot at the edge of the first opening. Proceed in a circular manner, slowly enlarging the opening and keeping it centered. A 3-mm opening is usually adequate and will not split peripherally in the posterior capsule.

Above all, avoid creating radial tears such as in the Maltese Cross method of capsulotomy.

If a patient has a severe contraction of the capsular opening, it would probably be a good idea to weaken it somewhat by YAGing a crescent-shaped segment out of the edge (Figure 7-11) or making small radial openings in the fibrotic capsular edge as described above.

Silicone implants will mark with the YAG more easily than PMMA implants. Although these are usually avoided by retro-aiming, some will occur. However, I have never seen any that created a visual disturbance.

Figure 7-10. Releasing tension in the anterior capsule with the YAG with the John method (John). (A) The laser surgeon should first create small V-shaped breaks in the anterior capsular ring with 2-10 laser shots. (B) Extend the relaxing cut no more than 5 mm. (C) A spiral YAG posterior capsulotomy is performed by the method of Shepherd. (D) Appearance post-YAG.

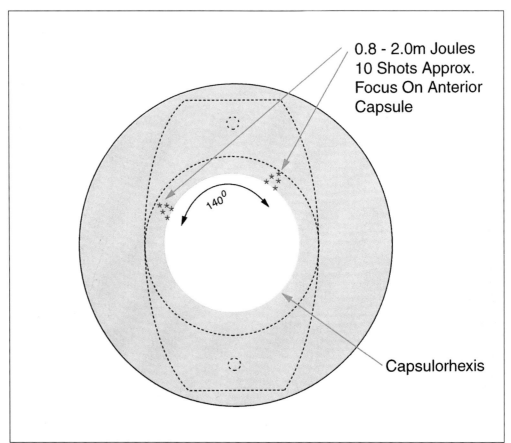

0.8 - 2.0m Joules 10 Shots Approx. Focus On Anterior Capsule

140°

Capsulorhexis

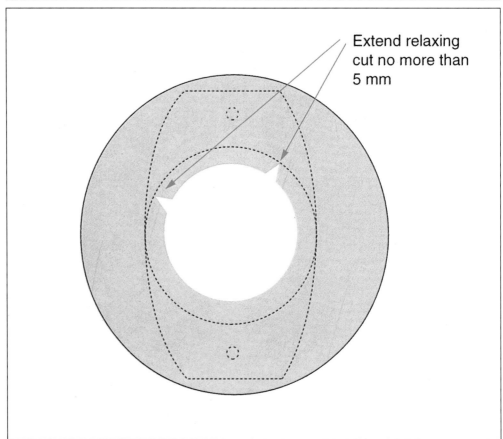

Extend relaxing cut no more than 5 mm

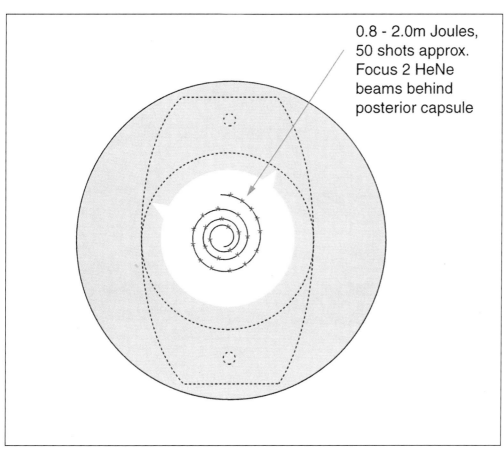

0.8 - 2.0m Joules,
50 shots approx.
Focus 2 HeNe
beams behind
posterior capsule

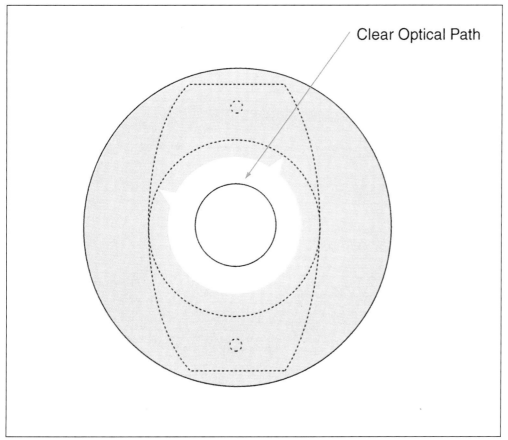

Clear Optical Path

Figure 7-11. Releasing tension in the anterior capsule with the YAG with the Shepherd method (John). (A) A crescent is removed from the edge of the capsule with the YAG. (B) The YAG enlargement leaves the circular rim intact. A spiral capsulotomy is then performed as shown in Figure 7-10C.

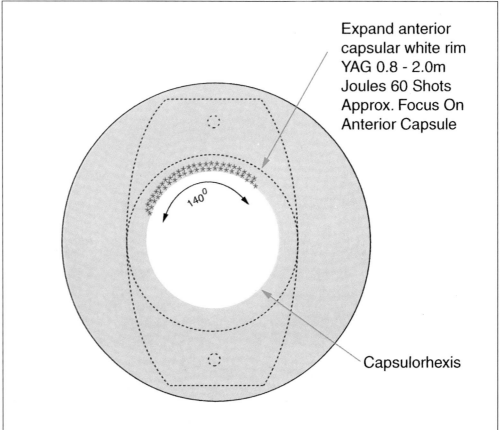

Expand anterior capsular white rim YAG 0.8 - 2.0m Joules 60 Shots Approx. Focus On Anterior Capsule

Capsulorhexis

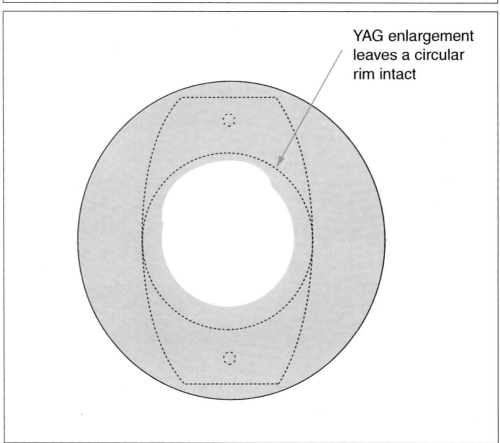

YAG enlargement leaves a circular rim intact

Capsular Phimosis

Caused by progressive contraction of the fibrosis associated with metaplastic lens epithelial cells, this complication is easily avoided. If it occurs, one should attempt to remove the fibrotic ring, or a large portion of it by YAG ablation.[8]

Shepherd Technique

1. The power settings are slightly lower, 1.2 to 1.4 millijoules.
2. The HeNe bean is aimed in front of the anterior capsule and implant. The two spots are focused on the anterior capsule. The joy stick is pulled back, separating the spots by a distance of two spot sizes.
3. Aim at the inside edge of the fibrotic ring and fire until there is a separation and then fire at the edge of the separation and extend the opening until a section of the ring or the whole ring falls free. It is unclear what happens to this segment. It disappears in a few days, either being absorbed or migrating behind the iris.

Avoid creating three or four radial openings as one does with PMMA implants. These tears can extend (under great stress) to and through the posterior capsule.

Decentration of Implants

While capsulorhexis is necessary to secure solid-plate implants, it is also at least a contributing factor in decentering some of them. The plate-haptic implant measures 10.5 mm in length and is therefore as large or larger than the vast majority of capsular bags. Some bags are larger, some by a significant amount. These are usually found in high myopes, and are more common when the white-to-white measurement is 13 millimeters or larger. Many of these patients have no problem with decentration, but if the capsulorhexis is asymmetric, there will be an unbalanced fibrotic force on one side of the implant because unequal amounts of capsule remain (Figure 7-12). These cases tend to decenter on the short axis. In these cases only implant a plate-haptic implant with the long axis parallel to these fibrotic forces, as described above.

A more ominous sign is decentration in the long axis. In this situation, the cause is one haptic in the bag and one out. It can occur if the surgeon has mispositioned the implant, but more commonly occurs with an undetected hole in the posterior capsule. The haptic can work its way through this opening and then into the vitreous. Treatment of decentration in the long axis is immediate lens exchange.

Treating Decentration—Shepherd Technique

Implants that are just decentered in the short axis or implants that are the wrong power can be handled in the following manner.

1. Reform the bag. The capsular bag can be reformed for at least several months following surgery. It has been performed as late as 18 months following surgery. The technique is to break the fibrous adhesions surrounding the haptic. Since the fibrotic bands do not attach to the silicone, a cannula with viscoelastin is inserted between the edge of the capsulorhexis and the implant and manipulated gently until most of the adhesions at the edge of the implant are severed. As one goes from central to peripheral the adhesions become less strong or non-existent. When most are gone, the lens is rotated 90 degrees from its original position. This final rotation will break the remaining adhesions. If the purpose of this technique was re-positioning, the surgeon can leave the implant in this position. I have never had one decenter secondarily.

2. If the purpose was lens exchange because of power differences, the original lens can be removed. The incision should be enlarged to 4.5-5.0 mm to remove the implant. Then the lens with correct power can be inserted. If this incision was clear corneal, I prefer to suture the wound if the size is 4.0 mm or larger. An 11-0 nylon running shoelace suture works well and causes no discomfort. It may be left in permanently or removed in six weeks

Anterior Fibrotic Membranes

Prevention is by far the most effective treatment for anterior fibrotic membranes. Scrupulous removal of all cortex, debridement of the posterior surface of the anterior capsule to remove many of the lens epithelial cells, and making a large capsulorhexis will prevent almost all of these complications. If faced with this problem, the surgeon should place the patient back on topical steroids every two hours during waking hours along with Atropine 1% four times daily. After a day or two the membrane should be disrupted with the nd:YAG laser.

Technique: The pupil is probably as widely dilated as it will get. Use an Abraham YAG contact lens. Set the power to 1.0 to 1.3 millijoules. Focus the HeNe beams together and then defocus by pulling the joy stick toward you until the beams are separated by a distance of two spot sizes. One can make a Maltese Cross opening in the central membrane, continue the steroids and Atropine, and the remainder of the membrane will absorb rapidly.

Anterior Implant Surface Pigmentary Deposits

In many ways anterior implant surface pigmentary deposits are the most troubling of the complications. Their cause is obscure. They are most common with combined procedures (cataract-trabeculectomy) but are found in patients on long-term miotic therapy, patients with chronic iritis, or anyone with a decreased blood-aqueous barrier. It appears that the pigment deposits that characterize the complication is a secondary development. The primary change seems to be a cobweb-like infiltrate of gray cells identified by some workers as giant cells. It is also possible that these giant cells are themselves secondary. Observation of the edge of the rhexis always reveals some proliferative activity. Could the initial problem be lens epithelial proliferation?

Pigmentary deposits usually appear in a relatively quiet eye, although some flare and cells may be seen. They can be

Figure 7-12. With an asymmetric capsulorhexis, there will be an unbalanced fibrotic force on one side of the implant because unequal amounts of capsule remain. These cases tend to decenter on the short axis. In these cases only implant a plate-haptic implant with the long axis parallel to these fibrotic forces (John).

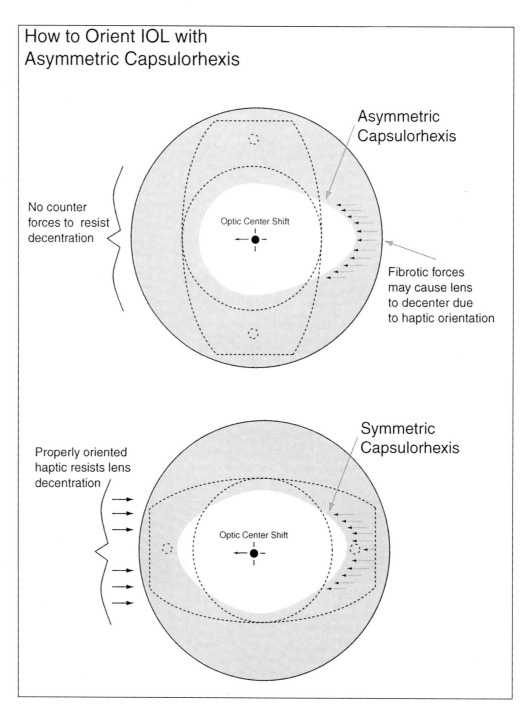

How to Orient IOL with Asymmetric Capsulorhexis

Asymmetric Capsulorhexis

No counter forces to resist decentration

Optic Center Shift

Fibrotic forces may cause lens to decenter due to haptic orientation

Symmetric Capsulorhexis

Properly oriented haptic resists lens decentration

Optic Center Shift

so dense as to decrease visual acuity four to five lines (Figure 7-13).

Treatment: This complication is treated similarly to the fibrotic membrane, but is apt to reoccur. For that reason, steroids/atropine drops should be a long term medication.

The pigment deposits are easily removed with the nd:YAG. I use the same settings and defocusing technique as for fibrotic membranes, but try to remove each individual pigment deposit and laser to the very edge of the capsulorhexis. Anterior synechia are common with this problem and these can be lysed with the laser at the same time.

REFERENCES

1. Shepherd JR: Continuous tear capsulotomy and insertion of a silicone bag lens. *J Cataract Refract Surg* 1989; 15:335-338.
2. Apple DJ, Kincaid MC, Mamalis N, Olson RJ: *Intraocular Lenses*, Baltimore, Williams and Wilkins, 1989.
3. Masket S: Post-operative complications of capsulorhexis. *J Cataract Refract Surg* 1993; 19:721-724.
4. Nishi O: Fibrinous membrane formation on the posterior chamber lens during the early post-operative period. *J Cataract Refract Surg* 1988; 14: 73-77.
5. Nishi O, Nishi K: Fibrin reaction following posterior cham-

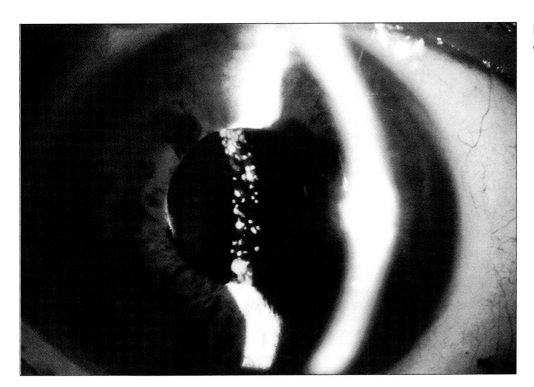

Figure 7-13. Pigmentary deposits (Shepherd).

ber lens implantation. *Implants Ophthalmol* 1988; 2:216-220.

6. Nishi O: Intercapsular cataract surgery with lens epithelial cell removal. Part II: effect on prevention of fibrinous reaction. *J Cataract Refract Surg* 1989; 15:301-303.

7. Miyake K, Maekubok Y, Nishi O: Pupillary fibrin membrane - a frequent early complication after posterior chamber lens implantation in Japan. *Ophthalmology* 1989; 96:1228-1233.

8. Hansen SO, Crandall AS, Olson RJ: Progressive constriction of the anterior capsular opening following intact capsulorhexis. *J Cataract Refract Surg* 1993; 19:77-82.

9. Choun-ki Joo, Jeong-ah Jeony, Jae-Ho Kim: Capsular opening contraction after continuous curvilinear capsulorhexis and intraocular lens implantation. *J Cataract Refract Surg* 1996; 22:585-590.

10. Nishi O, Nishi K, Sakka Y, Sakuraba T, Maeda S: Intercapsular cataract surgery with lens epithelial cell removal. *J Cataract Refract Surg* 1991; 17:471-477.

11. Shepherd JR: Capsular opacification associated with silicone implants. *J Cataract Refract Surg* 1989; 15:448-450.

12. Shepherd JR: Capsulotomy rate found lower for silicone than PMMA IOLs. *Ocular Surgery News* 15, Aug 1991.

13. Rentsch F. Baue H: Reduction of after-cataract by removal of lens epithelium. Presented at 1992 ASCRS symposium, San Diego.

14. Shah S, Spalton D: Natural history of cellular deposits on the anterior intraocular lens surface. *J Cataract Refractive Surg* 1995; 21:460-471

RECENT ADVANCES IN PHACOEMULSIFICATION SYSTEMS

CHAPTER 8

I. Howard Fine, MD, Richard S. Hoffman, MD

In the past several years there have been dramatic improvements in phacoemulsification technology involving every aspect of phacoemulsification systems from the phaco tip all the way down to the foot pedal. Improvements in the generation of ultrasonic power, fluidics, user interfaces, and tips and handpieces have been extremely advantageous to the cataract surgeon. It is because of these improvements that phacoemulsification has rapidly become the primary extraction technique in many parts of the developing world, despite the challenges of harder, darker nuclei.

ULTRASONICS

Advances in the generation of ultrasonic power stem from improvements in both the quality and quantity of crystals in the piezo-electric crystal configuration in systems such as the Alcon Series 20,000 LEGACY. The ultrasonic driver in the Legacy is controlled by a dedicated microprocessor which allows for exact control of ultrasonic power at all power levels. The turbosonic handpiece utilizes a four-crystal transducer design, which is capable of producing a much more standard and reproducible stroke length at each power setting regardless of the load (mass and density of nuclear material) at the phaco tip. Since the load is continually changing, the system must be able to adjust or else the cutting efficiency will be compromised. The Legacy is able to maximize efficiency utilizing a new complex control system, "constant admittance tuning," which matches the driving frequency of the console to the operating frequency at the phacoemulsification handpiece maintaining optimal power regardless of lens density.[1]

Some of the other advances affecting the ultrasonic generation of energy for phacoemulsification involve technology that harnesses options for judicious application of power such as the power modulations available on the AMO Diplomax System. Among these modulations are autopulse phaco, burst mode phaco, and occlusion mode phaco.

In autopulse phaco, the phaco handpiece will run in continuous power mode at high phaco power and will automatically change to pulsed power when the foot pedal is eased into lower powers. This setting is useful for grooving the central nucleus at higher powers in continuous mode while using the more delicate control of pulsed phaco at lower powers for extending the groove out to the periphery if desired. Burst mode phaco produces bursts of 40, 60, or 80 millisecond duration at preset ultrasound power levels when the foot pedal is placed in position 3. This mode is helpful for impaling the nucleus for chopping techniques and in quadrant removal where vacuum accompanied by intermittent bursts of power are commonly utilized. Finally, occlusion mode phaco allows for power modulation of the phaco handpiece in continuous, pulse, autopulse, burst, or power off modes depending on whether the phaco tip is occluded or unoccluded (Table 8-1). This setting allows for the judicious use of phaco power with programmable vacuum levels and aspiration rates.[2] All of these modulations allow for programmable changes in ultrasound energy delivered to the eye so that inappropriate energy that can result in increased chatter and less purchase of nuclear material can be avoided.

PHACOTMESIS

Other energy sources have been combined with ultrasound with the hope of enhanced efficiency. However, it is difficult to foresee whether these new technologies will find a market niche. PhacoTmesis combines high-speed mechanical rotatory power to ultrasonic linear oscillation with the achievement of some added safety for the iris, corneal endothelium, and

TABLE 8-1

HIGH VACUUM TUBING
PHACO POWER MODE
(Sculpting - Phaco 1)

Unoccluded	Occluded
Continuous	Continuous
Pulse 33%	Pulse 33%
Pulse 50%	Pulse 50%
Pulse 66%	Pulse 66%
Autopulse	Autopulse
Burst 40 ms	Burst 40 ms
Burst 60 ms	Burst 60 ms
Burst 80 ms	Burst 80 ms
Power OFF	Power OFF

posterior capsule. The Tmesis tip is covered by the irrigating silicone sleeve; thus there is no sharp oscillating or rotating tip exposed to touch or damage vital intraocular tissues. The Tmesis tip creates a pulverizing effect on the nucleus at a small distance just in front of the tip without the need for actual contact. In addition, the rotating tip creates a circular fluid current which combined with the aspiration flow causes a microscopic whirlpool effect that maintains the followability of the lens fragments within the pulverizing aspiration zone.[3] Although PhacoTmesis may provide added safety, it may be at the expense of efficiency.

LASER

In the constant search for improvements in cataract extraction, surgeons have begun investigating laser energy as an alternative energy source to ultrasound. Four ultraviolet (excimer) laser wavelengths have been investigated including 193 nm (argon fluoride), 248 nm (krypton fluoride), 308 nm (xenon chloride), and 351 nm (xenon fluoride). Use of the excimer laser for cataract removal appears to be hampered by limitations in fiber optic technology and safety concerns regarding possible injury to the surgeon and patient from ultraviolet excimer laser energy.[4] Concern regarding the safety of ultraviolet wavelengths has directed focus onto the infrared wavelengths as potential energy sources for cataract removal. The Nd:YLF 1053 nm picosecond laser has been shown to be effective in softening the lens and cortex by external ablation followed by internal standard irrigation and aspiration. The main disadvantage of this technique is that it requires a two-staged procedure since no intraocular device using this wavelength currently exists.[4]

Premier Laser Systems in conjunction with Dr. D. Michael Colvard have designed and manufactured an Erbium:YAG laser for cataract extraction which offers many advantages compared to ultrasound energy. The Erbium laser uses non-ultraviolet radiation and can be delivered through a fiberoptic delivery system, thus allowing cataract extraction in a one-staged intraocular technique. In addition, the Erbium laser can be used to perform a continuous curvilinear capsulotomy and ablates tissue without thermal injury. This laser offers a substantially gentler lens cutting mechanism with a shorter learning curve than ultrasonic phacoemulsification; potentially making small-incision cataract surgery more accessible to a greater number of surgeons around the world.[5]

The Nd:YAG laser, the energy source most commonly associated with intraocular applications, has been the most studied of all energy sources and is presently in clinical use as part of an FDA-sponsored study in the USA and in studies in other countries. The laser developed by Paradigm Medical Industries uses a solid-state pulsed Nd:YAG 1064 nm laser whose energy can be delivered through a fiber-optic intraocular delivery system. In this system, a columnated beam allows for a high energy density for efficient emulsification while permitting the beam to be confined within a metal-walled chamber.[6]

A Nd:YAG 1064 nm laser developed by Dr. Jack M. Dodick differs from the Paradigm laser in that the lens is not ablated by applying laser energy directly to the lens. In his system, the lens is disrupted by shock waves which are created by the laser striking a titanium target within the probe. The use of a titanium target greatly reduces the threshold needed for optical breakdown of lens material which allows for much lower energy use compared to the quantity of energy required without a target. In addition, the titanium target shields the surrounding intraocular structures as well as the eyes of the surgeon from direct laser light.[4]

Although these lasers are still restricted except under FDA-approved clinical trials, eventual approval for widespread clinical use by cataract surgeons worldwide has the potential of replacing ultrasonic phacoemulsification with a safer, more efficient laser energy source.

FLUIDICS

The most important recent advance in phacoemulsification fluidics involves high vacuum cassettes and tubing which allow use of much higher vacuums than were previously considered safe in an intraocular environment. These cassettes have resulted in the ability to utilize vacuum as an extractive instrument with a reduced need for the application of ultrasound energy. Using high vacuum cassettes, ultrasound is utilized mainly for fashioning segments of nuclear material in such a way that they continuously occlude the tip for evacuation by the vacuum. New pump systems make the achievement of vacuum smoother and more precise, and microprocessor controls help achieve stabilization of the anterior chamber. High vacuum tubing is generally thicker walled and contains a narrower bore than standard tubing, resulting in some restriction of movement of fluid through it. As a result, there is an inherent safety from down-sized tips and vacuum tubing so that with loss of occlusion at the tip, the added resistance to flow disallows fluid from moving rapidly through the tip and the tubing. This added resistance markedly reduces collapsing of the anterior chamber and vaulting of the posterior capsule.

In addition to high vacuum cassettes and the ability to utilize vacuum in extraction techniques, one of the more important changes in fluidics has been the programmable vacuum rise times available on several machines such as the AMO Diplomax and the Surgical Design Ocusystem II. In systems which utilize a peristaltic pump, the speed of vacuum rise following occlusion of the tip is directly proportional to the aspiration rate. Thus, a low aspiration rate will produce a slow vacuum rise time and a high aspiration rate will produce a fast vacuum rise time.

With occlusion-mode phaco, the AMO Diplomax has the ability to program an Occluded Aspiration Rate that is independent of the aspiration rate in the unoccluded state. With this ability the surgeon can program a low aspiration rate setting in the unoccluded state with a slow or fast vacuum rise time once occlusion occurs, or a high aspiration rate setting in the unoccluded state followed by a slow or fast vacuum rise time in the occluded state.[2]

This feature allows the surgeon to customize flow and vacuum rise times for each stage in the phacoemulsification procedure. For instance, sculpting can occur with a low aspiration rate and slow vacuum rise time allowing the surgeon adequate time to react if undesired occlusion takes place. During nuclear quadrant removal, a low aspiration rate with a fast vacuum rise time allows the quadrant to be seized under low flow without aspirating the surrounding epinucleus. Then once occlusion occurs, the vacuum will rise quickly allowing the quadrant to be extracted efficiently for emulsification.

Finally, a high aspiration rate and slow vacuum rise time can be programmed for safe and efficient removal of the epinucleus toward the tip without having to extend the tip out toward the periphery and once occlusion takes place, a slow vacuum rise time will aspirate the epinucleus in a slower, more controlled environment which is less likely to rupture the posterior capsule.[2] The sophistication of the AMO Diplomax allows the surgeon the option of choosing from any one of a number of power modulations or vacuum and aspiration flow rates in the unoccluded state to a wide variety of other parameters in the occluded state all during the same step within the cataract procedure.

Two additional innovations with respect to fluidics involve reverse-flow phacoemulsification first described by Dr. Charles Kelman. In this system the standard sources of irrigation and aspiration are reversed—gravity-fed fluid from the irrigation bottle is directed through the phaco needle and aspiration fluid exits the eye through the sideports in the silicone sleeve. Reverse-flow sculpting allows the phaco tip to safely sculpt very deeply without the risk of capturing and rupturing the posterior capsule since it is always being repulsed by the fluid flowing from the phaco tip.[7] Dr. Jack Singer's "phaco unplugged" utilizes a similar mechanism with appropriate placement of valves between the lines in the OcuSystem II.

USER INTERFACE

Improvements and changes in user interfaces have simplified the surgeon's life in the operating room and made phacoemulsification more efficient. Most new systems have the ability for multiple programmable features. The most sophisticated utilization of these systems allows separate programs to be set up for multiple surgeons in any one facility, different grades of nuclei by each surgeon, and different steps by any particular surgeon during the same procedure. A variety of graphics and clearly recognizable icons are available in many of the systems, expediting the programmable features of these machines.

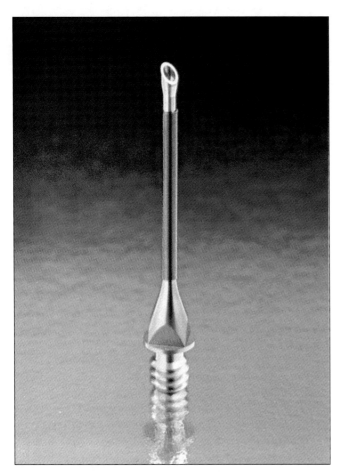

Figure 8-1. The MicroSeal Tip (Mackool system) contains a central titanium needle, surrounded by a Teflon fluid jacket, both of which are surrounded by a soft silicone sleeve.

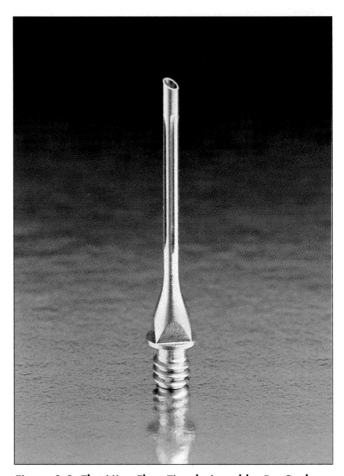

Figure 8-2. The MicroFlow Tip, designed by Dr. Graham Barrett, has spiral grooves in the outer wall of the phaco needle against which the silicone sleeve cannot be fully compressed.

The Alcon Legacy System has voice confirmation of changes in phaco programs, freeing the surgeon to respond once the program has changed without having to wait for a nurse or technician's confirmation. The foot pedal of the AMO Diplomax has a control for program changes so that a kick to the right takes the machine to a second program, another kick to a third program, and a kick to the left moves back one program. This frees the surgeon from having to communicate with the operating room staff and wait for confirmation of the change.

Many of the machines have complete setup programs that, through graphic and icon representation, enable the technician to automatically prime the machine and confirm its readiness. In addition, there are trouble-shooting programs which allow one to rapidly search for sources of trouble.

PHACO TIPS AND HANDPIECES

Probably the most widely expanding area in phacoemulsification instrumentation involves improvements in phaco tips.

Increasingly there has been an attempt to downsize tips and modify sleeves so that they are easier to insert through the phacoemulsification incision. In addition, much thought has been given to designing tips which will reduce the incidence of incisional burns and increase cutting efficiency.

Two phaco tips designed specifically to reduce incision burns are the MicroSeal Tip and the MicroFlow Tip. The MicroSeal Tip (Mackool system) contains a central titanium needle, surrounded by a Teflon fluid jacket, both of which are surrounded by a soft silicone sleeve (Figure 8-1). The soft, outer silicone sleeve is designed to deform to the shape of the incision, preventing incisional outflow. The inner, rigid Teflon jacket acts as a heat insulator and a cooling jacket. It prevents the silicone sleeve from being compressed against the titanium ultrasonic needle by the incision, thus preventing heat transfer from the vibrating needle to the incisional tissue.

The MicroSeal Tip has an added benefit in that it allows for a large expansion of the anterior segment space and dra-

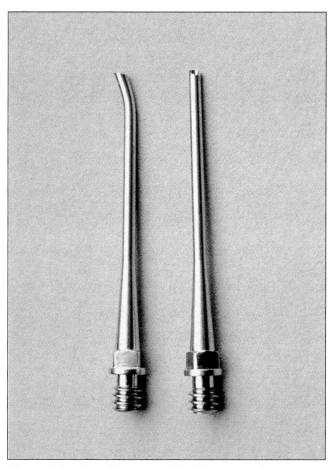

Figure 8-3. The Kelman tip, which has a 30-degree downward bend at the front portion of the needle, achieves increased non-axial vibration which produces considerable enhancement of the cavitational energy at the tip.

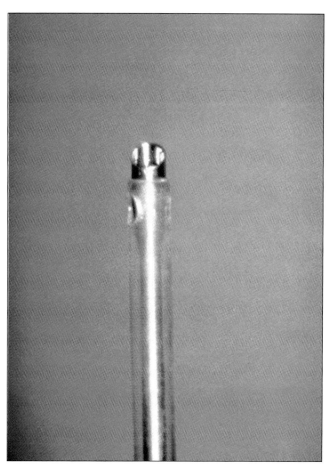

Figure 8-4. The Cobra Tip is widened distally and narrowed proximally with an inner bell configuration at the tip.

matically reduces the total volume traveling through the eye during a procedure. At the same time, it enhances followability because all fluid exits the eye through the phaco needle rather than creating turbulence by having competing currents through the phaco needle and through the incision.[8]

The MicroFlow Tip, designed by Dr. Graham Barrett, has spiral grooves in the outer wall of the phaco needle against which the silicone sleeve cannot be fully compressed (Figure 8-2). As a result, there is always some cooling fluid flowing around the needle in the grooves, even during instances when the incision may be compressing the sleeve against the needle.

Innovations for the phaco tip are now concentrating on designs to increase cutting efficiency. The Kelman tip, which has a 30-degree downward bend at the front portion of the needle, achieves increased non-axial vibration which produces considerable enhancement of the cavitational energy at the tip (Figure 8-3). This increased cavitation results in

greatly improved ability for cutting or grooving of nuclear material in advance or in front of the tip without a need for contact of the nuclear material by the tip itself. In very hard nuclei one can actually create grooving without any downward or forward force on the nucleus by the tip, which is obviously a great advantage in cases of weakened zonules, zonular dialysis, pseudoexfoliation, postvitrectomy, and traumatic cataracts.[1]

In addition, the shape of the Kelman tip has been useful for non-rotational grooving, since one can emulsify nuclear material in advance of contact by the tip as well as in the withdrawal of the tip from its distal position to its sub-incisional position. Gimbel has described using this tip in a sweeping motion so that grooving can be done keeping power on in both the forward and backward strokes of the handpiece, as well as in rotations of the handpiece to the right and left in the middle of the initial groove. In this manner, one can create cruciate

Figure 8-5. A tip with a V-shaped inferior surface to facilitate grooving.

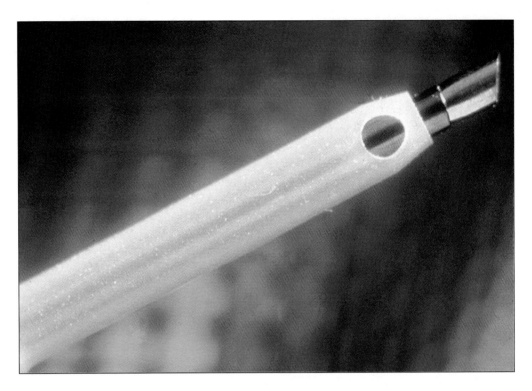

grooving, facilitating cracking of the four quadrants without challenging potentially weakened zonules.[9]

Surgical Design has created a unique innovation to the phaco needle which they have named the Cobra Tip. While most conventional phaco tips have a uniform thickness throughout their length, the Cobra Tip is widened distally and narrowed proximally with an inner bell configuration at the tip (Figure 8-4). This bell or funnel configuration creates much more surface area than conventional tips for acoustic wave generation, in addition to focusing the ultrasonic energy to a more localized area. This innovation allows for lower energy settings to be used, reducing potential damage to the corneal endothelium.[10]

Mastel Precision Instruments has worked with a variety of other changes in tip conformation, size, and finish in an attempt to improve performance. There is some feeling that changing the finish from highly polished to matte may result in an enhancement in cavitational energy. In addition, some tips have been fashioned with a V-shaped inferior surface to facilitate grooving while others have been designed with a sharpening of a portion of the tip itself so that a chisel-like configuration can facilitate grooving (Figures 8-5 and 8-6).

With the advent of chopping techniques for cataract extraction, there has been increasing interest in the development of zero-degree tips. The fine details of the shape and size of these tips are undergoing continued evaluation by many companies. There is no question that chopping procedures are facilitated by the zero-degree tip where good control requires adequate lollipopping of the nucleus by the

phaco tip. High cavitational energy tips tend to be associated with a widening of the tunnel as one tries to drive the needle in to lollipop the nucleus, resulting in a less firm hold on nuclear material. Mastel has designed a zero-degree square chisel tip which appears to facilitate lollipopping for chopping techniques (Figure 8-7). In addition, Microsurgical Technology has designed a unique tip called the Selbel Flathead phaco tip which claims to perform more rapid grooving and enhanced lollipopping of the nucleus for chopping procedures (Figure 8-8).

With the thought of continuing to improve the comfort of the phacoemulsification handpiece, Dr. Sam Masket has designed an "ergonomic tip." This tip is bent near the hub in such a way that the hand is in a more comfortable position above the plane of the needle during the course of phacoemulsification (Figure 8-9). Handpieces themselves are also undergoing change. These changes are mostly directed toward lighter weight and slimmer models, with a variety of contours on the surface that enable easy manipulation by the surgeon. There is also a tendency for companies to internalize the irrigation and aspiration lines within the handpiece in order to decrease the overall bulk created by externalized lines along the length of the handpiece.

CONCLUSION

As techniques for cataract removal have changed, phacoemulsification systems have also evolved in order to improve the safety and efficacy of modern cataract surgery. Concurrently, advances in phacoemulsification systems have

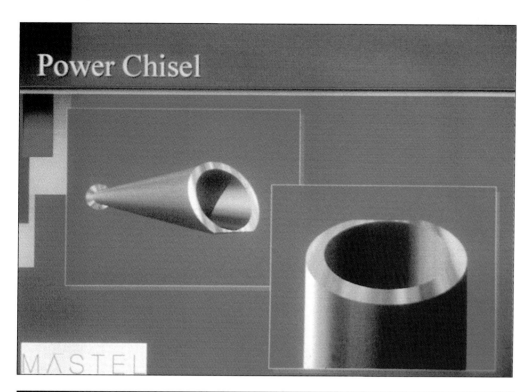

Figure 8-6. The chisel-like configuration of this tip facilitates grooving.

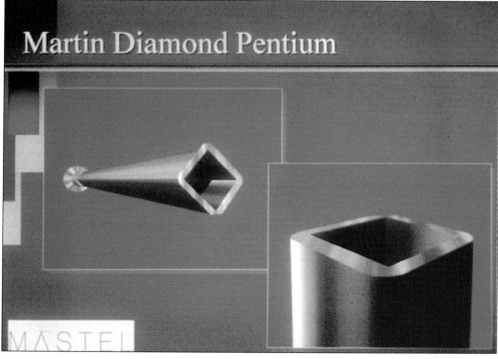

Figure 8-7. Mastel has designed this zero-degree square chisel tip which appears to facilitate lollipopping for chopping techniques.

allowed for advances to be made in lens extraction techniques. Improvements in the generation and judicious use of ultrasonic power in addition to the potential benefits of other energy sources allow for less traumatic removal of lens material with lower energy requirements. Likewise, sophisticated fluidic programmability with high vacuum cassettes and tubing allows phacoemulsification to be performed with more efficient use of energy under a more controlled intraocular environment than has ever been available in the past. Improvements in user interfaces have simplified the utilization of these machines by both the surgeon and support staff. Finally, design changes for tips and handpieces have

Figure 8-8. Microsurgical Technology has designed this unique tip called the Selbel Flat-head phaco tip, which claims to perform more rapid grooving and enhanced lollipopping of the nucleus for chopping procedures.

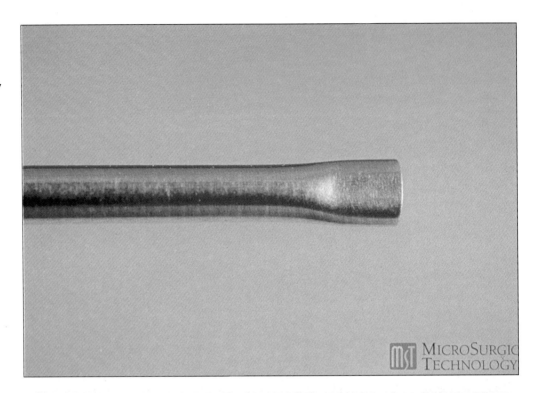

Figure 8-9. This tip is bent near the hub in such a way that the hand is in a more comfortable position above the plane of the needle during the course of phacoemulsification.

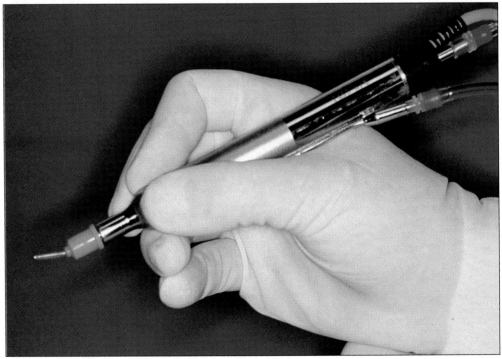

improved efficiency and comfort while potentially decreasing the incidence of serious wound complications such as incisional burns in clear corneal tissue. These advances and future improvements in phacoemulsification systems will likely result in increasing use of phacoemulsification as the primary technique for cataract extraction throughout the world as the procedure becomes even safer and easier to master.

REFERENCES

1. Fine IH. Alcon Series 20000 Legacy phacoemulsification system. In: Fine IH (ed), *Phacoemulsification: New Technology and Clinical Application*. Thorofare, NJ, Slack, 1996; 19-36.

2. Masket S. Thorlakson R. The OMS Diplomax in endolenticular phacoemulsification. In: Fine IH (ed), *Phacoemulsification: New Technology and Clinical Application*. Thorofare, NJ, Slack, 1996; 67-80.

3. Anis A. Phacotmesis. In: Fine IH (ed), *Phacoemulsification: New Technology and Clinical Application*. Thorofare, NJ, Slack, 1996; 131-143.

4. Dodick JM, Sperber LTD. Current techniques in laser cataract surgery. In: Fine IH (ed), *Phacoemulsification: New Technology and Clinical Application*. Thorofare, NJ, Slack, 1996; 146-153.

5. Colvard DM, Kratz, RP. Cataract surgery utilizing the Erbium laser. In Fine IH (ed), *Phacoemulsification: New Technology and Clinical Application*. Thorofare, NJ, Slack, 1996; 162-180.

6. Eichenbaum DM. Paradigm System: A laser probe for cataract removal. In Fine IH (ed), *Phacoemulsification: New Technology and Clinical Application*. Thorofare, NJ, Slack, 1996; 155-158.

7. Kelman CD. Reverse-flow phaco technique for safe nucleus sculpting. Proceedings from the Fourth Annual Ocular Surgery News Symposium: Cataract & Refractive Surgery, New York, 1995.

8. Mackool RJ. Storz Premiere/MicroSeal System description. In Fine IH (ed), *Phacoemulsification: New Technology and Clinical Application*. Thorofare, NJ, Slack, 1996; 83-100.

9. Gimbel HV, Chin PK. Phaco sweep. *J Cataract Refract Surg* 1995; 21:493-503.

10. Grabow HB. The Surgical Design Ocusystem II[ART]. In Fine IH (ed), *Phacoemulsification: New Technology and Clinical Application*. Thorofare, NJ, Slack, 1996;104-128.

ADVANCED PHACOEMULSIFICATION TECHNIQUE

CHAPTER 9

Howard V. Gimbel, MD, FACS, David Brown, MD, I. Howard Fine, MD, Hideharu Fukasaku, MD, William Maloney, MD, Jack A. Singer, MD, Spencer P. Thornton, MD, FACS, James P. Gills, MD

NUCLEOFRACTIS

The fundamental principle of most nucleofractis techniques is to fracture, segment, and remove the lens in the most efficient manner. The nucleus of the lens must be weakened sufficiently to facilitate a complete posterior plate fracture.

The first step is hydrodissection and hydrodelineation. While hydrodissection separates the entire lens (cortex and nucleus) from the capsule, hydrodelineation separates the soft epinuclear shell from the dense nucleus. Hydrodelineation begins the efficient segmentation for removal of the lens. The delineation process will assist in the fracturing of the lens into manageable pieces during phacoemulsification by forcing solution into the lamellar formation of the lens.

The key element to nucleofractis techniques is directly dependent on the anatomic relationship of the lens fibers and the lenticular sutures: the Y sutures. These sutures develop during the embryonic stage of growth, forming one suture anteriorly and one posteriorly. As the lens develops, these sutures branch out from their origin into increasingly complex patterns. Furthermore, epithelial cells lay down lens fibers in concentric layered patterns, eventually forming a lamellar structure resembling layers of an onion.

The historical development of nucleofractis, a term coined when the first such technique, divide and conquer, was described, has seen many variations of the technique described, all resulting in the safe and efficient removal of a cataractous lens. A common thread between many of these techniques is the removal of enough nuclear material, by sculpting, to obtain fractures which expedite the entire phaco process.

Gimbel Techniques

Divide and Conquer

Divide and conquer nucleofractis can be viewed as four basic steps: 1) sculpting until a thin posterior plate of nucleus remains, 2) fracturing of the posterior plate and nuclear rim, 3) breaking away a wedge-shaped section of nuclear material for emulsification, and 4) rotating the remaining nucleus for further fracturing and emulsification.

Sculpting must be performed to sufficiently debulk the nucleus before the posterior plate can be cracked. By nudging the lens inferiorly with the second instrument, the upper central part of the nucleus can be sculpted very deeply, to the point of sculpting directly parallel and close to the posterior capsule. This maneuver allows the tip to remove more of the upper part of the nucleus during sculpting and to reach the posterior pole of the lens very early for effective fracturing (Figure 9-1).

Multi-directional Divide and Conquer

Traditional sculpting techniques use a forward-backward motion of the phaco tip (perpendicular to the incision). Converting this motion to a lateral motion (parallel to the incision), the surgeon is able to safely sculpt deeper into the lens material. Ideally, the tip of the instrument is never occluded. With "phaco sweep", the surgeon can maintain a visual perspective of how deep the sculpting is proceeding by observing, beside the tip, the change in the red reflex; and because the tip is moving parallel with the posterior capsule, the surgeon will avoid inadvertently pushing the tip through the epinucleus, causing posterior capsule rupture (Figure 9-2).

Figure 9-1. The phacoemulsification process shows the nudging of the lens inferiorly with a second instrument (a spatula through a paracentesis at 3 o'clock) and slowly sculpting until the red reflex indicates passage into the epinucleus (Gimbel).

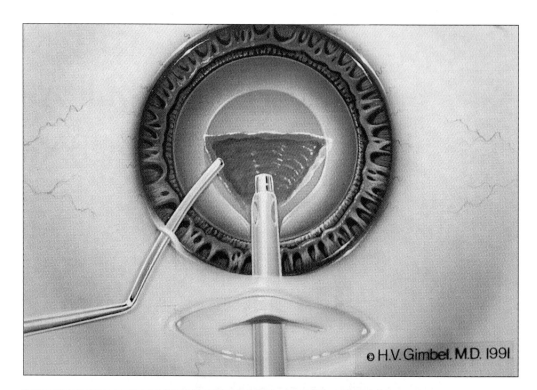

© H.V. Gimbel. M.D. 1991

Figure 9-2. Sweeping movement of the phaco tip shows the tip remains in a parallel plane with the main incision (Gimbel).

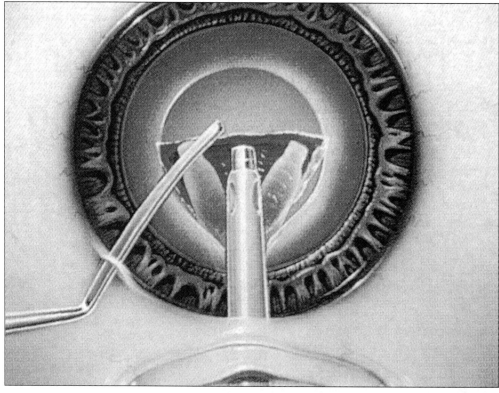

Once the surgeon has reached the posterior pole, the initial nuclear plate fracture—whether vertical, horizontal, or separating or chop—can be created. The surgeon has three tools available to accomplish this fracture: the phaco handpiece, the spatula, and the naturally occurring Y sutures of the lens.

With the multi-directional divide and conquer technique, the fracture is really a combination of separation and shearing. After phaco sweep and downslope sculpting, the spatula instrument pushes toward the 6-o'clock position, and the phaco tip pushes down superiorly and stabilizes or even pulls toward the incision, creating the horizontal fracture (Figure 9-3).

Then the multi-directional fracturing is accomplished

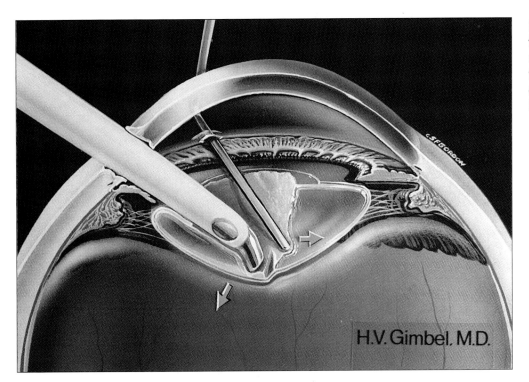

Figure 9-3. Horizontal fracture is accomplished utilizing the spatula, phaco tip, and the naturally occurring suture lines within the lens (Gimbel).

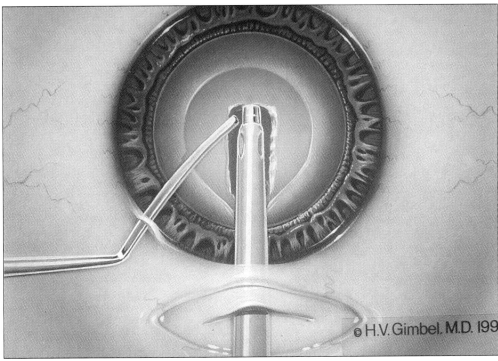

Figure 9-4. Sculpting is limited to a central trough or trench within the lens. Sculpting to the posterior pole can be accomplished if the trench is twice the width of the tip's sleeve (Gimbel).

without rotating the lens. With the natural fault lines in the lens, fracturing is accomplished very easily with simple, two instrument separation. The fracturing is enhanced by not only separation, but by shearing (pushing down on one segment), so fracturing occurs in two planes. The upper hemisection can be rotated 180° for similar fracturing, or it can be simply slid down into the central part of the capsule and approached from the equatorial side.

Trench Divide and Conquer

For trench divide and conquer, polar sculpting is limited to a central trough or trench (Figure 9-4). This technique is the preferred method for a very soft nucleus, where one has to maintain much of the nuclear material centrally that is firm enough to push against to obtain a fracture.

Figure 9-5. (A) During the fracturing process, the lens is nudged slightly inferiorly and stabilized with the second instrument (passed through the paracentesis). **(B)** The fracture is obtained with the two instruments pushing away from each other (phaco tip to 9 o'clock and second instrument to 3 o'clock). The lens can be removed in any fashion comfortable to the surgeon (Gimbel).

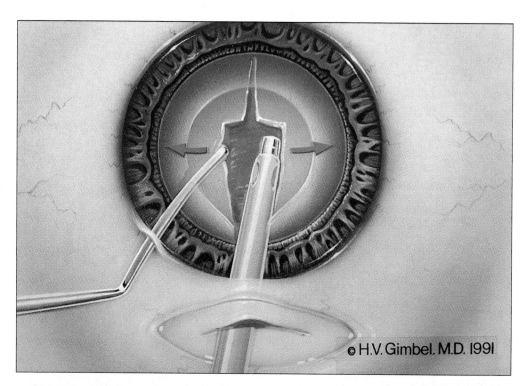

© H.V. Gimbel, M.D. 1991

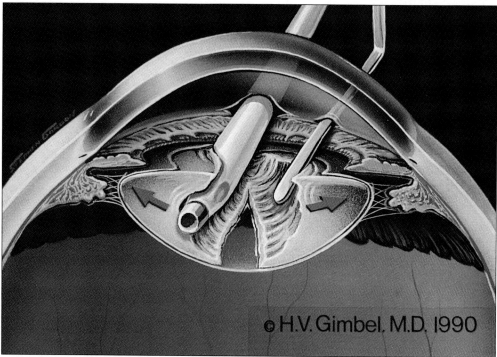

© H.V. Gimbel, M.D. 1990

For sculpting, the nucleus is nudged slightly inferiorly and stabilized with the spatula. The fracture is obtained with the two instruments pushing away from each other (spatula to 3 o'clock and phaco tip to 9 o'clock) (Figures 9-5 A&B).

In soft lenses the entire hemisection may be taken at one time. In more dense lenses each hemisection is fractured into two or four pieces by stabilizing the hemisection under the sideport with a spatula, engaging the remaining bulk of nucle-

us with the phaco tip and pushing with the phaco tip toward the initial fracture line. An anterior posterior shearing movement also helps to fracture.

Crater Divide and Conquer

A trench, trough, or groove is not used with dense, brunescent lenses, because it does not weaken the entire lens nucleus enough to easily fracture, and the resulting segments are

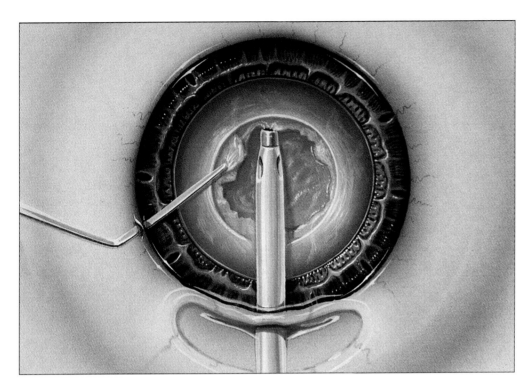

too large to manage safely. Instead a central crater is sculpted, leaving a dense peripheral rim (Figure 9-6). After the central core of the nucleus is removed, the fracturing process is accomplished by placing the chopping instrument under the anterior capsule at the 6-o'clock position. Meanwhile, the phaco tip is placed into the bulkhead of the nuclear rim. The vacuum of the tip is used to stabilize the nucleus. No ultrasound is used. The chopping instrument then pulls in a three-vector plane (Figures 9-7 A&B): toward the incision, slightly away from the phaco tip, and gently toward the posterior capsule. The result is a fracture through nuclear rim and any remaining, thinned nuclear plate. The nucleus is rotated for additional small segment fractioning. The entire lens is fractured before any pieces are removed, maintaining the distension of the capsule, which helps to prevent an inadvertent capsule rupture (Figure 9-8).

Cracking and Chopping Techniques

Singer Autocrack Phaco Using the Curved Diamond Cobra Tip

A new method of nuclear disassembly called autocrack phaco utilizes a curved diamond-shaped Cobra phaco tip (Figure 9-9) to crack the nucleus without chopping it with a second instrument. The focus of previous phaco chop and phaco crack methods have been on the "phaco-chopper" while the phaco tip was used mainly to hold onto the nucleus with high vacuum. The curved diamond Cobra tip is the first phaco tip designed to crack the nucleus without the use of a "phaco-chopper". Any second instrument can be used to manipulate the nuclear segments created by the Cobra tip.

The diamond shape of the phaco tip in relation to the 15° bevel and 30° curve of the needle combined with high vacuum and a triple infusion stream (Figure 9-10) create the conditions for autocrack phaco. Parameters are set at a flow rate of 25 cc/min, a vacuum limit of 200 mmHg, and linear phaco power of 10-50%. The Cobra tip is rotated 90° so its bevel is sideways (Figure 9-11A), and the tip is driven into the center of the nucleus using ultrasound (Figure 9-11B). Once the center of the nucleus is reached, foot switch position 2 is engaged and vacuum is allowed to build (Figure 9-11C). During the vacuum rise or shortly thereafter, the autocrack occurs (Figure 9-11D), and propagates forward from the phaco tip to the equator of the nucleus. The diamond shape of the Cobra tip acts as a wedge, or pointed snow plow, which cracks and splits the nucleus. The triple infusion stream then separates the nuclear segments and helps to propagate the crack along nuclear fault lines.

Then the second instrument is simply used to hold the nucleus steady while the Cobra tip is moved to the opposite side in order to complete the nuclear separation along the autocrack. The diamond shape of the tip acts like a miter and prevents rotation of the nucleus during separation, which can stress the zonules and capsule. The autocrack maneuver is then repeated on each heminucleus, and the quadrants are aspirated using high vacuum and low ultrasound energy.

Autocrack phaco works well with any nuclear density. In 4+ nuclear sclerotic cataracts, the autocrack may not propagate forward from the phaco tip as readily and may need some help from the second instrument.

When autocrack phaco is combined with cortical-cleaving hydrodissection and hydrodelineation, the method evolves

Figure 9-7. (A) The fracture is accomplished by placing the chopping instrument (passed through the paracentesis at 3 o'clock) under the anterior capsule at the 6 o'clock position. The phaco tip is placed into the bulkhead of the nuclear rim. The vacuum of the phaco tip will stabilize the nucleus. **(B)** The chopping instrument will be pulled in a three-vector plane: toward the incision, slightly away from the phaco tip, and gently toward the posterior capsule. While maintaining occlusion, the phaco tip moves in a three-vector plane: toward the 9 o'clock position, toward the incision, and toward the anterior chamber (Gimbel).

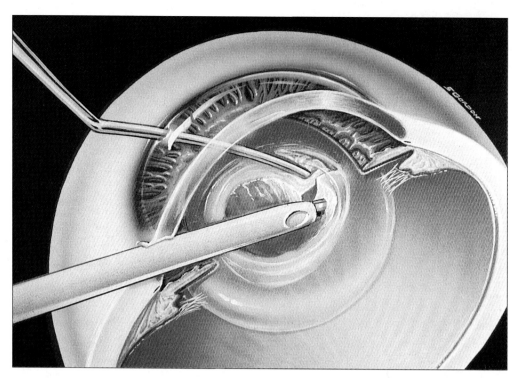

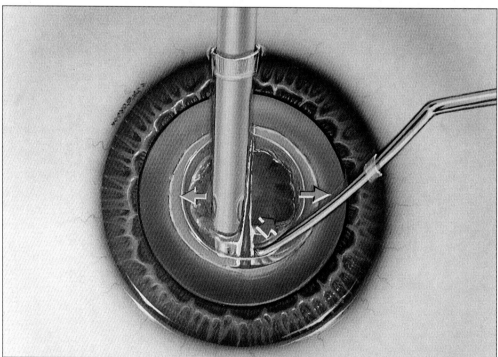

into autocrack and flip phaco. The epinucleus keeps the capsule bag on stretch while the nucleus and cortex are removed with the phaco tip.

Singer Tri-linear Phaco

Ultra-high vacuum levels of up to 500 mmHg enhance the hydrodynamic power of the aspiration system and improve cutting efficiency, which facilitates chopping and phaco-aspiration of dense cataracts. The use of ultra-high vacuum levels was enabled by programmable vacuum rise time (adjustable rise time, or ART), enhanced automatic surge prevention, and high vacuum tubing.

The addition of simultaneous linear control of power, flow, and vacuum (tri-linear phaco) enhances efficiency while maintaining safety. The initial flow rate is set high for followability, and a secondary flow rate is programmed to slow the vacuum rise curve for safety. A linear rise of vacuum

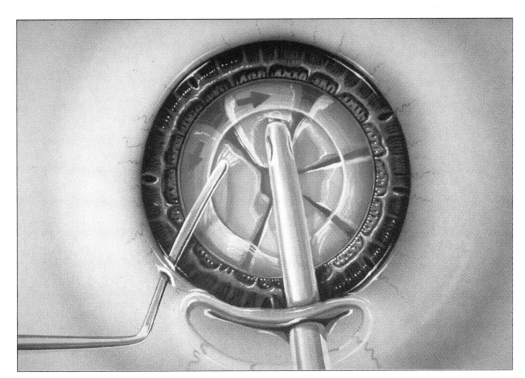

Figure 9-8. The entire lens is fractured into small segments before being removed (Gimbel).

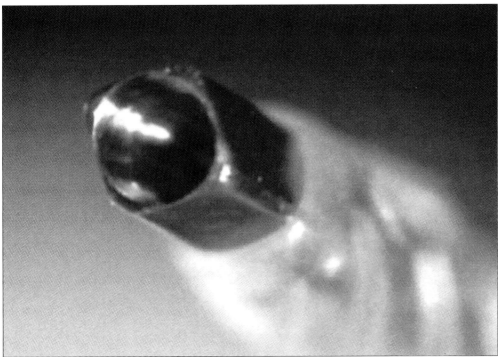

Figure 9-9. Diamond-shaped Autocrack Cobra phaco tip (Singer).

limit, ultrasound power, and flow rate in foot switch position 3 overrides the programmed settings to provide an infinitely variable surgeon-controlled climb to 500 mmHg.

Table 9-1 outlines the current Singer settings for the Surgical Design Ocusystem IIe^art. With these tri-linear settings, high vacuum limits and high flow rates are used in the background "as needed".

When the tip is not occluded, a relatively fast flow of 25-38 cc/min provides excellent followability, attracting mobile lens material to the phaco tip. After tip occlusion, the vacuum rises quickly to the programmed activation point of 50 mmHg, which activates the secondary flow rate of 3 cc/min, thus slowing the vacuum rate rise. As ultrasound power is added in a linear fashion, the lens material occluding the tip

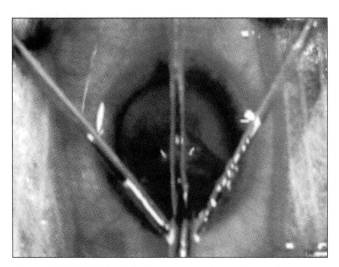

Figure 9-10. Triple-infusion stream from Curved Diamond Cobra tip (Singer).

TABLE 9-1	
CURRENT SURGICAL DESIGN OCUSYSTEM IIE SETTINGS FOR SINGER TECHNIQUE	
Power	10 to 50% linear
Flow	25 to 38 cc/min linear
Vacuum	200 to 500 mmHg linear
ART	50 mmHg activation point 3 cc/min secondary flow

is fragmented and aspirated. Therefore, high vacuum from 200 to 500 mmHg occurs only when emulsifying dense lens material that requires higher ultrasound power levels.

When the occlusion is broken, the vacuum drops below the activation point of 50 mmHg, and the flow rate increases to 25-38 cc/min. The higher flow rates occur only when emulsifying dense lens material that requires higher ultrasound power levels, which works to counteract the tendency of ultrasonics to push lens material away from the tip.

Fukasaku Snap and Split

The "Snap and Split" technique uses the concentrated potential energy released by snapping to easily and safely crack the nucleus. The technique uses a Snapper hook (Katena Products, Inc.) for the Snap and Split technique, which is much shorter and safer than the long phaco chop hook (Figure 9-12).

The key to the Snap and Split is concentrated energy along the meridional stress lines created by lens fibers. The lens fibers are formed by the differentiation and elongation of the lens epithelium at the equator. These lens fibers run meridionally around the equator of the lens from the posterior to the anterior lens surface (Figure 9-13). The juncture forms the Y sutures. It is important to mentally visualize these meridional fibers because these are the stress lines along which the vector forces created by snapping and the subsequent splitting will occur (Figure 9-14).

The epinucleus is first removed by aspiration, allowing visualization of the nucleus. Next, the nucleus is sculpted deeply adjacent to the center of the nucleus (Figure 9-15). The Snapper hook is placed adjacent to the phaco tip at the stress lines created by the lens fibers. The phaco tip is then buried into the nucleus with slight phacoemulsification and the nucleus fixated using high vacuum aspiration at 100, 125 or 150 mmHg depending on the hardness of the nucleus

(Figure 9-16). The Snapper hook and phaco tip are then moved in opposite, arc-like motions with the Snapper hook pulling and the phaco tip pushing (Figure 9-17), separating the nucleus in half (Figure 9-18).

I routinely use a high vacuum phaco technique. When I crack the cataract nucleus, the surgeon needs to grasp the center of the nucleus firmly with high vacuum in order to concentrate phaco energy efficiently. I use the NIDEK CV 12000 and depending on the hardness of the nucleus set the vacuum at 100, 125, 150 mmHg, ultrasound power at 70, 80, 90% and flow rate at 27, 28, 28 cc/min. High vacuum setting enables one to concentrate phaco energy in a discrete zone where it is most effective. With the Snap and Split technique, the phaco tip and Snapper hook are rotated tangentially past each other. The phaco tip moves forward with an arc-like tangential force, pushing the cracked portion away. The Snapper hook is then moved around the phaco tip, hooking the half portion away.

The nucleus is then rotated for quartering. The phaco tip is buried into the nucleus at the center of the half nucleus with slight phacoemulsification and the snapper hook is placed adjacent to the phaco tip at the stress lines of the lens fibers. The phaco power is magnified between the phaco tip and the snapper hook (Figure 9-19). The snapper hook is pressed into the nucleus. The snapper hook and the phaco tip are tangentially rotated past each other and snapped into quarters (Figure 9-20). Phacoemulsification and aspiration of the quartered fragments then proceeds with ease within the central safe zone. All manipulation occurs within the central 5-mm safe zone.

Phaco Burst

The original Snap and Split technique divides the nucleus with mechanical force between the phaco tip and Snapper hook. A refinement of the original Snap and Split technique uses concentrated phaco energy at the meridional stress line of the lens to literally burst a hard nucleus with magnified phaco power instead of mechanical power. Phaco burst power is magnified between the phaco tip and the Snapper hook in a contra-coup fashion (Figure 9-21). The nucleus is split with phaco burst power inside the nucleus tunnel at the meridional stress lines of the lens. When combined with the mechanical power between the snapper hook and phaco tip, the very

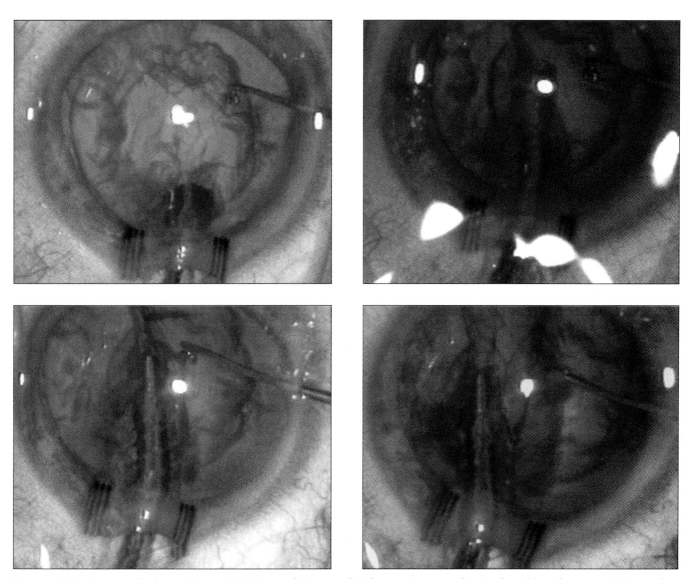

Figure 9-11. Autocrack phaco (Singer). (A) Curved Diamond Cobra tip is rotated so its bevel is sideways. (B) Curved Diamond Cobra tip is driven into the center of the nucleus using ultrasound. (C) Vacuum is allowed to build, the autocrack occurs and propagates forward from the phaco tip to the equator of the nucleus. (D) The nucleus is steadied while the Cobra tip is moved to the opposite side to complete the nuclear separation along the autocrack.

hard nucleus is easily divided. The combination of the two techniques I call Phaco Burst and Snap.

Snap and Split for the Small Pupil

The Snap and Split technique is ideal for the small pupil. Because all manipulation is carried out in the 5-mm central safe zone, the surgeons can always see the instruments and blind maneuvering beneath the iris is not necessary. Some surgeon use the iris retractor to enlarge the pupil. However, this can traumatize the iris and lead to inflammation. The Snap and Split technique is minimally traumatic with less post-operative inflammation and is very fast. A new, small pupil Snapper hook (Katena Products, Inc.) (Figure 9-22)

facilitates the technique in these cases. The outside of the hook can be used to push the iris aside non-traumatically while the inside surface of the hook is used to snap the nucleus. Implantation of the IOL in the bag can be ensured by pushing aside the iris with two Snapper hooks.

Three Keys to the Snap and Split

The three keys to success with the snap-and split technique are:

1. Using the specially designed Snapper hook. This hook is designed to be both safe and effective, with a short hook that will not damage the posterior capsule or the edge of the CCC.

Figure 9-12. The Snapper hook (bottom) for the Snap and Split technique is much shorter and safer than the long phaco chop hook (top) (Fukasaku).

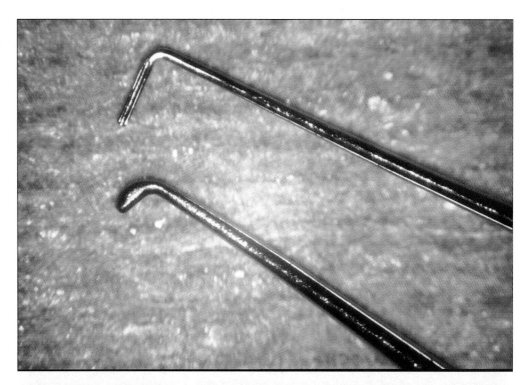

Figure 9-13. The lens fibers run meridionally around the equator from the posterior to the anterior lens surface. The juncture of these fibers forms the Y sutures. The lens fibers fun meridionally in this slit lamp view (Fukasaku).

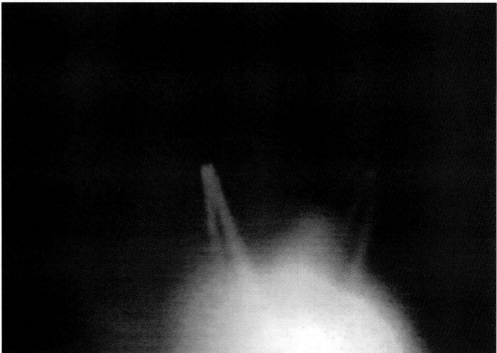

2. Deeply sculpting the nucleus and burying the phaco tip into the nucleus while fixating it with high vacuum, effectively creating a fulcrum around which the tangential vector forces created by snapping are magnified.
3. Pressing the Snapper hook into the nucleus next to the phaco tip and cracking the nucleus with opposite arc-like forces. Visualizing the meridional stress lines of the lens helps ensure the correct arc-like, tangential motion.

NUCLEAR FLIPPING

The Fine Chip and Flip technique, in which the nucleus is phacoemulsified around the edges until it can be safely flipped over, introduced a new dimension in phacoemulsification. More recent flipping techniques utilize other developments in phacoemulsification. The culmination of these techniques is the Maloney Supracapsular Phaco, in which the

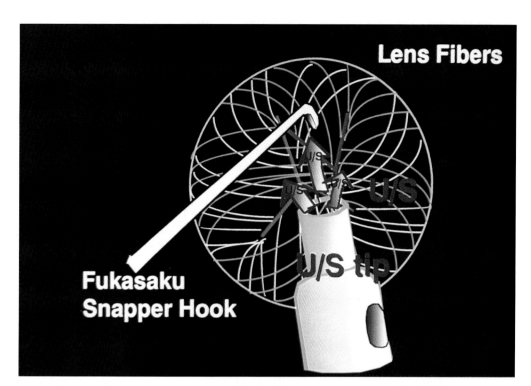

Figure 9-14. It is important to mentally visualize the stress lines. Use concentrated phaco energy at the meridional stress lines of the lens to burst a hard nucleus with magnified phaco power (Fukasaku).

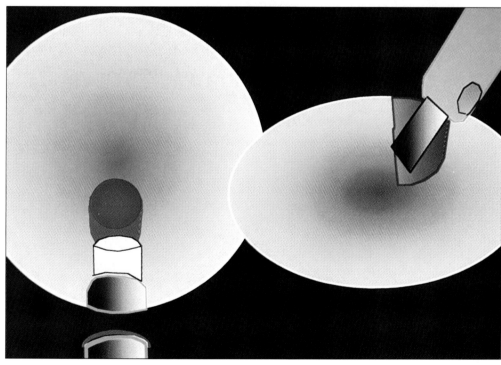

Figure 9-15. The nucleus is sculpted deeply adjacent to the pole of the lens (Fukasaku).

nucleus is first flipped and then actually removed from the bag for phacoemulsification.

Fine Chop and Flip

The chop and flip technique is designed to take advantage of various new technologies available through the Alcon 20000 Legacy, including high vacuum cassettes and tubing, multiple programmable features, and the Mackool microtip combined with the Duovisc Viscoelastic System.

A sideport incision is made to the left with a 1-mm trifaceted knife. Utilizing the soft-shell viscoelastic technique described by Steve Arshinoff, MD, from Toronto, Viscoat is placed into the eye through the sideport incision. It fills the anterior chamber but allows the eye to remain soft. Provisc is instilled on top of the center of the lens capsule under the Viscoat. Provisc forces the Viscoat up against the cornea, cre-

Figure 9-16. The Snapper hook is placed adjacent to the phaco tip at the stress lines created by the lens fibers. The phaco tip is buried into the nucleus with slight phacoemulsification. Phaco burst power is magnified between the phaco tip and the Snapper hook in a contra-coup fashion to split the nucleus at the stress line (Fukasaku).

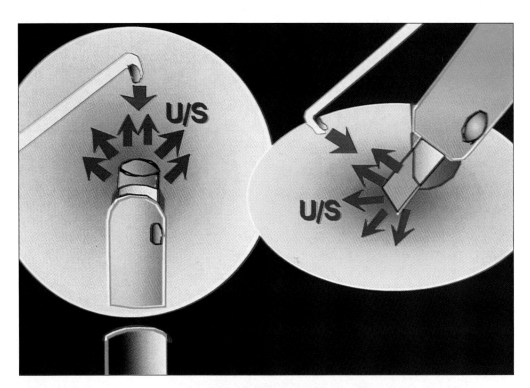

Figure 9-17. The Snapper hook is pressed into the nucleus next to the phaco tip. Arc-like tangential forces with the Snapper hook and the phaco tip will crack the nucleus (Fukasaku).

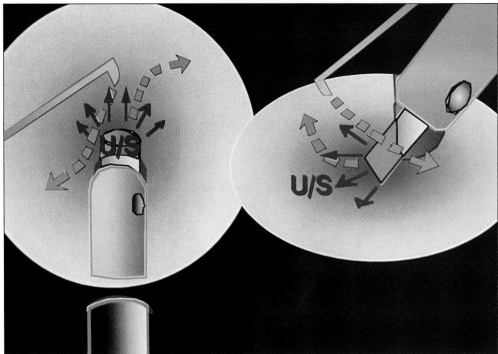

ating a soft shell which helps to stabilize and maintain the anterior chamber. Additionally, Provisc is a much less adhesive viscoelastic and prevents any tendency for iris prolapse during the hydro procedure.

After cortical cleaving hydrodissection and hydrodelineation, the nucleus should rotate easily within the capsular bag. The 30° bevel down Mackool/Kelman microtip is used to aspirate the epinucleus uncovered by the capsulorhexis. The Fine/Nagahara chopper is placed in the golden ring and is used to stabilize the nucleus by lifting slightly and pulling toward the incision slightly (Figure 9-23), after which the bevel-up phaco tip lollipops the nucleus in pulse mode at 2 pulses/second (Table 9-2). This pulse rate minimizes ultrasound energy into the eye and maximizes the hold on the nucleus as the vacuum builds between pulses. Because of the decrease in cavitational energy around the tip at this low pulse

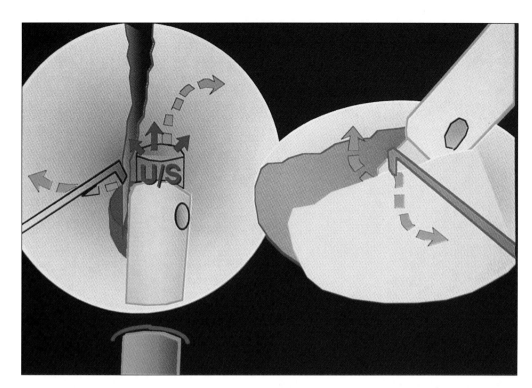

Figure 9-18. The Snapper hook and phaco tip are moved in opposite, arc-like motions with the Snapper hook pulling and the phaco tip pushing (Fukasaku).

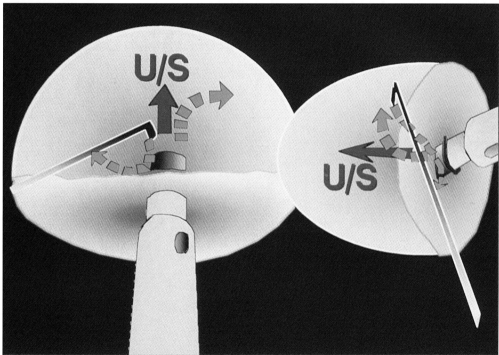

Figure 9-19. The nucleus is rotated for quartering and the phaco tip is buried into the nucleus at the center half of the nucleus to fix-ate. The Snapper hook is pressed into the nucleus to the phaco tip with slight phacoemulsification (Fukasaku).

rate, the tunnel in the nucleus in which the tip is embedded fits the needle very tightly and provides an excellent hold on the nucleus, thus maximizing control of the nucleus during scoring and chopping (Figure 9-24).

The Fine/Nagahara chop instrument is grooved on the horizontal arm close to the vertical "chop" element, with the groove parallel to the direction of the sharp edge of the vertical element. In scoring the nucleus, the instrument is always

moved in the direction that the sharp edge of the wedge-shaped vertical element is facing (as indicated by the groove on the instrument), thus facilitating scoring. The nucleus is scored by bringing the chop instrument to the side of the phaco needle.

The nucleus is chopped in half by pulling the chopper to the left and slightly down while moving the phaco needle to the right and slightly up. Then the nuclear complex is rotated.

Figure 9-20. The Snapper hook and phaco tip are tangentially rotated past each other and snapped into quarters. All manipulation occurs within the central 5-mm safe zone (Fukasaku).

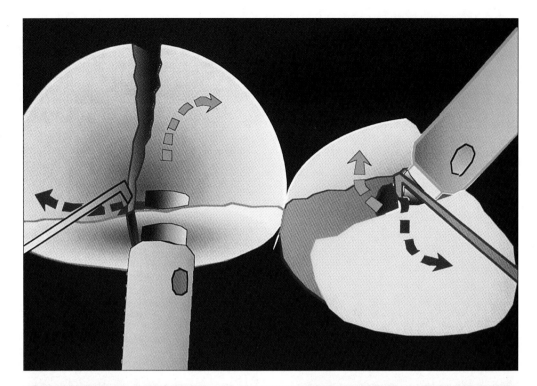

Figure 9-21. Phaco burst power is magnified between the phaco tip and the Snapper hook in a contra-coup fashion. The concentrated phaco energy bursts a hard nucleus at the stress lines of the lens fibers (Fukasaku).

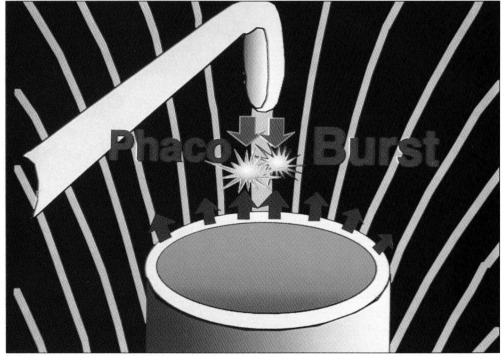

The chop instrument is again brought into the golden ring (Figure 9-25), the nucleus is again lollipopped, scored, and chopped, with the resulting pie-shaped segment now lollipopped on the phaco tip (Figure 9-26). The segment is then evacuated, using high vacuum and short bursts of pulse mode phaco at 2 pulses/second (Figure 9-27).

The nucleus is continually rotated so that pie-shaped segments can be scored, chopped, and removed essentially by the high vacuum, assisted by short pulses of phaco. The short pulses of ultrasound energy continuously reshape the pie-shaped segments which are kept at the tip, allowing for occlusion and extraction by the vacuum. The size of the pie-shaped segments is customized to the density of the nucleus with smaller segments for denser nuclei. With the low pulse rate, the nuclear material tends to stay at the tip rather than chatter, as vacuum holds between pulses. The chop instrument is used to stuff the

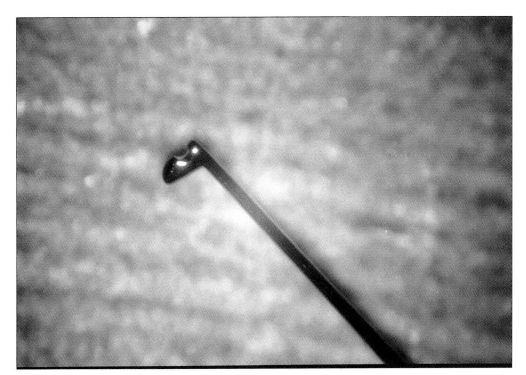

Figure 9-22. The small pupil Snapper hook (Katena Products, Inc.) has two features: the outside of the hook can be used to push the iris aside non-traumatically, while the inside surface is used to snap the nucleus (Fukasaku).

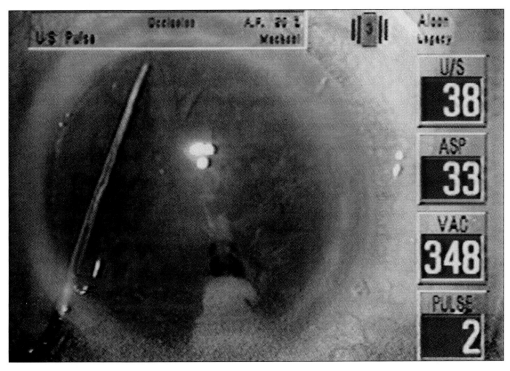

Figure 9-23. Stabilization of the nucleus during lollipopping for the initial chop (Fine).

segment into the tip or to keep it down in the epinuclear shell.

After evacuation of the first hemi-nucleus, the second hemi-nucleus is rotated to the distal position in the bag and the chop instrument stabilizes it while it is lollipopped. It is then scored (Figure 9-28) and chopped. The pie-shaped segments can be chopped a second time to reduce their size (Figure 9-29), if they appear too large to easily evacuate or removed without chopping a second time.

There is very little tendency for nuclear material to come up into the anterior chamber with this technique. Usually it stays down within the epinuclear shell, but the position of the endonuclear material can be controlled by the chop instrument. Following evacuation of all of the endonuclear material (Figure 9-30), the epinuclear rim is trimmed in each of three quadrants, mobilizing cortex as well. As each quadrant of epinuclear rim is trimmed, the cortex in the adjacent cap-

TABLE 9-2
PARAMETERS FOR FINE CHOP AND FLIP

MacKool System Hi-Vac (Alcon Legacy) Phaco Parameters				I & A	
Memory Mode	Chop Mem 1 pulse	Trim Mem 2 pulse	Flip Mem 3 pulse	Cortical Mem 1-3	Viscoat Mem 4
Power	50	35	35	surg vac	surg as
Aspiration	28/33	20/18	22	38	60
Vacuum	350	180	180	500+	500+
Mode	pulse 2/sec	pulse 7/sec	pulse 7/sec	cont irrig	cont irrig
Bottle ht	78	72	72	70	70
AMO Diplomax Hi-Vac Phaco Parameters			**I & A Control/Surg Vac Control**		
	Chop phaco 1	Trim phaco 2	Flip phaco 3 pulse	Cortical Clean-up	Viscoat Removal
Power	60	60	60		
Aspiration Cont Flow	26/30	32/26	32/16	10	30
Vacuum	50/250	40/90	70/150	500	500
Mode	multi-burst	multi-burst	multi-burst	cont irrig	cont irrig
Bottle ht	32	32	32	28	28

Figure 9-24. Completion of the initial chop (Fine).

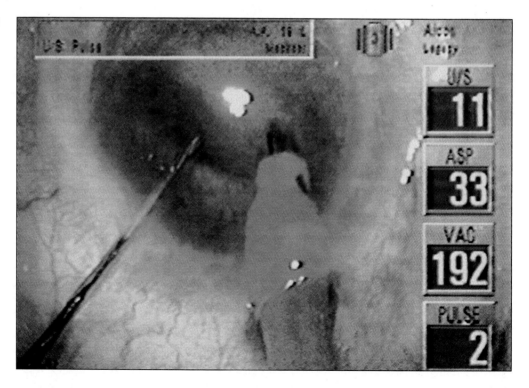

sular fornix flows over the floor of the epinucleus and into the phaco tip. Then the floor is pushed back to keep the bag on stretch until three of the four quadrants of epinuclear rim and forniceal cortex have been evacuated. It is important not to allow the epinucleus to flip too early, thus avoiding a large

amount of residual cortex remaining after evacuation of the epinucleus.

The fourth epinuclear rim quadrant is then used as a handle to flip the epinucleus (Figure 9-31). As the remaining portion of the epinuclear floor and rim is evacuated from the eye,

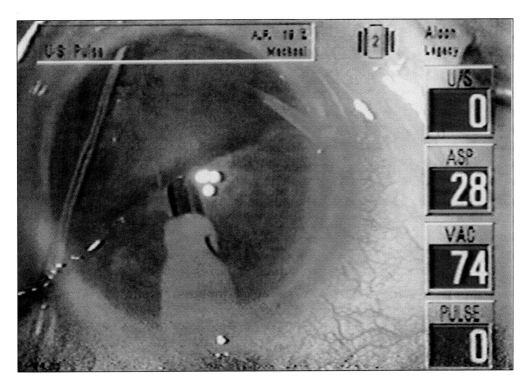

Figure 9-25. Stabilization of the nucleus prior to commencing the second chop (Fine).

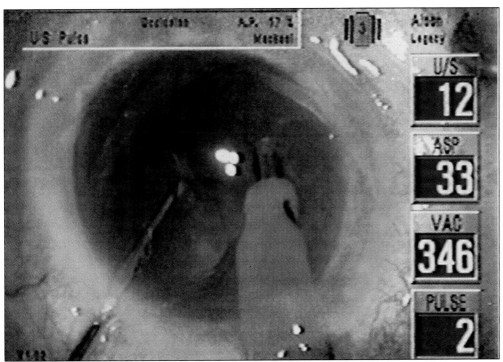

Figure 9-26. Pie-shaped segment adherent to the phaco tip following completion of the second chop (Fine).

usually all of the cortex is evacuated with it (Figure 9-32). Residual cortex is viscodissected into the capsular fornix and evacuated with residual viscoelastic, the posterior capsule being protected by the optic of the IOL.

Continuing with the Arshinoff soft-shell technique, the capsular bag is filled with Provisc, and Viscoat is injected into the center of the capsular bag to help stabilize the anterior segment and to blunt movement of the IOL as it is implanted

into the eye. Mobilization of Viscoat is greatly facilitated, as it is encased within the much more highly cohesive Provisc, and less time is necessary to evacuate residual viscoelastic.

Brown Phaco Flip

When fluid from the hydrodissection floats the nucleus out of the bag, phacoemulsification can proceed in the iris plane, allowing the case to be completed much more quickly and

Figure 9-27. Mobilization of the first pie-shaped segment (Fine).

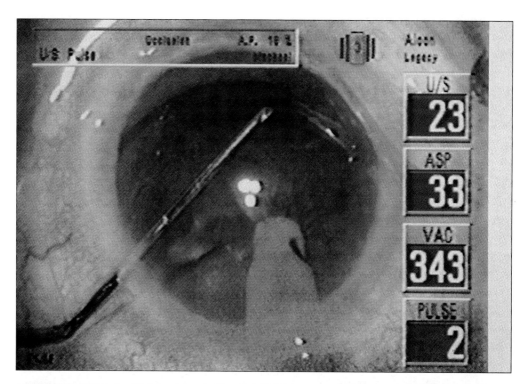

Figure 9-28. Scoring of the second hemi-nucleus (Fine).

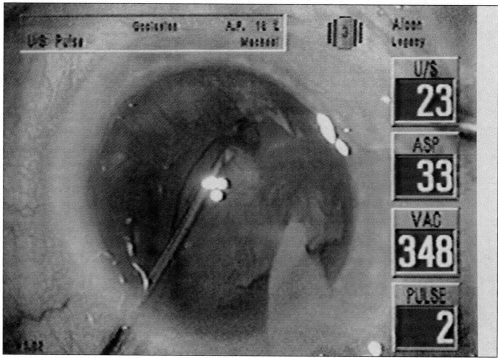

easily. Unfortunately, this levitation does not always occur, and even when it does, the lens frequently slips back into the bag before phaco can be completed. The phaco flip technique is a simple method to turn the nucleus upside down so that it can not slip back into the bag as easily.

The most important step is a large continuous curvilinear capsulorhexis (CCC) of at least 5 mm in diameter and preferably 6 mm and complete hydrodissection to separate the nucleus and epinucleus from the capsule. Use a blunt 25-gauge olive-tip cannula (Storz Ophthalmics) to direct balanced salt solution between the capsule and the cataract until a fluid wave passes between the nucleus and the epinucleus (Figure 9-33). If there is not complete hydrodissection, insert the cannula underneath the opposite side of the capsulorhexis and repeat the hydrodissection.

After hydrodissection, use the same cannula to gently push

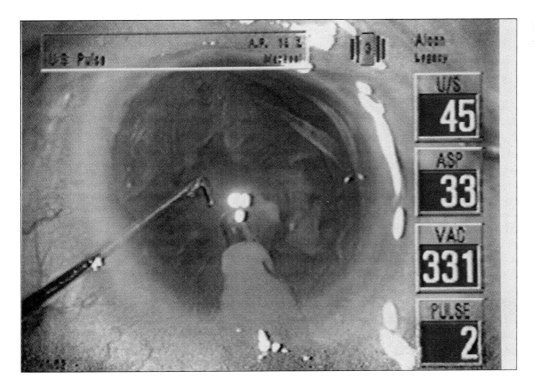

Figure 9-29. Mobilizing the final quadrant (Fine).

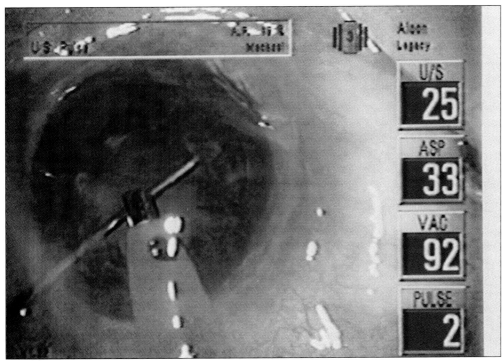

Figure 9-30. The epinuclear shell being rotated for trimming (Fine).

down the nucleus at the superior and inferior poles, rocking it back and forth to help free up any remaining attachments. Then, use the cannula to rotate the nucleus in the bag, first in a clockwise direction, and then in a counterclockwise direction (Figures 9-34A-D).

Once the nucleus is freely spinning in the bag and there are no attachments, gently press down on it with the olive-tip cannula and use a rotating motion to flip the nucleus over and bring it forward into the anterior chamber. It is important to totally invert the nucleus, thus preventing it from falling back into the capsular bag (Figure 9-35).

After the lens is out of the bag, proceed with a two-handed iris-plane phaco and then use a 0.4-mm I/A tip for cortical cleanup. I use a STAAR phaco XL6 with aspiration set at 30, vacuum at 80 and power at 100, with a 30° oval phaco tip.

Figure 9-31. Flipping of the epinucleus (Fine).

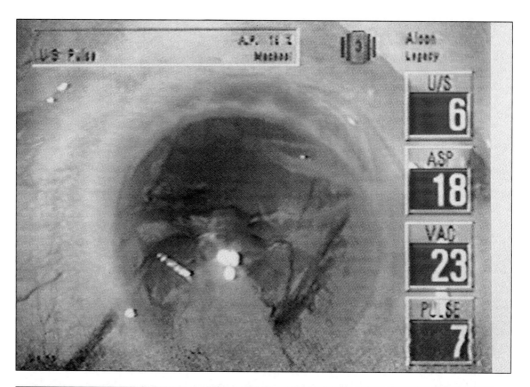

Figure 9-32. Empty capsular bag following flipping of the epinucleus (Fine).

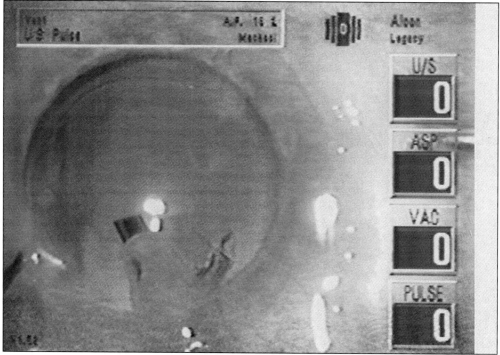

Maloney Supracapsular Phaco

The arrival of capsulorhexis forced phaco into the capsular bag. The resulting capsular confinement of the phaco process has led to a total reconceptualization of the process into nuclear disassembly. All of these disassembly techniques have converged into either cracking or chopping.

There are two important factors that may lead phaco out of

the bag into the supracapsular space. First is the trend toward larger capsulorhexis. The second is the new generation of phaco machines with significantly greater fluid capabilities.

Phaco has evolved to a safe and efficient, but somewhat labor intensive, process. Current techniques use the concept of "balanced flow"; that is, sufficient flow to mobilize just the disassembled portion of the cataract without disturbing the adjacent capsule. A need to stay within the boundaries of this

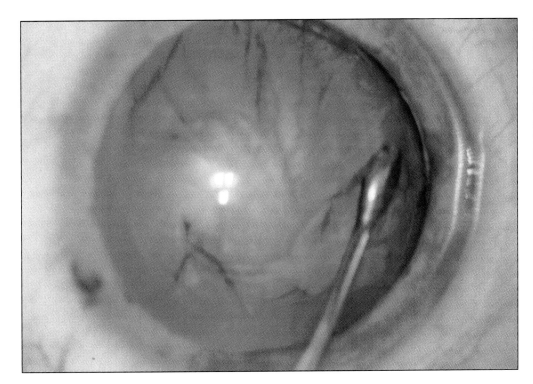

Figure 9-33. A blunt 25-gauge olive-tip cannula (Storz Ophthalmics) is used to direct balanced salt solution between the capsule and the cataract until a fluid wave passes between the nucleus and the epinucleus (Brown).

delicate balance has prevented full use of the fluid capabilities of new phaco technology. Peak-flow phaco requires the process be done in the supracapsular space, above the capsule but beneath the iris.

The key to performing supracapsular phaco is tilting the nucleus and flipping it over and out of the bag (Figure 9-36). This maneuver requires a larger capsulorhexis of 5 to 6 mm. The lens tilt usually occurs spontaneously during hydrodissection. If it does not, the nucleus can be rotated with the hydrodissection cannula to free any cortical attachments before repeating hydrodissection. Failure to achieve a lens tilt can be due to either insufficient fluid during hydrodissection, or a small capsulorhexis. Occasionally a very soft nucleus will refuse to tilt. If lens tilt is not achieved, the case can simply be converted to any endocapsular technique.

Nuclear transposition is unquestionably the most dramatic maneuver in this technique. To begin, the hydrodissection cannula is used to gently depress the posterior pole of the tilted nucleus further and then initiate a sweeping motion, which is guided in the correct direction by the contour of the posterior capsule. The cannula is withdrawn slightly but maintains contact with the same surface of the nucleus and then, still guided by the posterior capsule, continues a smooth uninterrupted turnover until the nucleus has reached a position just beyond

the vertical midline. The hydrodissection cannula is removed.

Viscoelastic is steadily instilled between the newly exposed underside of the partially overturned nucleus and the endothelium, while the cannula slowly continues the transposition of the nucleus until it is reoriented horizontally, but now fully upside down. The viscoelastic cannula adjusts the final position of the inverted nucleus completely within the supracapsular space, which lies behind the iris but above and completely external to the collapsed capsular bag. Viscoelastic is supplemented according to nuclear density and surgeon preference.

Upon completion of nuclear transposition, any preferred phaco method of cracking, chopping or sculpting can be used. The inversion of the nucleus enhances followability and removal to the supracapsular space allows higher aspiration flows, increasing efficiency.

SUMMARY

Whether performed within the capsule or in the supracapsular space, phacoemulsification has evolved to a technique of nuclear disassembly, or nucleofractis. The specific technique used to separate the nucleus—cracking, splitting or chopping—depends on factors such as hardness of the nucleus, maturity of the cataract, and surgeon preference.

Figure 9-34. (A,B,C,D) After hydrodissection, the same cannula is used to gently push down the nucleus at the superior and inferior poles, rocking it back and forth to help free up any remaining attachments. Then, the cannula is used to rotate the nucleus in the bag, first in a clockwise direction, and then in a counter-clockwise direction (Brown)

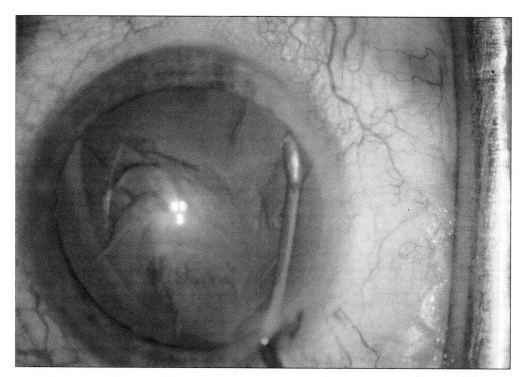

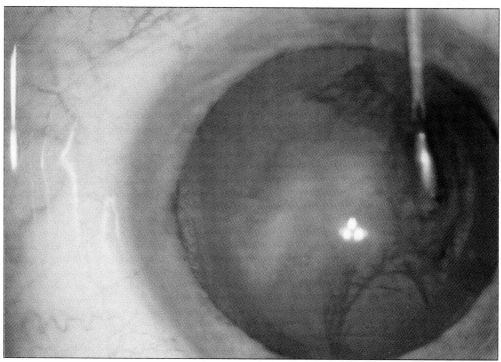

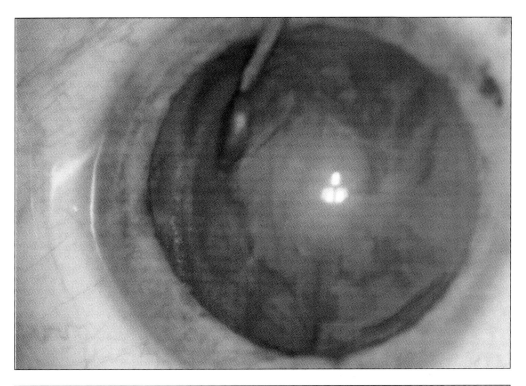

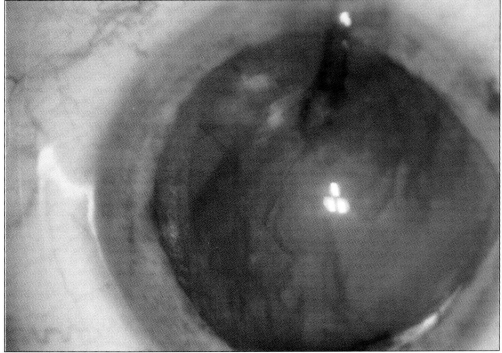

Figure 9-35. It is important to totally invert the nucleus, thus preventing it from falling back into the capsular bag (Brown).

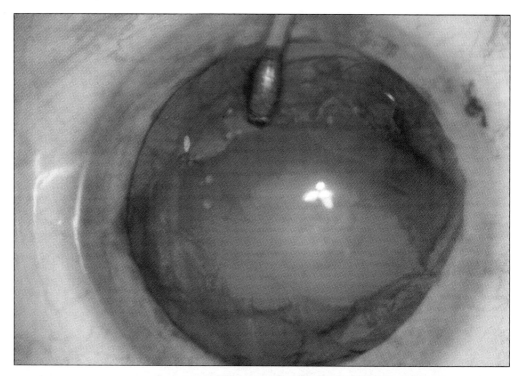

Figure 9-36. The key to performing supracapsular phaco is tilting the nucleus and flipping it over and out of the bag (Maloney).

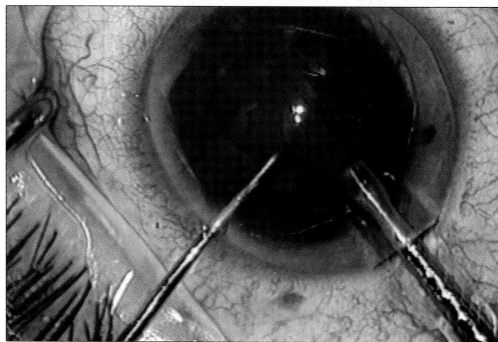

AVOIDING THE COMPLICATION CASCADE

Robert Fenzl, MD

Most complications are not isolated events, but instead result from a cascade of unforeseen events that begin early in the case and slowly develop to a final, climactic disaster. Complications are an inevitable part of cataract surgery. The old adage that the only physician without complications is the one that doesn't do surgery is as true today as it has ever been.

The real question is how can we eliminate preventable complications and decrease the frequency of unavoidable complications by proper planning and meticulous adherence to detail? Most surgeons are so fixated on their final error that they are never able to determine the origin of the disaster. In most cases, there is a series of 3-5 errors that precede the actual complication. I call this series of errors the *Complication Cascade*.

To better identify the early problems that culminate in a serious complication, periodically review the videos of a sampling of cases—especially those in which a complication occurred. If this review is not possible, ask a colleague to observe a series of cases.

As discussed in Chapter 1, patient selection, managing expectations, and proper IOL calculation are key to patient satisfaction. While a poor refractive result is not technically a complication, it can be as significant to the patient as any other complication seen in eye surgery, and therefore an optimal refraction should be given as much attention as the actual surgical endeavor.

SETTING-UP FOR THE SURGERY

When a surgeon experiences persistent problems in surgery, as often as not, the set-up of the OR table and improper positioning of the patient is the culprit. Obviously, a patient who is comfortable and well positioned on the operating table is important for successful cataract surgery, but it is surprising how often the patients are actually uncomfort-

able or poorly positioned. This problem has only been enhanced by the transition to a temporal approach. Unfortunately, many surgical beds do not allow easy access of the surgeon to the temporal aspect of the patient's eye.

The patient should be properly positioned on the surgical table, allowing the surgeon easy temporal access. There must be ample room between the table and the surgeon's legs to maximize comfort. The patient's head should be positioned so that the orbit is perpendicular to the plane of the visual axis of the microscope. Hyperextension or underextension of the chin inhibits the red reflex and causes problems with visualization of the inferior or superior part of the eye. Lateral rotation can cause the eye to disappear into the nasal canthal area, or pooling of BSS.

Preparing for Astigmatic Keratotomy

Additional preparation is required when performing astigmatic keratotomy at the time of cataract surgery. During the preoperative evaluation, a mark is made on the limbus at the steep axis with a low temperature, disposable cautery. Preoperative marking decreases the possibility of off-axis placement of the relaxing incision. Important data, such as the preoperative keratometry measurements, the corneal topography, and the preoperative refraction, should be easily visible from the microscope. The surgical keratometer is invaluable for performing astigmatic keratotomy and special care should be taken to position the patient's head to maximize visibility of the keratometer reflex.

Cataract Incision Placement

There are several factors to consider when performing limbal relaxing incisions combined with a Langerman-style hinge clear corneal incision. The angle between the primary incision and the paracentesis port and individual anatomical differences must be considered to maximize surgeon accessi-

Figure 10-1. Patch graft following corneal burn.

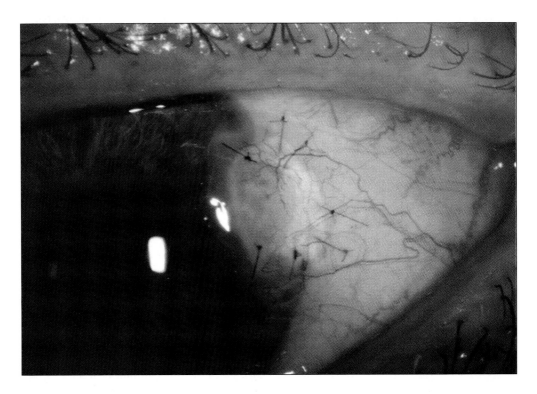

bility. Poor planning can lead to an improperly placed incision or paracentesis port resulting in uncomfortable hand position. Poor positioning can cause complications later on.

One of the most common errors occurs when the cataract incision is positioned directly adjacent to the surgeon's body, i.e., a 9:00 incision when the surgeon is also positioned at 9:00, forcing the surgeon to use uncomfortable and inefficient hand positions. Also, when the incision is placed directly in front of the surgeon, tubing from the hand piece will frequently bump the surgeon's chest, which could cause the tubing to become disconnected from the hand piece and result in complications such as loss of chamber depth.

Paracentesis Placement

The second most common positioning error is placement of the paracentesis port 90° away from the incision. This angle creates problems during maneuvers such as cracking because it is difficult to efficiently utilize the phaco and secondary instrument at this angle. A 45-60° angle between the incision and paracentesis port maximizes maneuverability. The ideal angle may vary slightly for each individual, but it is absolutely necessary that the incision be placed to optimize surgeon comfort and individual patient anatomy.

SURGICAL INCISION

Setting up the Architecture

The wound is frequently the initiator of a complication cascade. Serious problems during phacoemulsification often originate from poor wound architecture coupled with poor planning.

Length of Tunnel

Whether clear corneal, "near clear", or scleral pocket, the incision should extend at least 1 mm—and preferably 1.5 mm—into the cornea for the incision to be architecturally sound. If the tunnel is less than 1 mm, iris prolapse can occur from inflow of fluid. In addition, constant chaffing from the phaco tip can damage the iris. If the internal incision is longer than 1.5 mm, visualization becomes impaired from corneal distortion when the phaco tip is depressed into the nucleus. Impaired visualization can cause the surgeon to maneuver the tip poorly and there is often significant postoperative corneal edema. Certainly bending the cornea in these cases can be equally as traumatic as direct contact with the endothelium.

A thick anterior lip seldom leads to complications. However, incisions that are too deep can cause early entrance into the anterior chamber and are often associated with iris-related complications. Conversely shallow wounds with thin anterior lips are easily torn during manipulation of both phaco and I & A.

Paul Ernest has shown that the incision seals best when it is square. This holds true for all types of incisions.

Wound Width

Small, tight wounds compress the phaco sleeve. Corneal burns may occur in cases where a hard nucleus requiring high power is coupled with a tight wound (Figure 10-1). In some cases, the sleeve can be compressed to such an extent that inflow is compromised. The anterior chamber then shallows, especially when sweeping from one side of the anterior chamber to the other. This shallowing heightens the possibility of a complication related to tip design. The problem may also occur during I & A.

While wider wounds may alleviate the problem of sleeve compression and heat generated in the tip, wounds that are too wide are also associated with certain problems. When the wound is too wide, the surgeon is often forced to work in a shallow chamber due to excess fluid outflow around the tip through the wide wound. There is also a greater tendency for ocular contents to be drawn inadvertently to the tip. Increasing the bottle height provides a limited deepening of the anterior chamber. Occasionally, the wound must be partially sutured before proceeding to improve wound architecture.

Fitting the Pieces Together

While the points listed above may seem obvious and inconsequential for routine surgery, they are important to remember when changing incision technique. Innovation results from incorporating new techniques into our personal strategies. Each new technique must be viewed as a puzzle piece that must fit securely with the other pieces. Just as pieces of different puzzles are not necessarily compatible, cataract techniques frequently are not either. For example, before deciding to adopt a colleague's high vacuum phaco technique, one must first be familiar with the type of phaco unit, settings, tip size and architecture of the wound used with the technique before proceeding.

Not all phaco tips are necessarily compatible with every incision technique. Many surgical complications are the result of combining the use of a new phaco tip with an incompatible incision. For example, when changing to a turbo tip, the incision must be downsized accordingly. Conversely, if the incision size is decreased without changing from a standard phaco tip to a turbo tip, corneal burn, sleeve compression and interruption of inflow are all potential problems.

CAPSULORHEXIS

The capsulorhexis is probably the most stressful part of cataract surgery for most ophthalmologists. A successful capsulorhexis sets the stage for smooth, uncomplicated surgery while unsuccessful capsulorhexis may increase the incidence of complications and necessitate a change from standard technique, increasing the risk of problems later on in the case.

Before performing the capsulorhexis, the surgeon should assess several factors. The factors that should be considered at the outset include: pupil size, density of the cataract, style and material of intraocular lens to be used, the patient's age, and the presence or absence of pseudoexfoliation. It is also important to note the presence of a posterior polar cataract or any loss of zonular support. Most of these factors can be noted during the preoperative examination, but they can all usually be apprised during assessment of the eye under the microscope.

Though some surgeons perform the capsulorhexis under air or BSS infusion, better control of this critical step is attained by the use of viscoelastic. While the choice of viscoelastic ultimately depends on the surgeon's preference, it is the instrument used to make the capsulorhexis, whether bent needle or cystotome, that dictates which viscoelastic is most appropriate. A thinner viscoelastic is more suitable to push the capsular edge forward with a bent needle or capsular forceps. If capsular forceps are used, a thicker viscoelastic is preferred because the increased viscosity maintains the chamber more consistently, especially important because of the larger incision required to facilitate forceps. Pushing the capsular edge through thicker viscoelastic is not an issue with the use of forceps as it is with a bent needle or cystotome.

It is critical that chamber depth be consistently maintained. A shallow chamber results in a tendency of the torn edge of capsule to extend peripherally into the zonules, preventing completion of a continuous tear capsulorhexis. Conversely, an exceedingly deep anterior chamber causes the capsular edge to remain centrally, resulting in a small capsulorhexis with its inherent problems.

Capsulorhexis technique should be customized to the physician and is most effective when the physician's comfort is considered foremost. The diameter of the capsulorhexis is dependent on which phaco technique is used. Generally, the capsulorhexis should be approximately 5 mm in diameter. However, if the entire nucleus is to be phacoemulsified outside of the bag—whether in front of the anterior capsule in the posterior chamber, or actually in the anterior chamber—a slightly larger capsulorhexis should be performed.

Certain risks are associated with a small capsulorhexis. The risk of complications increases due to capsular stress near the wound by the phaco tip, which may lead to zonular disruption and/or phaco contact with the capsule 180° from the incision. This in turn can cause a tear in the anterior capsule. In addition, a small capsulorhexis has a higher tendency to form anterior capsular fibrosis complicated by contraction.

Special Situations

If a patient has known zonular dehiscence, a combination of both a bent needle or cystotome and capsulorhexis forceps can be used to direct forces away from the area of zonular disruption as much as possible. Obviously, in cases of pseudoexfoliation, extreme care should be taken by taking multiple, small grabs to decrease the force exerted on the zonules. The capsulorhexis should be at least 5 mm in diameter to minimize zonular traction.

In cases of posterior polar cataracts, a significantly larger capsulorhexis should be performed if possible, allowing anterior prolapse of the nucleus early during phacoemulsification. In a significant percentage of these cases, the cataract is fused to the posterior capsule and may disrupt the capsular integrity early in the case.

When a patient has a small pupil, care must still be taken to create a 5 mm capsulorhexis. A 5 mm capsulorhexis can be made if the pupil is of reasonable size and reactive. If the surgeon does not wish to stretch the pupil, the tear can be extended beyond the pupillary margin while viewing the visible cap-

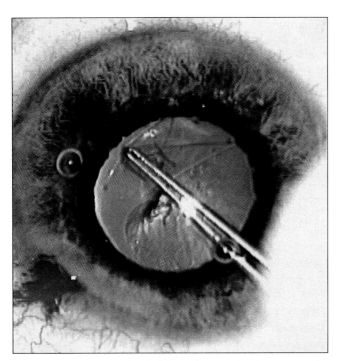

Figure 10-2. A 5-mm capsulorhexis is made by extending the tear beyond the pupillary margin.

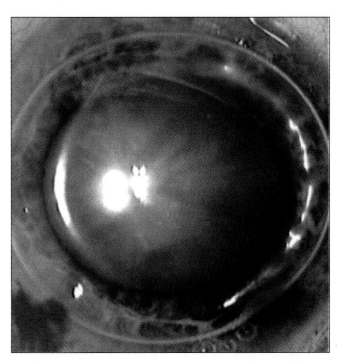

Figure 10-3. Aqueous is removed and replaced with an air bubble.

sule to determine the extent of the peripheral progression of the tear (Figure 10-2). In most cases, a 5 mm capsulorhexis can be consistently performed if the pupil is at least 3.5 mm. When possible, it is more desirable to stretch the pupil so there is an adequate view of the impending capsulorhexis.

The patient with white, mature cataract presents the most difficult scenario for performing a capsulorhexis. Not only is the capsule very friable in these cases, but it can be very difficult to distinguish the capsule from the lens itself. Several techniques have been recommended to maximize visualization for capsulorhexis, but both require significantly more skill than when working with a patient with a good red reflex. The techniques described below make capsulorhexis easier in these cases by improving visibility and contrast of the anterior capsule.

The first technique is described by James P. Gills, MD elsewhere in the book (see Chapter 18). He uses a Grieshabor light pipe to produce tangential illumination across the anterior chamber while performing the capsulorhexis. For this technique, the microscope light is turned off. The surgical assistant uses the light to follow the leading edge of the capsule and improve the surgeon's visibility.

My preference is to use a solution of injectable fluorescein dye diluted 50% with BSS to tint the capsule and improve contrast.

Two paracentesis ports are made. The aqueous is removed and replaced with a single air bubble (Figure 10-3). The cataract wound should not be made at this point to make the

air bubble easier to maintain. A tuberculin syringe containing the fluorescein is placed through one of the stab incisions. The cannula tip must be irrigated well to avoid staining the entire paracentesis and cornea with dye. A minute amount of fluorescein is placed on the anterior capsule and painted across the capsule with the cannula (Figure 10-4). After the cannula has been removed, one should wait approximately 2 minutes before proceeding to allow the fluorescein to permeate into the capsule. The air is then replaced with viscoelastic and standard capsulorhexis is performed. The contrast created by the fluorescein dye greatly improves visibility of the anterior capsule and allows the surgeon to create a more flawless capsulorhexis in the patient with a white cataract.

If an anterior capsular extension occurs during capsulorhexis, one should immediately convert to a can opener capsulotomy. Remember that can opener tears must be multiple and in all quadrants—even in the area where continuous curvilinear capsulorhexis was partially performed. If the can opener tear is not performed around the entire circumference of the capsule, all forces will be directed toward the areas of the can opener tears. If done in this manner, there is a high probability of extending the tear around to the posterior capsule. If multiple small tears are made with the standard can opener technique—including the areas where the capsule was torn successfully—it is less likely that forces will be directed to any one area, and the probability of posterior extension decreases. Also remember that once a can opener tear has been performed, the force the capsule can tolerate during pro-

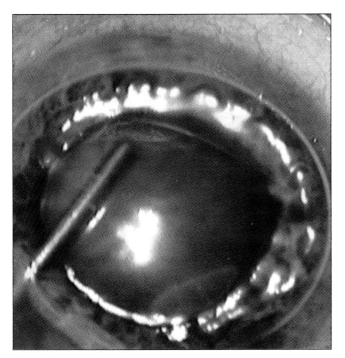

Figure 10-4. Fluorescein is painted on the capsule.

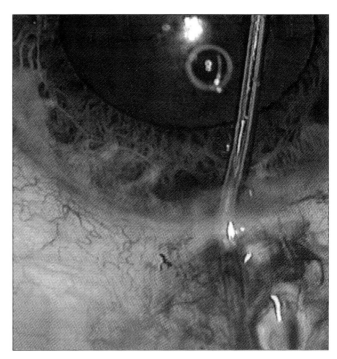

Figure 10-5. The wound is depressed to express viscoelastic before hydrodissection.

cedures such as cracking are significantly reduced. Care should be taken during any endeavor that stresses the capsule.

If a plate silicone lens is the standard routine and the anterior capsule is compromised, immediately instruct the operating room staff that another style lens is necessary. A plate-haptic silicone lens should never be placed in any capsule where integrity has been compromised. My preference in this situation is a three-piece silicone lens to avoid enlarging the 2.5 mm incision. An acrylic lens could also be used in this situation with only minimal enlargement of the incision.

HYDRODISSECTION

For nearly all modern phacoemulsification techniques, hydrodissection and possibly hydrodelineation are necessities. Freeing the nucleus so that it can rotate freely without traction on the capsule is a critical step in all but a few phaco techniques. Different approaches to the procedure have been suggested as well as altering the size and design of various irrigating tips, but the most critical issue is that there is complete cleavage, allowing free rotation of the nucleus.

One of the most common problems encountered during hydrodissection results from not expressing enough viscoelastic from the anterior chamber before hydrodissection (Figure 10-5). The added fluid forced into the capsule can easily blow out a fragile posterior capsule. Even if viscoelastic is adequately removed from the anterior chamber, forceful irrigation of BSS can cause this very devastating complication. This event is more common when a small capsulorhexis

has been performed, since there is less area for fluid leakage and greater pressure is forced into an intact bag.

The second most common complication is incomplete lens mobility because of inadequate hydrodissection. Difficulty rotating the lens during later stages of phaco can lead to zonular stress and a possible capsular tear. Lack of lens mobility also increases the need for lens manipulation and the likelihood of a posterior capsular tear from the phaco tip or secondary instrument.

The third and probably least common complication is inadvertent irrigation of fluid in front of the anterior capsule. This fluid is forced through the zonules and into the posterior chamber. Rapid and significant shallowing of the anterior chamber ensues from the pressure of the fluid behind the lens. While this complication is uncommon, it can be a very difficult one to deal with since the eye becomes extremely hard, despite a very shallow, formed anterior chamber. Proceeding becomes very difficult and can actually worsen the situation.

Rather than continuing, allow time for the fluid to re-diffuse anteriorly, which can be facilitated by the use of hyperosmotics such as Mannitol to draw the fluid from the eye. Occasionally vitrectomy is necessary to deepen the anterior chamber. In some cases, it is necessary for the patient to leave the operating room and return hours or even a day later to complete the case. The surgeon should always consider this option rather than proceeding and possibly worsening the situation.

Lastly, in the cases of a posterior polar cataract often found in relatively young patients, hydrodissection should be done with great care if at all, because in a significant portion of these cases, the cataract is incorporated into the posterior capsule. During hydrodissection, this "plug" is released, allowing entrance of the lens material into the vitreous cavity at a very early stage of surgery. If one is able to visualize that the cataract is not incorporated into the capsule, gentle hydrodissection can be done. If not, thorough sculpting of the nucleus without hydrodissection and only limited delineation is recommended.

Sculpting should be carried as deeply as possible without disrupting the central posterior cataract. Only after the lens has been removed as thoroughly as possible in situ should the remaining material be mobilized using high vacuum. The last part of the remaining epinucleus can be removed with I & A. This technique allows removal of the largest percentage of the lens before possible disruption and loss of integrity of the posterior capsule can occur.

PHACOEMULSIFICATION

Avoiding the Pitfalls

Whether the surgeon flips, chips, cracks, divides and conquers, or uses any other phacoemulsification technique, certain principles should be kept in mind to prevent complications. Special care should be taken at this stage if there were any previous problems because the complication cascade climaxes during the final stages of the procedure.

Before even introducing the phaco tip into the eye, it should be tested first to ensure that the ultrasound is functioning properly, and the irrigating and aspiration lines are also functioning and well secured to the unit. In addition to the inconvenience of discovering that a malfunctioning tip was placed in the eye, or that one of the lines is not working, there is the possibility that these scenarios could lead to a complication. Frequent removal and insertion of instruments increases the incidence of stripping Descemet's membrane.

When the tip is first placed into the eye, the unit should be set at position 2 for a number of reasons. The first is to verify that all lines are clear and secure, but even more importantly, if the unit immediately goes to phacoemulsification, especially if the eye is full of viscoelastic, the tip may become obstructed. This problem is more common with the small diameter turbo tips that also restrict inflow and can lead to immediate and severe corneal burn.

A number of studies have shown that the cracking techniques now in vogue usually require less phaco time and power. However, cracking is associated with a slightly higher risk of additional manipulation with a second instrument that may be poorly visualized at times. For many, this concern outweighs the advantages. No matter what the case, the phaco tip should be kept visible at all times.

If a central groove is to be made for a divide and conquer technique, it should be made as deeply as possible. Creating the groove does not require either high vacuum or high aspi-

ration if small layers are taken with each pass. It is safer to create a deep groove using several small passes than with one deep pass. Initiating power can cause a sudden corneal burn if the lens is thick and viscous in nature, if the tip is buried too deeply in the nucleus, or if the anterior chamber is still full of viscoelastic. After the lens has been divided, regardless of technique used, the unit should be turned to a higher vacuum power. Be careful when changing vacuum that the level is consistent with the fluidics specific to the unit and size of the phaco tip that is being used. For example, many units are unable to maintain chamber depth after the tip is cleared with vacuum levels as low as 100 mm Hg, while other units can maintain chamber depth with vacuum level of 500 mm Hg if a small tip or turbo tip is used. If any of the variables mentioned are not appropriately combined, capsular rupture or endothelial damage can occur very rapidly. Never mix and match setting and techniques without full knowledge of the properties and fluidics specific to your unit.

An example of a mismatch is using zero vacuum phaco during sculpting. If large amounts of cortex are taken and there is no vacuum to clear the tip, corneal burns can occur rapidly and may significantly impact the outcome—especially if a clear corneal incision is used. The risk of corneal burn is greatest when using a small diameter turbo tip. A zero vacuum setting with these tips may actually read 30 mm Hg or more on the machine because of the increased resistance created by smaller tips.

When bite-sized chunks of nucleus are available for the tip and the vacuum has been increased, a low phaco power is used to purchase the material and cause the tip to be buried in the nuclear fragment. At this time, the phaco power should immediately be removed, otherwise purchase of the piece will be lost.

The piece of nucleus should be brought into the center of the chamber with the tip always facing the piece of nucleus to be emulsified. If phaco is performed out of the bag—whether the entire nucleus is brought between the anterior capsule and iris, or the entire nucleus is brought into the anterior chamber (a technique popularized by David Brown, MD) the tip is placed under the nucleus. In this technique, a highly angled tip is used to phaco under the cataract, leaving a bowl of material anterior to protect the endothelium. In a crack or chop technique where pieces are removed, the tip should be turned toward the piece. Turning the tip 90° so power is directed equally away from the endothelium and the capsule is most efficient (Figure 10-6), although on occasion it is more effective to turn the bevel down toward the posterior capsule. The tip should rarely be turned bevel up for in-the-bag phaco. If it is, it should be done for a very limited time.

Because most of the techniques currently used require high vacuum levels to acquire and emulsify the nucleus, tips with low angulation are most effective. A tip with no angulation is difficult to use; 15° is the most efficient angle for a high vacuum setting. Highly angled tips are best used when working from the posterior aspect of the lens to the anterior and high vacuum is not needed.

The phaco power should only be on during the period when the nucleus is actually being emulsified. While this sounds obvious, phaco power is often wasted when there is no contact between the nucleus and the phaco tip, or after a piece has been emulsified and another piece is being maneuvered to the tip. Breaks in power should also be frequent to clear previously emulsified material and allow fluid to egress the bore so the tip can cool. Breaking the power is done most efficiently in the pulse mode. Short breaks in emulsification allow the vacuum to work efficiently and to maneuver better purchase of the lens material to the tip.

During phacoemulsification, the area between 4:00 and 5:00 of the inferior capsule is the most vulnerable. If hydrodissection or hydrodelineation is not thorough, attempts to remove material from this area can lead to anterior or posterior capsular rupture. It is also possible to create traction on the equatorial capsule under high flow or aspiration and to weaken the zonules in this area.

The highest risk of capsular rupture, while infrequent, occurs at the very end of phacoemulsification. At this point, small chips or pieces of nucleus may remain in the eye. Attempting retrieval—especially if the body of the tip has not been cleared of any trapped remaining nucleus—can create a surge when vacuum is released and cause contact with the posterior capsule. Contact between the posterior capsule and the phaco tip can quickly destroy perfectly executed phacoemulsification. Another common time for contact to occur between the phaco tip and capsule, though rare, is when thick nuclear material is removed with phaco rather than I & A. While techniques that utilize the phaco tip for removal of the nucleus and cortical material may be very efficient and economical, using the phaco tip for I & A increases the risk of posterior capsular rupture.

Protecting the Cornea

While it is generally unwise to deviate from standard procedure during phaco, special cases occasionally arise where modification of the routine phaco technique is advantageous to protect the cornea. There are two specific techniques that can be utilized to greatly increase the success of the procedure by using additional viscoelastic during phacoemulsification.

James P. Gills, MD introduced the first application to me. In this simple technique, viscoelastic is added through the paracentesis port during the early stages of phaco. The frequency depends on the degree of endothelial deficiency. I add viscoelastic as frequently as every couple of seconds to as little as one or two additional injections above the routine use. If the endothelial cell count ranges from 800-1500 cells per mm^2, I add an additional layer of viscoelastic at the end of the crack or chop to provide an additional buffer when the chips are brought into the central pupil area. When the endothelial cell count is less than 800 cells per mm^2, I use the viscoelas-

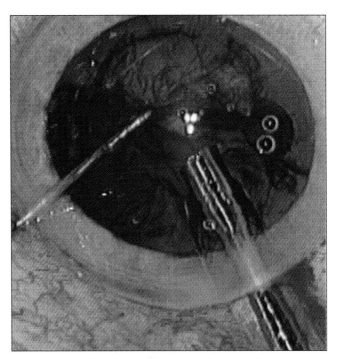

Figure 10-6. The phaco tip is turned 90° to direct power equally from the endothelium and posterior capsule.

tic cannula as my secondary instrument after the crack or chop and inject additional viscoelastic frequently to make sure the anterior chamber is sufficiently deepened at all times to protect the endothelium (Figure 10-7).

Patients with endothelial cell counts below 500 cells per mm^2 can tolerate phacoemulsification without undergoing simultaneous corneal transplantation when additional viscoelastic is injected during phaco. In fact, I have operated on several patients using this technique with uncountable cells with no corneal decompensation to date. This technique works well for those patients with stromal thickening, but no noticeable epithelial edema. These patients are frequently able to avoid or prolong a corneal transplant when viscoelastic is judiciously used during the procedure to protect the fragile endothelium.

It is equally important to provide extra protection for the healthy cornea when the nucleus is very dense. High power and long phaco times are known to adversely affect the endothelium. The same technique used for Fuch's Dystrophy can be applied to these cases. We seldom find corneal edema on the first postoperative exam when this technique is used.

IRRIGATION AND ASPIRATION

As with phacoemulsification, the I & A tip should be examined to make sure that all lines are secure and functioning before the tip is placed into the eye. It should be confirmed that the unit was changed to the I & A setting to provide proper aspiration and vacuum. Again, individual techniques may

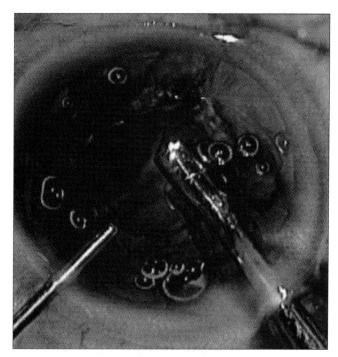

Figure 10-7. Injection of viscoelastic during phaco to protect the compromised cornea.

vary, but with lower aspiration levels and the use of a peristaltic pump, the unit should be placed underneath the anterior capsule in the No. 1 position with irrigation only. It should then be turned to position No. 2, engaging aspiration, grasping the cortex and stripping it to the center for removal.

As with phacoemulsification, the area of the capsule between 4:00–5:00 seems most vulnerable to complication. If the surgeon is right-handed and the incision is shifted slightly right, the area in question is 180° from the incision. Whether a straight or angled tip is used, the I & A port is usually directly up against the anterior capsule. Grabbing the capsule and stressing the zonules is very possible at this position. For this reason, the tip should be turned approximately 10°-15° so there is less likelihood of grasping the anterior capsule. Slowly progress around the capsule from the starting point, making sure the tip is never turned more than 30°, which generally keeps the tip pointing toward the cortex but also provides added safety from grabbing the anterior capsule. At the same time, the tip is not turned posteriorly toward the posterior capsule where capsular rupture is inherently possible. Always remember that the highest incidence of posterior capsular rupture is during I & A and not phacoemulsification.

For most surgeons, the most difficult cortex to remove is directly under the incision. The use of an angled tip can improve accessibility, but care must be taken to avoid downward rotation of the tip toward the posterior capsule. Capsular rupture and zonular lysis most frequently occur when removing cortex under the incision. If cortex is very difficult to

remove in this area, two additional techniques can be used. First, use a cannula to irrigate and a second to aspirate either through the primary incision or the paracenteses, which loosens the cortex for easy removal. The second technique is to leave the cortex and insert the lens implant. Once inserted, the lens is then rotated several times in the bag to loosen the cortex. Additionally the lens provides the extra security of keeping the posterior capsule back. The cortex can then be easily removed.

If the surgeon is comfortable with both high vacuum and high flow and/or aspiration levels, the technique described for cortex removal can be modified slightly. With a 500 vacuum setting and 18 for aspiration with the Surgical Design Unit, the cortex is easily drawn toward the tip even from a distance. Therefore, I seldom put the I & A tip underneath the anterior capsule, but instead, hold it at the edge. The high flow and high vacuum allows me easily to draw the cortex from a much greater distance between the tip and the delicate capsule. The downside is that the high aspiration and high vacuum levels allow little margin for error. If contact does occur between tip and capsule, capsular rupture is possible. Capsular rupture is uncommon when the aspiration and vacuum settings are lower. When a small amount of cortex is left on the posterior capsule, some surgeons have a tendency to retrieve it with the I & A tip in the routine settings. I would strongly recommend against this practice. Most machines have settings specifically intended for central cortex retrieval and they should be used for this endeavor.

CAPSULAR POLISHING

Although I know of no statistics that show a positive correlation between polishing the posterior capsule and decreased incidence of posterior capsular opacification, my clinical impression is that it at least delays the process. Decreasing the epithelial load and providing the patient with a crystal clear capsule certainly has its advantages. I've made it a part of my standard procedure in hope of delaying the process of capsular opacification and possibly lowering the incidence.

INTRAOCULAR LENS

Since I routinely use silicone plate IOLs, I will concentrate on avoiding complications when using these lenses, although I will briefly discuss how to avoid difficult situations when other lenses are used.

To decrease the problem of postoperative pressure spikes, I have used an anterior chamber maintainer as described by James P. Gills, MD during lens insertion (Figure 10-8). There is no question that it greatly decreases the likelihood of residual viscoelastic. Residual viscoelastic left in the eye commonly causes pressure spikes within the first few hours after surgery, which can be devastating in patients with already compromised optic nerves or vessels.

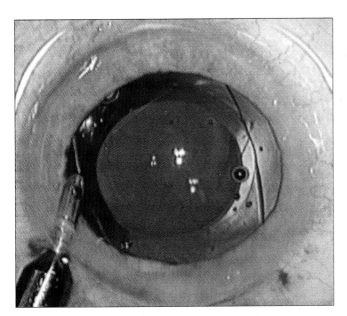

Figure 10-8. The anterior chamber maintainer.

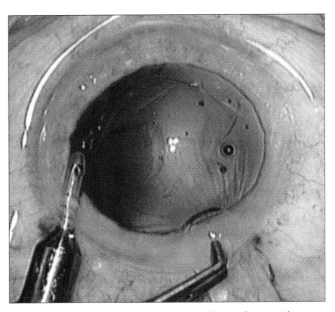

Figure 10-9. Insertion of foldable silicone lens with modified injector cartridge.

IOL Insertion

There are several reasons for inserting silicone lenses with injectors rather than folding with forceps. I prefer an injector because it allows placement of the lens through the smallest possible incision. As James P. Gills, MD, will discuss elsewhere (see Chapter 18), modification of the injector allows placement of the lens without wound stretch through a 2.5 or even smaller incision, creating a more astigmatically neutral incision (Figure 10-9). A reliably neutral incision allows us to correct pre-existing astigmatism at the time of surgery.

In addition to these advantages, a silicone lens in a cartridge is never in contact with the external structures of the eye. Whether folding silicone or acrylic lenses, or inserting a single-piece PMMA lens, the lens itself is in contact with tears, lashes, conjunctiva and other external ocular structures. Lenses inserted through an injector have a far lower chance of contamination with bacteria and foreign material during insertion.

This does not mean that a single-piece PMMA lens is not the lens of choice in certain conditions. These conditions specifically include: inadequate capsule for capsular fixation, anticipated vitreo-retinal surgery in the near future, or when a lens needs to be sutured to the iris because of lack of posterior capsular support.

If there is significant loss of capsular support and an anterior-chamber lens is not appropriate, data so far in several studies have shown that a peripherally iris-sutured posterior-chamber lens has a lower complication rate than the sclerally-sutured posterior-chamber lens. The technique is easy and should be learned by those who wish to place posterior-chamber lenses in eyes with no capsular support.

Check the Lens Position

When implanting a plate silicone lens, care must be taken to ensure that the intraocular lens is indeed capsular fixated. Because of the transparency of the capsule, optic and haptics of the lens, it is may be difficult to ascertain whether the lens is truly posterior to the anterior capsule or merely floating in the ciliary sulcus. Always use an instrument to check the lens fixation by depressing the lens and noting whether the anterior capsule is actually anterior to the lens. The I & A tip is very effective for this purpose.

Even though I use an anterior chamber maintainer, some viscoelastic is used in the injector. After the lens is injected, I use the I & A tip for the dual purpose of removing the viscoelastic used for lens insertion and checking the lens position simultaneously (Figures 10-10 A&B).

Strategies for the Non-intact Capsule

When using a plate silicone intraocular lens, the integrity of the capsule and zonules must be assessed before electing to use a plate silicone IOL. The anterior/posterior capsule must be flawless if a plate IOL is used. Loss of zonular integrity will cause a differential fibrosis of the bag, which increases the probability of IOL shift and glare. Loss of capsular integrity leads to compression of the lens. In a very high percentage of cases, the lens is pushed through the weakened area and displaced either through the anterior capsule, or forced through the posterior capsule and into the vitreous.

The possibility of this complication should also be considered in the patient where a vitrectomy within the first three months after cataract surgery is a known possibility. If a vitrectomy will be necessary or likely within the first three

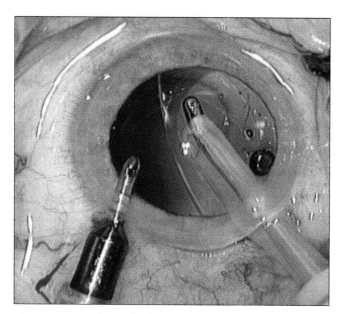 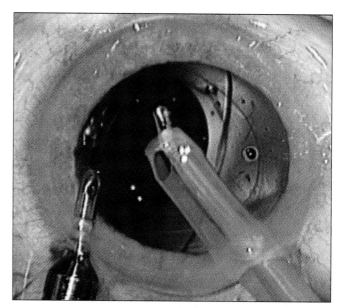

Figure 10-10A & B. The lens is checked for capsular fixation and viscoelastic is removed simultaneously with the I&A tip.

months after cataract surgery, a possibility of capsular disruption exists during vitrectomy. This scenario will likely end in mal-placement of the IOL into the vitreous. YAG capsulotomies in patients with plate lenses should be performed no earlier than two months postoperatively, and preferably three, to reduce the likelihood of compressing the lens through the posterior capsule opening and into the vitreous.

In any case where the capsular bag is not intact, a foldable three-piece silicone intraocular lens or a single-piece PMMA lens should be used instead of a plate silicone lens. I prefer to use three-piece silicone lenses unless the capsular bag has been too disrupted to support the IOL in the bag, and sulcus fixation is required. Also, if the possibility of vitreo-retinal surgery using gas is planned soon after cataract extraction, a one-piece, PMMA IOL should be used to provide a more rigid, stable platform in front of the gas. This should be standard procedure for patients undergoing macular hole closure after cataract extraction.

There are times when a three-piece silicone intraocular lens is my lens of choice. I prefer to use injectors with these lenses but they have always been frustrating because they provide very limited control of the IOL as it emerges into the eye. These lenses tend to emerge from the injector cartridge rapidly and uncontrolled. It can be devastating to watch a small capsular rent extended during IOL insertion after diligently working to preserve as much of the capsular integrity as possible.

Recently, I have had great success with Allergan's new Unfolder. I rarely advocate the use of any particular instrument, but the Unfolder provides smooth and easy insertion of three-piece silicone lenses in cases where I normally would have been forced to use a PMMA lens after enlarging the incision. My preference for three-piece silicone lens haptic material is polyamide (such as the STAAR AQ2003). But I am willing to deal with polypropylene and the disadvantage of easy loss of memory associated with this material for the advantages of the Unfolder.

WOUND CLOSURE

After phacoemulsification and lens insertion have been successfully completed, do not let your guard down. Continue to watch for potential hazards. Wound closure is extremely important because hypotony in the early postoperative period from wound leak may be the reason why surgeons converting to clear corneal incisions have frequently noted an increase in the incidence of endophthalmitis. Overinflation can lead to intraocular pressure spikes resulting in complications. For this reason, we routinely check the intraocular pressure of our patients before leaving the recovery room. Sam Masket, MD has also shown in a recent survey of ASCRS members that one of the positive characteristics of cataract surgeons reporting low incidence of endophthalmitis is the use of antibiotics in the irrigating solution. Not only should antibiotics be used in the irrigating solution, but also as an intracameral injection at the end of the cases to assure maximum safe concentrations.

Care, forethought and planning are the greatest deterrents of complications. If we remember the concept of the complication cascade, many complications can be avoided. When problems are encountered, taking the time to review surgical videos or observation of cases by a colleague will be help to identify the complication cascade more easily. Then we will have learned how to better avoid complications in the future.

REFERENCES

Perry P: Collective outcomes analysis of cases submitted under the American Board of Eye Surgeons Cataract Certification Program. Presented at the 1997 Annual Meeting of the American Society of Cataract and Refractive Surgery, Boston.

Powe NR, Oliver OD, Geiser SC: Synthesis of the literature on visual acuity and complications following cataract extraction with intraocular lens implantation. *Arch Ophthalmol* 1994;112:239-252.

Kahn M, Obstbaum SA: Complications of cataract surgery and their management. In *Management and Care of the Cataract Patient.* Weinstock FJ (ed), Blackwell Scientific Publications Inc. 1992, 185-197.

Cionni RJ, Osher RH: Complications of phacoemulsification surgery. In *Management and Care of the Cataract Patient.* Weinstock FJ (ed), Blackwell Scientific Publications Inc. 1992, 198-211.

Acheson JF, McHugh JD, Falcon MG: Changing patterns of early complications in cataract surgery with new techniques: a surgical audit. *Br J Ophthalmol* 1988; 72:481-4.

MANAGEMENT OF INTRAOPERATIVE COMPLICATIONS

Michael E. Snyder, MD, Robert J. Cionni, MD, Robert H. Osher, MD

Although cataract surgery by phacoemulsification is highly successful, even in the most experienced hands complications occur. The best approach to management of complications is thorough preparation followed by careful execution of a decisive plan. This chapter reviews a wide variety of surgical complications, their evolution during the surgical procedure, and approaches to intraoperative surgical management. Of course, the best management of complications is to avoid them. However, when unpreventable untoward events occur, a well thought out, carefully executed plan can maximize the patient's visual result.

PATIENT RELATED PROBLEMS

In phacoemulsification cataract surgery, regional and, more recently, topical anesthesia have largely supplanted general anesthesia, thus the patient is an active participant in the procedure. The patient's role in cataract surgery is to remain still during the procedure. In cases of topical anesthesia, the patient is also responsible for looking in the appropriate direction, usually directly into the microscope. Complications can occur when patients move their head, body, or eye, cough, or squeeze their eyelids.

Patient movement is often related to a patient's surprise at an unexpected sensation, which can be at the time of periocular injection, or at any time during the surgery when topical anesthesia is utilized, as patients may have sensations which, while not painful, may certainly be unexpected. Patients for which the surgery is planned under topical anesthesia should be fully educated and carefully selected. We prefer not to use topical anesthesia for patients who tend to be "squeezers" in the office, young athletes (who have an exaggerated oculocardiac reflex), or patients with whom the surgeon cannot communicate during surgery either because of hearing difficulties or language barriers.

One effective way to limit patient movement in the operating room is to provide proper education in advance about what will be experienced so that the level of anxiety will be low. Additionally, patients should be instructed not to speak during the procedure unless they are having discomfort to limit unintentional head movement.

Some patient movement can be related to discomfort in the back, arms or legs. Careful attention to patient comfort before surgery begins may prevent fidgeting related to aches or cramps. Some kinds of movement can be related to involuntary tremors or nervous ticks. Many times, taping the forehead will serve as a satisfactory reminder and help stabilize the patient's head. However there are rare instances where general anesthesia should be considered from the start. When patients become oversedated they may fall asleep and might awake with a start. The best way to keep patients from waking up suddenly is to keep them from falling asleep.

If patient movement begins to interfere with the procedure, the first approach should be to remove the instruments from the eye. With most carefully constructed phacoemulsification wounds, the wound will be secure by the self-sealing tunnel and the problem can be addressed calmly. When speaking with the patient, the surgeon should sound calm and in control. If patients sense the surgeon's anxiety they may become more anxious as well, further limiting their ability to cooperate. The anesthesiologist or anesthetist may be very helpful in alleviating patient discomfort or anxiety. However it is best to avoid oversedation. In the rare cases of extreme patient movement that cannot be alleviated, if the wound is self-sealing, one can always convert to general anesthesia to complete the case safely.

Patient coughing is often related to a dry mouth. Instructing the patient to swallow may alleviate a tickle in the throat, or, occasionally, a cough drop may be helpful.

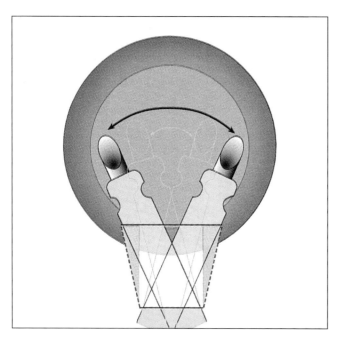

Figure 11-1. When an overly long tunnel results in an oar lock phenomenon, enlarging the internal portion of the tunnel can improve phacoemulsification probe mobility within the anterior chamber.

In cases under topical anesthesia, excessive globe movement can impair the safe completion of cataract surgery. If the patient is unable to hold the eye steady, or if they are perceiving discomfort from the surgery, augmenting the anesthesia with a subtenon, peribulbar, or retrobulbar block may be helpful, which can be accomplished quite safely when a self-sealing wound is present. Instillation of intraocular unpreserved 1% lidocaine may alleviate some patients' sensations and discomfort[1] (see Chapter 2).

If positive pressure from attempted eyelid closure hampers the procedure, an orbicularis block can be administered through the plastic drape.

COMPLICATIONS RELATED TO THE INCISION

Several factors may influence the placement, type, and technique for construction of the incision for phacoemulsification. There are currently many approaches discussed in detail elsewhere in this book, for constructing self-sealing, astigmatically predictable wounds. Careful wound construction can save much difficulty later in the case.

We feel that the first criterion to consider in choosing wound placement should be adequate surgical exposure and approach. A prominent superior orbital rim or brow should sway the surgeon toward a temporal approach. A difficult view or difficulty in accessing the wound over a steep brow may make a straightforward case exceedingly difficult.

Entry Into Suprachoroidal Space

When making a scleral tunnel, if the groove is too deep, the incision may enter the suprachoroidal space with possible suprachoroidal hemorrhage or effusion leading to hypotony. A guarded blade will usually prevent the incision from becoming deeper than planned.

When the surgeon recognizes an entry into the suprachoroidal space, there are three options for management. Deep radial sutures affixing the inner scleral layer to the posterior edge of the wound will preserve that operative site. Alternatively, the entire groove can be closed with interrupted sutures and the wound site can be repositioned to either side and started again, or a clear corneal incision can be created in front of the scleral wound.

Premature Entry

In a scleral-tunnel incision, if the tunnel is too short, the anterior chamber is entered too posteriorly and iris prolapse can occur, causing damage to the iris which can significantly increase the difficulty of the case and may lead to other complications (see section on iris prolapse, below). The initial tunnel should extend into the clear cornea before wound entry. If an early entry is detected quickly and is near the level of the iris insertion, consideration can be given to reconstructing a new wound to either side of the first incision.

If a clear-corneal incision is too short, it may not be secure at the end of the surgery, despite stromal hydration, which may necessitate the placement of a single interrupted radial suture or a horizontal mattress suture, though the latter is more difficult to perform with a clear corneal incision.

The Tunnel is Too Long

When the corneal or scleral tunnel is too long an "oar lock" phenomenon can occur, making manipulation of the phaco instrument inside the eye difficult. If this problem occurs, the internal portion of the wound can be enlarged, which will allow easier movement of the handpiece, taking special care not to enlarge the total incision width (Figure 11-1).

An overly long tunnel may also cause dimpling and distortion of the cornea, limiting the view, stressing the endothelium, and making the surgery more difficult. If this problem occurs, the tunnel can be recreated with an earlier entry. When this maneuver is used, special care must be taken not to catch instruments on the internal corneal lip (Figure 11-2).

The Wound is Too Small

Safe phacoemulsification requires a wound that is properly matched to the equipment being used. If the wound is too small, several potential complications may occur. A tight wound will not allow adequate movement of the phaco handpiece and the globe will therefore move excessively, making the phacoemulsification extremely difficult.

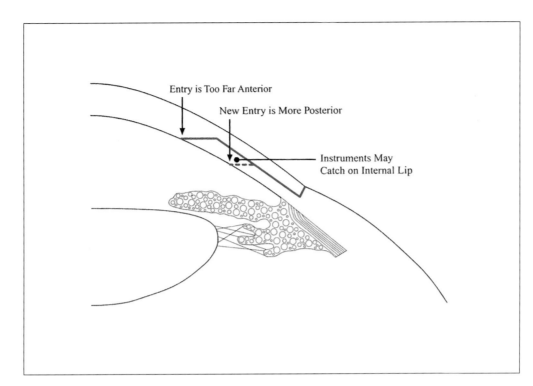

Figure 11-2. To decrease the length of a corneal tunnel, a second, earlier, entrance into the anterior chamber can be created. Special care should be taken to avoid catching instruments on the internal lip which is created.

A tight wound also risks scleral or corneal burn if the infusion is compromised by an overly snug fit. Some newer phaco tip designs allow a tighter fit while helping to prevent a crimped infusion. One can detect an overheating phaco tip early if, after a pulse of phaco, a burst of whitish "lens milk" is seen. A tight wound is recognized quickly and the keratome can be used to enlarge it slightly to accommodate the phaco instrument. If scleral or corneal thermal burn occurs, the wound should be enlarged for completion of the case and the wound should be closed with horizontal mattress sutures, affixing the posterior tunnel roof to the anterior tunnel floor.[2,3]

Attempts to pull the roof of the tunnel back to the groove will likely lead to high induced astigmatism and it will be difficult to prevent a leaky wound. Most commonly, after several weeks, the corneal tissues will relax to lessen the induced astigmatism from corneal collagen shrinkage. If necessary, astigmatic keratotomy can be performed at a later time, at least three months after surgery.

A tight wound may also increase the risk of Descemet detachment. (See Descemet detachment section, below).

The Wound is Too Big

If the keratome entry is too large for the phaco handpiece selected for the case, excessive fluid outflow will occur, leading to continued shallowing of the anterior chamber, which can be remedied by placing an interrupted suture at one side of the wound to reduce its width.

DESCEMET DETACHMENT

Occasionally, Descemet's membrane can become detached from the posterior corneal stroma during cataract surgery. This problem is most often related to the edge of the membrane becoming caught on an instrument as it is being inserted through the wound or paracentesis. Too small a wound with a tight fit will increase the risk, while a well constructed wound and deep anterior chamber at the time of phaco entry into the anterior chamber will minimize this occurrence. An instrument should never be forced through a tight wound. A slight posterior direction and pressure during insertion of the instruments on entry into the anterior chamber can help prevent catching the edge of Descemet's. Additionally, the bevel of the phaco should be facing upward as the tip is passed through the wound. Special attention should be given when implanting an intraocular lens, as the edge of the haptic, inserting forceps, or injector device can also catch on Descemet's membrane edge.

When a Descemet tear or detachment is noted, efforts should be directed toward repositioning the membrane and to limiting the extension of the detachment. A small detachment may be repositioned by pressing slightly on the posterior wound edge, causing an egress of fluid. An air bubble placed into the anterior chamber can be very helpful in repositioning and splinting a larger detachment.[4] This maneuver offers the additional advantage of creating an air-fluid interface at the membrane, making visualization easier. Some investigators have experimented with expansile gases such as C3F8 and SF6.[5,6]

Use of viscoelastic agents has been described for repositioning a detachment. However they should be used with caution. If viscoelastic material separates the stroma from the membrane it can be exceedingly difficult to reattach. In a

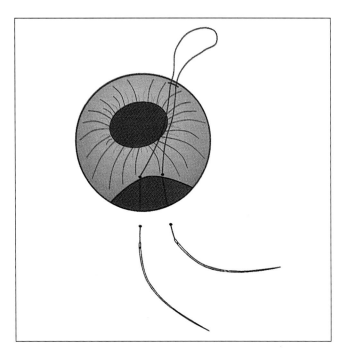

Figure 11-3. Iridodialysis repair is achieved by passing a double armed 10-0 prolene suture transcamerally, engaging the peripheral iris margin, and exiting through the sclera at the iris root. The knot is tied externally and rotated internally.

larger detachment or if there is some traction on Descemet's after repositioning, a full thickness 10-0 nylon corneal suture can be placed parallel, but a millimeter or two central, to the internal wound entry, splinting the membrane in position. If the tear does not extend centrally, the suture can be passed in a radial fashion, entering through clear cornea central to the hinge of attachment. If there are no scrolled edges, some Descemet detachments will reattach spontaneously, though it may take a few months.[7,8]

If the detachment is at the wound and quite small, the tear may be peeled away in a similar fashion to capsulorhexis to prevent a loose edge from enlarging during the case. This maneuver effectively removes endothelial cells, however, so should be used only when the defect is very small.

Rarely, Descemet's membrane can become detached by viscoelastic injection into the sub-Descemet's space. If this occurs, a large air bubble placed into the anterior chamber via a paracentesis from a site where attachment is still present will aid in visualization of the extent of detachment. The viscoelastic can be expressed by creating a direct opening through the cornea and overfilling the anterior chamber. Alternatively, the viscoelastic can be removed by a large bore, blunt cannula, such as a Simcoe cannula, with no irrigation. Attempts to irrigate out the viscoelastic would likely be met with increased detachment of the membrane.

IRIS PROLAPSE

Prolapse of the iris can lead to numerous other complications including pupil irregularity, miosis, iris atrophy, uveal incarceration in the wound, iridodialysis, intraocular hemorrhage, and cystoid macular edema resulting from prostaglandin release. A properly constructed incision with its internal entry in clear cornea will help prevent iris prolapse, while a posterior entry will invite its occurrence. Care should be taken to avoid excessive injection of fluid or viscoelastic agents into the eye since acute elevation of the intraocular pressure can cause iris prolapse.

The surgeon should try to identify the cause of the iris prolapse and alleviate the underlying problem. If spontaneous iris prolapse occurs with sudden, unexplained anterior chamber shallowing, suprachoroidal hemorrhage should be suspected and all instruments should be removed from the self-sealing incision, the iris should be left where it is, and the hemorrhage should be addressed when the globe integrity is secured (see section on suprachoroidal hemorrhage, below).

If iris prolapse is resulting from excessive intraocular pressure, the tendency to prolapse may be reduced by eliminating sources of external pressure, such as repositioning the lid speculum or, in the case of lid squeezing during topical anesthesia, adding an orbicularis block to the eyelid. The intraocular pressure can be reduced by aspirating a small amount of aqueous or viscoelastic from a separate incision site. Iris tissue can be gently reposited using a small amount of viscoelastic or a blunt iris spatula using very small sweeping strokes via a paracentesis incision. If this maneuver is unsuccessful, a peripheral iridectomy can neutralize the pressure gradient between the anterior and posterior chambers and facilitate iris repositioning.

If the prolapse results from a posterior entry, one can occasionally get by with performing the hydrodissection and hydrodelineation via the paracentesis site, then, once placing the phaco safely in the anterior chamber, keeping the phaco tip in place, thus keeping the incision "plugged". If these measures are not successful, one may consider moving the incision to another location. Repeated iris manipulation may result in a flaccid, frayed iris. Intraocular miotic gently delivered directly to the pupillary margin with a cannula may help pull the iris tissue away from the wound. This maneuver, of course, will constrict the pupil and should not be attempted prior to lens removal. Overly aggressive attempts at repositing the iris without alleviating the cause of prolapse may result in an iridodialysis or excessive bleeding.

IRIDODIALYSIS

Exuberant manipulation of the iris when attempting to reposit the iris may occasionally tear the iris away from its insertion resulting in an iridodialysis. A large iridodialysis can hinder completion of the cataract surgery and can make intraocular lens implantation more difficult as well.

Postoperatively, an unrepaired iridodialysis may result in pseudopolycoria and, possibly, monocular diplopia. Additionally, the floppy iris leaflet may result in peripheral anterior synechiae. Repair is directed toward repositioning the iris root to its native place of insertion at the scleral wall.[9,10]

Our preferred method for repair is to place one or more double-armed, horizontal mattress sutures via a paracentesis in a transcameral fashion engaging the iris root and passing the suture through the sclera at the iris insertion (Figure 11-3). The suture is tied externally and the knot is rotated internally. We prefer a 10-0 prolene suture with long, curved needles for this maneuver.

INTRAOCULAR HEMORRHAGE

Intraocular hemorrhage can limit the surgeon's ability to visualize the anterior segment structures, thereby increasing the difficulty of the surgery. In addition, there are postoperative consequences. Blood may accumulate between the IOL and the posterior capsule or it may pass through the zonules into the vitreous. Although intraocular hemorrhage will usually absorb, it may delay visual recovery, stimulate posterior capsule opacification, prevent pupillary movement by clot formation leading to posterior synechiae, or, rarely, result in corneal blood staining.

There are two primary sources for intracameral hemorrhage, the iris and the scleral tunnel. The best way to avoid iris bleeding is to not touch uveal tissue. If manipulation of the iris causes a break in the major or minor iris circle, the best treatment is to firm up the globe with adrenalized balanced salt solution to tamponade the bleeding. When hemorrhage occurs from the scleral wound, increasing the ocular tension alone may halt the bleeding. Point cautery to the feeder vessel away from the wound can also stop the bleeding, though it may distort the wound and compromise its self-sealing architecture. It is best to try to evacuate the blood before clot formation occurs by gently depressing the posterior lip of the wound with a cannula. Alternatively, the blood may be aspirated and exchanged for balance salt solution either through a paracentesis or via the primary wound. A simultaneously irrigating and aspirating device will maintain the closed system and reduce the likelihood of hypotony and recurrence of the bleeding. Maintaining a high-normal intraocular pressure at the completion of the procedure will seal the anterior lip of the wound more tightly, preventing entrance of blood into the anterior chamber.

COMPLICATIONS RELATED TO ANTERIOR CAPSULOTOMY

Continuous tear capsulorhexis is much stronger and resistant to peripheral extension. Moreover, if a tear in the posterior capsule occurs, there is a much greater likelihood of being able to stabilize an implant in the posterior chamber.

Peripheral Extension (Capsulotomy Too Large)

Controlling the direction of a continuous tear capsulotomy requires a balance of the forces acting on the anterior capsule. When the anterior lens surface is more convex, the natural tension from the zonules will direct the tear more peripherally. The anterior lens surface may be more convex, and therefore at a greater risk for peripheral extension in a number of situations including a shallow chamber or positive pressure. The youthful eye has a more elastic capsule which also increases the risk of peripheral extensions. In these settings, making a smaller capsulorhexis may increase the margin of safety. The opening can be enlarged later in the case if it becomes necessary. Deepening the anterior chamber to create a flatter anterior lens surface tends to facilitate the capsulorhexis procedure. If the viscoelastic escapes as the cystotome or forceps are placed into the anterior chamber, the surgeon can select a more highly retentive viscoelastic or perform the capsulorhexis with a bent needle or cystotome placed through a small paracentesis to facilitate maintaining a deeper anterior chamber. It is best to try to redirect the tear by folding the capsule completely over on itself and establish the tension forces in the direction you wish the tear to follow (Figure 11-4). The surgeon should overcome the reflex to pull the capsule centrally, which may force the tear to extend to the equator.

Occasionally, the anterior capsule tear will extend too far peripherally to allow its recovery. Persistent heroic attempts to force the tear centrally may cause it to extend around the equator into the posterior capsule. The surgeon should return to the starting point and proceed with a second tear in the opposite direction, or convert to a can-opener capsulotomy. In these cases, the phacoemulsification should be performed with great caution, taking special efforts to avoid any undue stress on the zonules or expansion of the capsular bag, which may encourage the tear to extend beyond the equator. If using a divide and conquer approach, extreme caution should be exercised when cracking the quadrants, as this technique places significant forces on the capsular bag. By contrast, the chop technique may divide the nucleus with less force. A stable chamber should be carefully maintained during both phacoemulsification and cortical aspiration. The cortical cleanup should be performed gently and lastly in the area of the peripheral extension. The IOL should be inserted into the bag with minimal force. The haptics should be oriented as far from the extension as possible. If it appears that IOL placement in the bag may be placing undue stress on the capsule, sulcus fixation may be preferable.

Capsulotomy Too Small

A smaller capsulotomy makes nuclear manipulation more difficult. There are a number of maneuvers that may facilitate nuclear removal, including endocapsular phacoemulsification, phaco-chop, debulking the nucleus and prolapsing the remaining portions using a second instrument, or debulking the nucleus and then enlarging the capsulorhexis.

Figure 11-4. (A) If the tension on the capsule (long arrow) is directed centrally in attempting to redirect a peripherally extending tear, the tear will likely extend further peripherally (short arrow). **(B)** If the anterior chamber is deepened and the capsule is folded over, the capsule will follow the direction of the tension forces applied and the peripheral extension can be redirected.

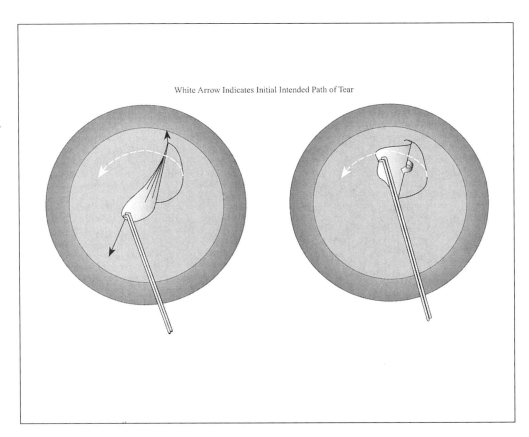

White Arrow Indicates Initial Intended Path of Tear

Figure 11-5. A right-angled irrigation and aspiration tip is helpful in removing subincisional cortex, particularly if the capsulotomy is small.

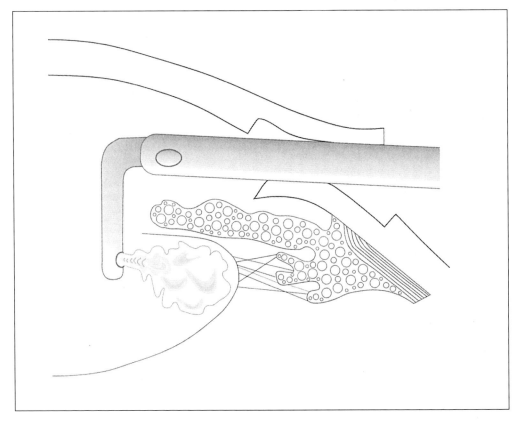

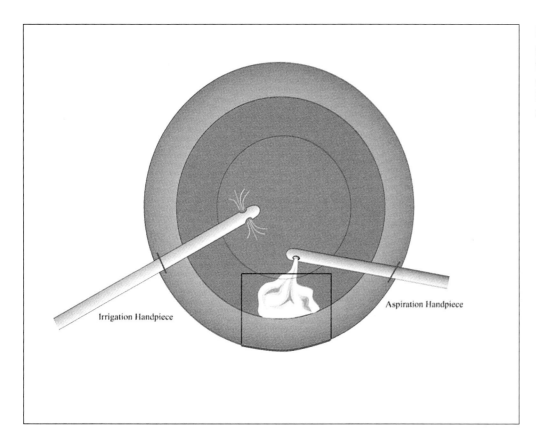

Figure 11-6. Bimanual irrigation and aspiration can facilitate removal of subincisional cortex, particularly if the capsulorhexis is smaller than usual.

A small capsulotomy also makes aspiration of subincisional cortex more challenging. This can be facilitated by use of a right-angled or J-shaped irrigation-aspiration tip (Figure 11-5), manual aspiration with a cannula, or bimanual irrigation-aspiration using two paracentesis stab incisions (Figure 11-6).[11]

Hydrodissection in cases with too small of a capsulotomy may result in an acute pupillary block glaucoma with devastating visual consequences.[12] This even should be considered one of the rare but true intraoperative emergencies. Prevention is directed at early detection; if during hydrodissection the lens appears to be moving forward, gently depressing the lens within the bag using the cannula will allow the fluid to escape around the equator, thus preventing the blockage. Once the syndrome has occurred and the pressure has dramatically increased, efforts should be rapidly directed to relieving the intraocular pressure, which can be done by distorting the capsulotomy to allow egress of the fluid, depressing the lens, or bluntly exploring the epinuclear space with a cannula to create a pathway for the fluid to escape. If the pressure cannot be quickly alleviated by these maneuvers, urgent intravenous administration of 50 cc of 25% mannitol should be given, provided that no significant medical contraindications exist.

A small capsulotomy may lead to the postoperative complications of capsular block syndrome,[13,14] or capsular contraction.[15,16] Capsular block occurs when some viscoelastic is trapped in the capsular bag by a tight adhesion of the anterior surface of the implant against the internal rim of the anterior capsulotomy. Osmotic forces draw fluid in, over-expanding the capsular bag and moving the implant forward with a resultant myopic shift. An anterior or posterior capsulotomy relieves the osmotic imbalance, thereby resolving this complication.

Capsular contraction occurs when the centripetal forces of the anterior capsular fibrosis overcome the centrifugal forces of overly lax zonules, which can limit the capsular opening to a tiny pinhole, limiting vision and requiring anterior capsulotomy. A large capsulotomy is far less likely to result in capsular contraction.[17] Use of an endocapsular ring or a one-piece PMMA implant may help prevent capsular contraction, while silicone lenses may encourage capsular contraction.[18]

Enlarging a small capsulotomy is safest under the protection of viscoelastic and following IOL implantation. An oblique nick is created in the capsular edge and the tear is guided around with a forceps (Figure 11-7). Superior enlargement is more difficult because a nick must be created with a sharp blade since reverse cutting scissors are not widely available. If available, side-cutting vitreoretinal scissors may be used through a sideport paracentesis.

COMPLICATIONS RELATED TO HYDRODISSECTION

Overly aggressive hydrodissection alone can result in a posterior tear and dislocation of the nucleus.[19,20] Hydrodissection is particularly dangerous in patients with posterior lenticonus. Posterior polar cataracts may be associated with a weakened or

Figure 11-7. A small capsulorhexis can be enlarged by creating an oblique nick in the capsular margin, then enlarging the tear with a Utrata forceps.

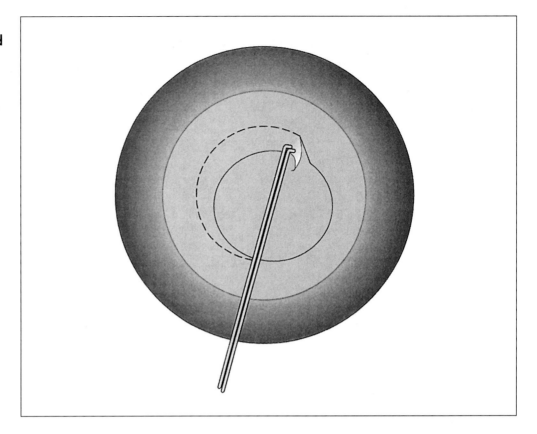

defective posterior capsule which may be more vulnerable to injury, even with usually safe maneuvers.[21] Gentle, limited, or no hydrodissection may be safest to prevent rupture of these most fragile capsules, while gentle, limited viscodissection may offer a greater degree of control.

COMPLICATIONS RELATED TO THE PHACOEMULSIFICATION

A variety of complications can occur during phacoemulsification and are discussed below.

Insertion of the Handpiece

Insertion of the phacoemulsification tip can strip Descemet's membrane, chafe the iris stroma, or even cause an iridodialysis. These complications are more likely to occur in eyes with positive pressure or anatomically shallow chambers in which there is less room between the iris and cornea. If the phaco tip is inserted bevel down, there will be less likelihood of iris damage. However a bevel-down technique somewhat increases the risk of a Descemet detachment.

The technique must be modified for cases with iris prolapse. First, the iris must be carefully reposited before attempting to place the phaco tip in the eye. Viscoelastic should be placed over the iris in the area of the wound and to either side. The tip can be placed into the anterior chamber with the irrigation off. If the surgeon attempts to enter the eye with irrigation on, recurrence of the prolapse will inevitably occur. Once inside the anterior chamber, irrigation can be resumed.

Excessive Globe Movement

An incision that is too tight may lead to globe movement with each stroke of the handpiece. A scleral tunnel that is too long may limit the view by rotating the eye away from the operative wound when the phaco handpiece is in place. If the surgeon's movement are adjusted so that the wound site acts as a fulcrum, globe movement can be reduced.

Shallow Anterior Chamber

The presence of a shallow anterior chamber makes phacoemulsification extremely difficult. Wound-related complications and damage to the iris are more likely. Additionally, the anterior capsulorhexis has a much greater tendency to extend peripherally. The use of a highly retentive viscoelastic will most often suffice in deepening the anterior chamber adequately. Combined with particular caution to entry of instruments through a more anterior wound site, an excellent outcome can be attained.

In some instances such as phacomorphic glaucoma, viscoelastics alone may not achieve an adequate working space in the anterior chamber. In these instances, intravenous mannitol may be helpful in reducing the vitreous volume and increasing the anterior chamber working space. Rarely, in the nanophthalmic eye, a single port, dry vitrectomy can be performed through the pars plana to decompress the vitreous cavity.

The sclerotomy is created with a 20 gauge microvitreoretinal blade 3.5 mm posterior to the 11:00 limbus and the vitrector is set on low aspiration, low vacuum, and a high cutting rate. Additional viscoelastic is simultaneously added to the anterior chamber via a paracentesis until an adequate anterior chamber space is achieved, resulting in successful phacoemulsification.

Anterior Chamber Collapse

With sudden collapse of the anterior chamber, the posterior capsule or corneal endothelium may be damaged. Each occurrence of collapse risks further damage and may promote pupillary miosis. Maintenance of a steady anterior chamber depth and volume requires a balancing of fluid inflow and outflow.

Insufficient Inflow

There are several possible reasons for unsatisfactory inflow. The bottle height may be too low, the tubing or cassette may be kinked or damaged, or the irrigation stream may not be activated due to inattentiveness to the foot pedal. Occasionally, a tight wound may pinch the irrigation sleeve around the phaco needle. If raising the bottle height does not improve the chamber depth, then inspection of the tubing and machine should be undertaken.

Excessive Outflow

A large (leaky) wound will allow fluid to escape around the phaco needle. If leakage is noted a suture should be placed to decrease the size of the open wound. A more subtle problem is a tendency for the surgeon to elevate the handpiece which causes the wound to gape and the chamber to collapse. The surgeon should pay special attention to the forces being placed at the wound, particularly in deep orbits where access to the wound may be difficult.

External Compression of the Globe

Any external force may cause an increase in posterior pressure and fluid egress. The forces may be related to surgical instrumentation, high anesthetic volumes or hemorrhage within the orbit, pressure from the eyelid speculum, or eyelid squeezing by the patient under topical anesthesia. The offending factor should be sought out and remedied.

Inappropriate Fluidic Parameters

Since chamber maintenance requires a balance between inflow and outflow, machine settings and capabilities are critical to maintaining an even balance. The surgeon should be familiar with the particular machine being used and its capabilities. When the phaco port is occluded and the ultrasound energy suddenly clears the tip, the potential energy stored within the tubing is transmitted to the tip and chamber collapse may occur. Some potential energy is also stored within the stretched fibers of the sclera. The higher the bottle, the higher the intraocular pressure, and more potential energy is available. This energy is also released when occlusion is broken, augmenting the tendency for chamber shallowing or collapse. Some phacoemulsification techniques requiring higher vacuum settings should be performed only with equipment that is properly designed for these tasks.

Several instruments alleviate this problem by a number of different solutions. Some machines have a microprocessor which senses the pressure within the tubing and shuts down the pump before a surge can occur. Another manufacturer designed cassettes which have a stiffer tubing that does not store as much potential energy, hence less tendency for postocclusion surge. Other slightly more cumbersome alternatives focus on different venting systems and second irrigation systems with anterior chamber maintainers. If an appropriately equipped system is not available, then the surgeon should select a lower flow, lower vacuum, lower aspiration technique.

Suprachoroidal Hemorrhage

Whenever sudden, unexplained anterior chamber shallowing occurs, suprachoroidal hemorrhage should be suspected. (Please see separate heading on suprachoroidal hemorrhage, below).

Positive Pressure

The presence of positive pressure makes phacoemulsification much more challenging and can lead to a number of complications. The depth of the anterior chamber decreases thereby diminishing the working space, which may cause the nucleus to prolapse into the anterior chamber and force the surgeon to use an anterior chamber phacoemulsification technique, increasing the risk of endothelial damage. As the vitreous face bulges forward, the posterior capsule becomes convex, making a capsular tear much more likely. Cortical aspiration and intraocular lens placement is also more difficult. When positive pressure is encountered, the surgeon should attempt to identify the cause and take appropriate actions to relieve or mitigate it if possible. The following paragraphs review some of the causes of positive pressure and ways to manage them.

Positive Pressure From External Compression

Any factor which transmits pressure to the scleral wall will result in positive pressure during the surgery. The eyelid speculum, or the eyelids themselves, may be inadvertently pressing on the anterior sclera, which, in turn, transmits this pressure to the vitreous and results in positive pressure. If the eyelid speculum is found to be the culprit, repositioning or selecting a different style of speculum may be necessary. The eyelids may directly compress the globe if the palpebral fissure is particularly narrow, or, in the case of topical anesthesia, if the patient is squeezing the eyelids. The former may require a lateral canthotomy to release the tension, while lid squeezing may be addressed by alerting the patient to relax the lids, or adding an orbicularis block through the drape.

Positive Pressure From Globe Distortion

A taut bridle suture may also induce positive pressure by distorting or compressing the anterior sclera. We rarely use bridle sutures, as we have found that with phacoemulsification, globe positioning is better achieved by careful positioning of the hands and instruments. Placement of a superior bridle suture may, in fact, rotate the globe downward, reducing the view for the procedure.

Positive Pressure From Increased Orbital Pressure

Any increase in orbital pressure will be directly transmitted to the posterior sclera, then to the vitreous, and positive pressure will ensue. The orbital pressure can be increased by several sources. First, excessive amounts of anesthetic volume delivered to the orbit will increase pressure. If during the administration of a block increased orbital pressure becomes obvious, further anesthetic infusion should be limited. Orbital hemorrhage will create positive pressure by a similar mechanism. When hemorrhage is significant, it is sometimes necessary to delay the surgery, as discussed elsewhere in this chapter. When positive pressure from increased orbital pressure is discovered during the case, cautious use of intravenous mannitol may reduce the vitreous volume and allow the case to continue more safely. This solution, however, only mitigates the problem and does not resolve it entirely.

A Valsalva maneuver can also increase orbital volume by decreasing venous return, leading to engorged orbital vessels. The cause of the Valsalva may be related to anxiety, the need to cough, discomfort, or a full bladder. When the cause is identified, the instruments should be removed from the eye and the appropriate measures taken to alleviate the inciting problem before the case continues. Orbital veins may also be engorged in obese patients, similarly resulting in positive pressure. Placing the patient in the reverse-Trendelenburg position may be very helpful.

Positive Pressure Causes Intrinsic to the Globe

Young patients generally have a less rigid, more elastic scleral wall, which may induce positive pressure. An eyelid speculum which lifts the lids away from the globe may help support the scleral wall, slightly reducing this tendency. In these cases hyperosmotics may dehydrate the vitreous gel, promote scleral collapse, and paradoxically increase positive pressure. Eyes with an anatomically small anterior segment also have a tendency toward positive pressure.

Choroidal volume may be increased from Valsalva by the same mechanism described above for the orbital vessels. Choroidal hemorrhage or effusion will also result in positive pressure. Management of this complication is addressed in this chapter under a separate heading.

Positive pressure also results from any increase in the vitreous volume. Irrigation fluid can track through intact zonules, a posterior capsular break, or a zonular dialysis. While higher bottle elevation increases the water pressure in the anterior chamber and increases the risk for fluid movement posteriorly, a lower bottle height can help prevent positive pressure. Vitreous overhydration can also result from inadvertent placement of the hydrodissection cannula into the ciliary sulcus.

Special Techniques in Positive Pressure Management

When the cause of positive pressure is not entirely reversible, some maneuvers may help in completing the surgery more safely. First, an increased anterior chamber depth can be achieved by decreasing both aspiration and vacuum settings. If the etiology of the positive pressure is not due to vitreous overhydration, the infusion bottle can be raised. Short bursts of phaco will lead to less aspiration than longer bursts and, consequently, a deeper, more stable chamber. Placing a second instrument behind the phaco tip in order to physically restrain the convex posterior capsule can make a rent less likely. With excessive chamber collapse, cortical removal can be accomplished using a "dry" manual technique with the help of viscoelastic material. Intraocular lens implantation may be facilitated by additional instillation of a retentive viscoelastic agent via a second incision prior to or during lens insertion. As noted above, intravenous hyperosmotics may occasionally be helpful in some instances, but should be avoided whenever scleral collapse is suspected.

In rare instances, positive pressure may threaten completion of surgery. An emergency pars plana vitreous aspiration may be indicated, although it is imperative to confirm the absence of a suprachoroidal hemorrhage. Because the pars plana vitreous removal maneuver carries additional risk, it should be used only when other more conservative alternatives have been exhausted. Finally, if all attempts to alleviate the positive pressure fail, or if suprachoroidal hemorrhage is present and the case cannot proceed safely, it might be necessary to close the wound and complete the case at a later time.

Iris Injury

Either direct contact with the iris or uveal prolapse through the incision can result in iris injury during phacoemulsification. Trauma to the iris may result in a flaccid iris with pigment epithelial defects, synechiae, and an abnormal pupil. Release of prostaglandins from the damaged iris may cause intraoperative miosis and post-operative cystoid macular edema.

Careful technique and adequate dilation are the most effective ways to avoid iris injury. Preoperative topical nonsteroidal drops and epinephrine added to the balanced salt solution will maintain the maximum pharmacological dilation possible. When the pupil is too small, several techniques to achieve dilation exist including pupil stretching,[22,23] multiple radial sphincterotomies, iris hook retractors,[24,25] and pupillary expanding rings.[26]

Surgeons should be very familiar with the fluidic parameters of their technique, as inadvertent aspiration of the iris margin may be more likely with increasing aspiration flow rate. In techniques which utilize a higher vacuum setting, the phacoemulsification machine should be equipped with adequate special safeguards against post-occlusion surge.

Once the pupillary sphincter tone has been compromised and the iris becomes flaccid, the tissue is more likely to be drawn to the aspiration port. A second instrument such as a Kuglen hook can be used to retract the iris, preventing further injury. Moreover, entry of the ultrasound or irrigation and aspiration tips may be accomplished through a viscoelastic agent. Once the tip is within the eye, infusion may be initiated safely.

Posterior Capsule Tears

A posterior capsule tear is probably the most frequent serious complication encountered by cataract surgeons. An opening in the posterior capsule may increase the risk of cystoid macular edema and retinal detachment.[27]

As with all other complications, prevention is the best approach, for which we prefer lower parameters and meticulous surgical technique. For example, we use a second hand sideport instrument placed behind the nuclear material to prevent the posterior capsule from coming up to the phacoemulsification tip. Yet when a posterior capsule tear does occur, proper management can preserve an excellent visual outcome in most cases.[28]

Some types of cataract are more prone to posterior capsular tears, and special precautions may be undertaken. The young patient with a cataract generally has a very soft nucleus and the instruments may more readily contact the capsule, resulting in a tear. Fluidic parameters should be particularly low on these patients so that the lens material, and possibly capsule, are not aspirated too quickly, offering the surgeon more precise control and more time to react.

Posterior Capsule Tears With Nuclear Material Still Present

If nuclear material remains, it should be removed either with phacoemulsification or by converting to an extracapsular procedure. The following paragraphs discuss approaches to fragment removal. However it should be noted that if vitreous prolapse is already present and the nuclear fragments are admixed in vitreous, then the vitreous should be addressed first. Manipulation of nuclear pieces that are attached to vitreous puts undue stress on the vitreous base and increases the risk for retinal detachment.[29]

The phacoemulsification should be completed with a very low flow system and low infusion to help prevent overhydrating the vitreous or forcing the nucleus posteriorly. A second instrument should be used to support the nuclear fragments, reducing their likelihood of falling through the break. The surgeon can provide posterior support for nuclear material via the pars plana, as described by Charles Kelman, M.D.[30]

A sclerotomy is created to allow entry of a spatula which can support the nucleus from behind. Even safer is to prolapse the nucleus out of the bag into the anterior chamber where emulsification or expression can be completed. If the fragments can be brought anteriorly, a Sheets glide may help to protect the capsular opening. This technique should be used with caution, as the manipulation of a trimmed Sheets glide within the anterior segment may compromise the capsular support for a PC-IOL. Ultrasonic energy should be applied in short bursts, adjusting the vacuum upwards to retain maximum control. The pulse mode of some instruments may be helpful. When the phacoemulsification is complete, the anterior chamber depth should be maintained by instilling viscoelastic through the paracentesis before the phaco tip is withdrawn, preventing chamber shallowing and reducing the risk of vitreous prolapse.

Conversion to an extracapsular technique is suited for cases in which one or two large pieces remain. If the surgeon chooses to enlarge the wound, several factors must be considered. First, the wound must be at least large enough to remove the largest fragment in one piece. Second, the control of a closed system will be lost with all of the attendant problems of an open limbal wound. If the wound is a scleral tunnel wound, the peritomy should be enlarged and the groove and tunnel increased with a crescent blade. The internal wound is enlarged with the keratome, taking care to cut on the in-stroke and not the out-stroke of the blade, to preserve the wound architecture. Viscoelastic should be placed under the nuclear fragments, which are retrieved by a lens loop. Attempted nuclear expression will likely result in vitreous prolapse and increase the risk of posterior dislocation of the nuclear material.

Conversion of a clear-corneal tunnel to a larger, extracapsular wound is much more challenging. First, a groove should be extended to the maximum length of the intended enlargement, regardless of whether or not a one-, two-, or three-planed incision was used initially. A keratome blade can be used to enlarge the tunnel, ideally trying to reduce the length of the tunnel while enlarging (Figure 11-8). The more anterior entry to the clear-corneal surgery makes retrieval of lens fragments more difficult. If nuclear pieces get caught in the chamber angle under the floor of the tunnel, they can be moved with judicious use of viscoelastic material via a paracentesis site. When closing the wound, care should be taken to prevent the internal floor of the tunnel from sagging and failing to seal down, requiring several sutures (Figure 11-9).

Posterior Capsule Tears With No Nuclear Material Present

If the tear occurs after the nucleus has been removed, or the nucleus has been safely removed by one of the above approaches, the surgeon must then turn the attention to tear containment and cortical aspiration. Once again, a low-flow situation will help prevent vitreous hydration and prolapse. A manual "dry" cortical stripping under viscoelastic should pro-

Figure 11-8. When enlarging a clear corneal incision for conversion to an extracapsular technique, the keratome blade should be positioned with its cutting surface parallel to the tunnel internal edge, as shown. The tunnel length will become shorter as the width increases.

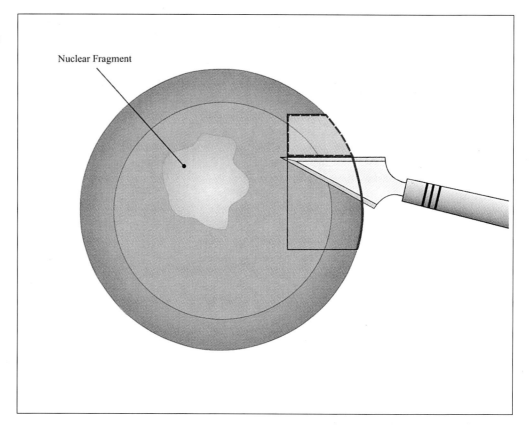

Nuclear Fragment

Figure 11-9. In closing an enlarged corneal tunnel, it is important to ensure that the sutures engage the posterior edge of the wound to prevent internal wound gape.

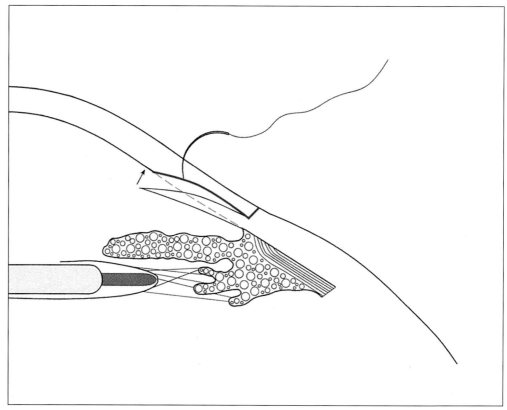

ceed from the equator toward the tear, avoiding any stress which may extend the tear. Alternatively, a gentle, low-flow Simcoe or automated aspiration may be used with caution. While complete cortical removal is often possible, heroic attempts to remove every last bit of cortex should be avoided. Overzealous attempts may lead to an enlarged tear or vitreous prolapse and may compromise PC-IOL placement.

If the tear is small and central, the surgeon may be able to carefully convert the tear into a continuous posterior capsulorhexis,[31] which can be accomplished only if the surrounding capsule is clean of cortex. This maneuver is challenging and should be attempted only by those who feel highly comfortable with capsulorhexis.

Posterior Capsule Tears and Vitreous Prolapse

When vitreous prolapse through a capsular tear is present, the surgeon's goals should be directed toward removing the vitreous from the anterior segment, maintaining capsular support for a posterior chamber implant, and limiting the risk of retinal complications. The likelihood of achieving these goals decreases with increased manipulation of the vitreous. Therefore, early detection of vitreous prolapse is key to a successful outcome. Whenever a posterior capsule break is identified, one of the surgeon's first maneuvers should be to determine the presence or absence of vitreous. As mentioned earlier, keeping the handpiece in the eye to maintain a closed system should be accompanied by reducing the infusion as a viscoelastic agent is injected into the anterior segment. The posterior capsule becomes concave and the chamber remains deep as the handpiece is withdrawn. Careful inspection of the anterior segment will identify any abnormal peaking of the pupil margin or the margin of the capsular break. If there is suspicion of vitreous prolapse, a cautious, slow sweep of the anterior chamber with a cyclodialysis spatula may elucidate tiny movements of the pupil, capsular margin, or remaining nuclear material distant from the direct touch of the instrument. If vitreous material is confirmed, any further manipulations should be deferred until the vitreous has been removed.

Several techniques for vitrectomy are available. The standard weck-cel limbal vitrectomy may offer the benefit of simplicity, but at the cost of limited control, and has the significant disadvantage of pulling the vitreous away from the vitreous base, thereby increasing the risk for retinal tears and detachment. Additionally, vitreous is drawn toward the wound where it may further interfere with subsequent maneuvers such as IOL placement. If a vitreous strand is not detected, it may lead to traction around the pupil margin postoperatively, increasing the chance of cystoid macular edema from Irvine-Gass syndrome.[32]

The weck-cel anterior vitrectomy is also much more likely to enlarge the capsular break and compromise support for an implant. We find the weck-cel useful only for the diagnostic purpose of detecting whether or not vitreous is present at the wound margin, and recommend against this technique

when a therapeutic vitrectomy is indicated. Special efforts are taken not to pull on the vitreous. A Vannas scissors should always be available in the opposite hand to immediately cut any engaged vitreous if the surgeon chooses to check the wound and finds vitreous gel to be present.

Automated vitrectomy techniques with a specially designed cutter offer a much increased margin of safety over weck-cel vitrectomy. Most vitreous cutters designed for anterior segment machines have a coaxial irrigation sleeve. This irrigation sleeve, in fact, can hydrate the vitreous as the cutting occurs, increasing the vitreous volume to be removed and, simultaneously, repelling the vitreous that the surgeon desires to engage by the force of the irrigation stream. We prefer to use a bimanual vitrectomy approach in which the sleeve is slid off the vitrector shaft and the irrigation line is placed into the anterior chamber and directed away from the vitrectomy site, achieving a stable anterior chamber, a constant intraocular pressure, and preventing hydration of the vitreous. A 21-gauge butterfly cannula placed through the paracentesis stab incision serves well for this purpose. The cutting rate should be relatively high, while the irrigation, aspiration, and vacuum levels should be relatively low.

The vitrector device can be placed into the eye via the cataract tunnel wound or via a pars plana sclerotomy incision. While both methods can achieve vitrectomy with good control, the pars plana approach offers some notable potential advantages, despite its greater technical demands. When the vitrectomy is performed via the pars plana approach, the vitreous is being drawn out of the anterior chamber space, as desired, and puts less tension on the vitreous base, while a limbal approach pulls vitreous forward through the tear, creating more tension and increasing the chance of enlarging the tear. Additionally, the vitrector device is much less likely to disturb any of the anterior chamber structures if it is not being placed through the anterior chamber. A vitrectomy through the cataract incision also may distort the cornea, limiting the view and gaping the wound, particularly with clear corneal incisions. A recent article demonstrated that the pars plana approach is more successful in removing subincisional vitreous.[33]

The pars plana vitrectomy in this setting begins by removing all instruments from the anterior chamber and injection of either viscoelastic agent or balanced salt solution. A conjunctival relaxing incision is made to allow access to the sclera 3.0 mm behind the limbus, and cautery is applied. For a superior cataract incision, the 11:00 meridian provides more comfortable hand positioning than going directly behind the wound. When operating temporally, the pars plana incision may be located slightly inferotemporally. A sclerotomy is created with a 20-gauge microvitreoretinal blade and the tip is visualized through the pupil after it has passed through the sclera into the pupillary space. The vitrector handpiece (with the irrigation sleeve removed) is placed through the sclerotomy taking special care not to force it through the wound. The vitrector tip is placed a few millimeters behind the posterior

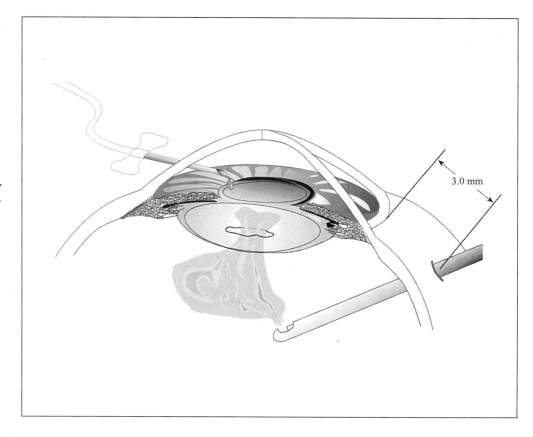

Figure 11-10. Anterior vitrectomy through a pars plana approach is achieved using a pars plana sclerotomy 3.0 mm posterior to the limbus with irrigation via a 21-gauge butterfly needle placed through the paracentesis. The vitreous is pulled away from the capsular opening by the vitreous cutter.

3.0 mm

capsular tear and the foot pedal is engaged, drawing the vitreous out from the tear (Figure 11-10). The handpiece should be held relatively still with only slow movements to change location. The edges of the capsule and other engaged anterior segment structures will wiggle with each cycle of the blade until the vitreous has been removed from the area. Once no anterior segment movement is detected and vitreous is no longer seen in the anterior segment, the vitrectomy is complete. The vitrector should be slowly removed and cutting performed at the scleral wall externally before the sclerotomy is closed with a 7-0 vicryl figure-of-eight suture.

A "dry" (no irrigation) vitrectomy is another useful technique when limited vitreous has extended through the capsular tear.[34] The anterior segment is filled with a viscoelastic agent to maintain the convexity and clarity of the cornea while tamponading the vitreous. The automated vitrector is advanced through the viscoelastic material into the capsular tear. Cutting is initiated, selectively removing the anterior vitreous behind the tear and severing the connecting base of the prolapsed strand. This technique minimizes the volume of the vitreous that is removed while precisely controlling the tear borders. The viscoelastic material maintains a stable anterior segment.

Once vitrectomy is complete, removal of remaining lens material can be achieved. As mentioned previously, the equatorial cortex should be removed first and the cortex around the tear should be stripped toward the tear so as not to increase the size of the opening.

Dropped Nucleus

Occasionally, when the posterior capsule has been violated, nuclear fragments remaining in the anterior segment may dislocate into the vitreous, especially if the infusion pressure has been at higher levels. If the fragments are suspended in the anterior vitreous, one may place some viscoelastic behind them for temporary support, then perform a limited bimanual vitrectomy to sever any engaged vitreous strands before pulling the fragments back into the anterior segment. The irrigation cannula can be used to support the pieces during vitrectomy. Manipulation of nuclear fragments which are entangled in vitreous gel may cause untoward traction on the vitreous base, perhaps resulting in retinal detachment or dialysis. If nuclear material dislocates posteriorly into the vitreous cavity, attempts to float the nucleus upward following a generous vitrectomy are sometimes successful. However, it may be best to temporarily ignore the lost nucleus, clean up the prolapsed vitreous, remove the cortex, and implant an intraocular lens. Retinal consultation for secondary removal of the lens material via a three-port pars plana vitrectomy with phacofragmentation can be scheduled in the early postoperative period. Heroic efforts to "catch" a falling nucleus or retrieve a fallen nucleus from the anterior segment approach have been associated with an increased risk of retinal complications and poorer ultimate visual outcomes.[35]

Placement of an intraocular lens implant may be undertaken, unless the fragment is large and hard, making pars plana phacofragmentation less likely to be successful and

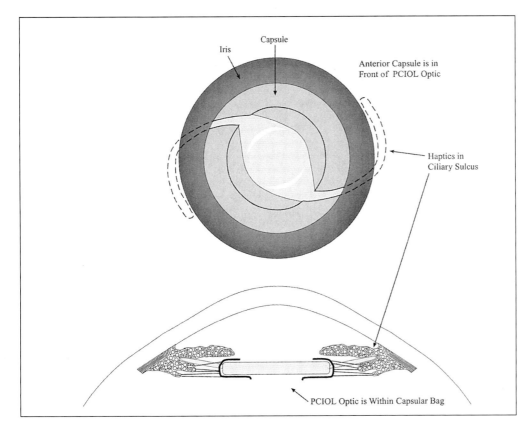

Iris

Capsule

Anterior Capsule is in
Front of PCIOL Optic

Haptics in
Ciliary Sulcus

PCIOL Optic is Within Capsular Bag

Figure 11-11. In cases where sulcus fixation of the intraocular lens haptics is required, the lens optic can be prolapsed through an intact capsulorhexis to achieve a posterior capture, providing additional stability and centration to the posterior chamber implant.

necessitating lens removal via a limbal incision, perhaps with the aid of a liquid perfluorocarbon. The cataract surgeon should understand his retinal specialist's philosophy concerning IOL placement prior to proceeding with lens implantation. If the eye is left aphakic, the anterior segment surgeon may accompany the vitreoretinal specialist to the operating room for secondary intraocular lens implantation.

Intraocular Lens Implantation

Stable and lasting placement of a posterior chamber implant in the presence of a capsular tear requires clear visualization of the capsulozonular anatomy. After viscoelastic material is instilled, a collar button or Kuglen hook can be used to retract the iris and to explore the remaining capsular support. The most desirable location and orientation of the lens should become evident.

A small posterior capsule tear may be converted into a posterior capsulorhexis, decreasing the chance of extension during IOL implantation. With a small tear, particularly if a posterior capsulorhexis has been achieved, in-the-bag implantation of an IOL can be accomplished. Dialing maneuvers may exert undue stress on the capsular bag and extend the tear. A trailing haptic compression maneuver or use of a foldable implant lens that unfolds slowly may be more gentle to the remaining capsular support structures. If the capsular tear is larger, sulcus fixation of a PC-IOL can be achieved. Viscoelastic material placed between the iris and anterior capsulorhexis facilitates implantation. The IOL power should be

reduced by 0.5 diopters from the capsular bag calculation.[36]

When the anterior capsulorhexis is intact and its diameter is less than that of the IOL optic, the haptics can be placed in the sulcus and the optic can be prolapsed posteriorly into the capsular bag (Figure 11-11). This maneuver increases support, facilitates centration, and helps to prevent pupillary capture. When this maneuver is planned, the capsular bag calculation of implant power should be used.

When capsular support for a posterior chamber implant is not adequate, several options are available. An IOL can be sutured into the ciliary sulcus using either one or two scleral fixation sutures,[37] the implant can be affixed to the peripheral iris with McCannel sutures,[38] or, in elderly patients with no other anterior segment or angle pathology, anterior chamber implants may be utilized. A prophylactic peripheral iridotomy should be performed to prevent iris bomb and pupillary block.

COMPLICATIONS RELATED TO INTRAOCULAR LENS IMPLANTATION

Several problems may occur in the process of implanting the intraocular lens. These complications may be related to the IOL haptic, the optic, the implanting forceps, or the lens injector devices. Generally, polymethylmethacrylate (PMMA) lenses are easier to implant. The most common complication is breakage of the trailing haptic during IOL placement. If this occurs the implant is removed and exchanged for another, similar lens.

Foldable intraocular lenses can present some unique challenges. Occasionally, the haptic of a three-piece implant lens can become bent during the insertion process, which can occur with either forceps implantation or injector systems. If a severe kink is noted after implantation, or worse, a haptic breaks, late decentration of the implant is possible with capsular fibrosis, despite adequate centering at the time of surgery. Therefore, these lenses should be exchanged immediately. Lens exchange may also be necessary if the lens optic is damaged by the injector device, or if cracks develop in the central optic of an acrylic lens.[39]

Lens exchange, however, presents a special problem when the optic is larger than the wound. There are several ways to overcome this problem. One approach is to enlarge the wound. However doing so carries the disadvantage of compromising the initial wound architecture and self-sealing nature. The surgeon can remove the implant from the initial wound by bisecting it and removing it in two pieces, accomplished by suspending the optic in the mid anterior chamber with a viscoelastic agent and cutting the optic in half with long Vannas-style scissors.[40]

The foldable lenses, however, tend to be slippery and may tend to escape the jaws of the scissors, much like pinching a watermelon seed; a sideport instrument or a forceps may be required for additional stabilization. A snare device has recently been introduced to split the lens with a wire loop, thereby avoiding this difficulty. Alternatively, the lens optic can be cut at least half way across and, if the surgeon grabs the haptic, the optic will usually deform through the wound and exit the eye in one piece.[41] An acrylic implant can be folded within the anterior chamber over a spatula introduced via a separate paracentesis located 180° opposite the incision, then explanted intact.[42]

If a foldable lens is inadvertently inserted upside-down, the anterior chamber can be filled with viscoelastic material and the lens somersaulted into proper orientation.[43]

While implanting the IOL, the leading haptic, the lens forceps, or the lens injector may catch on the edge of Descemet's membrane causing detachment. Therefore, special care should be taken. Trying to force an IOL through too small an incision increases this risk.

Placement of a plate-haptic silicone IOL in the presence of a capsular tear is contraindicated, as there is a tendency for these lenses to dislocate into the vitreous cavity.

ZONULAR DIALYSIS

Zonular dialysis may be present prior to surgery as a result of either trauma or in association with one of several specific disorders such as Marfan Syndrome, Weil-Marchesani Syndrome, or homocystinuria. Phacodonesis, iridodonesis, vitreous in the anterior chamber, or visibility of the lens equator may provide important clues to zonular instability. Exfoliation syndrome also results in weakened zonules.[44]

When a known zonular dialysis exists preoperatively, the surgeon should attempt to place the incision so that it will not be necessary to cross over the area of zonular dehiscence with the phacoemulsification tip. Although the capsulorhexis may be more difficult when loose zonules are present, a slow-motion technique assisted by viscocleavage and a fractioning technique will usually allow safe removal of the nucleus. Occasionally, the capsular bag can be locally stabilized in the meridian of dehiscence by placing flexible iris retractors around the capsulorhexis margin.

Of course, zonular dialysis also occurs from intraocular manipulations during surgery. Prompt recognition and avoidance of further trauma is the best initial management. A highly retentive viscoelastic agent may tamponade the hyaloid face, helping to prevent vitreous prolapse into the anterior chamber. As mentioned previously, a low bottle height will limit the tendency towards vitreous overhydration. Low aspiration settings may help prevent chamber fluctuations, vitreous prolapse, and unintentional traction on the remaining zonules. When zonular dialysis is present, cortical aspiration should be performed by either a dry technique or gentle irrigation and aspiration, directing all forces tangentially to help prevent "unzipping" of the remaining zonules. An endocapsular ring is a remarkable device to keep the capsular bag open and evenly distribute the forces on the zonules, making implantation of an intraocular lens into the capsular bag possible.[45]

When placing a lens into the capsular bag, there is some debate regarding the optimal orientation of the IOL haptics with some surgeons advocating parallel to the dialysis, while others prefer perpendicular to the dialysis. Orientation is not a concern if an endocapsular ring has been placed. Once positioned, the lens should be gently moved in each direction to assure that centration is secure. In cases where sulcus fixation is chosen, the haptics should be oriented as far from the dialysis as possible. Prolapse of the optic into the capsular bag provides additional support.

When the zonular dialysis is large, alternative methods of IOL fixation should be considered.

SUPRACHOROIDAL HEMORRHAGE

Suprachoroidal hemorrhage is a dreaded complication for all ophthalmic surgeons. Several risk factors for suprachoroidal hemorrhage are known, including advanced age, systolic hypertension, atherosclerosis, intraoperative tachycardia, anticoagulation, uveitis, glaucoma, and axial myopia.[46-48]

The risk of suprachoroidal hemorrhage may be reduced by altering the use of anticoagulants in the preoperative period. However this reduction in risk should be carefully weighed against the possible medical consequences of discontinuing the aspirin or coumadin. Intraoperatively, systolic hypertension and tachycardia should be carefully watched for and managed.

When choroidal hemorrhage does occur, prompt diagnosis may prevent disastrous consequences. Warning signs include unexplained shallowing of the anterior chamber, a disturbance in the red reflex, or positive pressure. If suprachoroidal hemorrhage is suspected, all instruments should be removed from the eye immediately. The self-sealing cataract incision adds a great deal of control to this potentially devastating condition. Viscoelastic agents or balanced salt solution instilled through a paracentesis will help tamponade the bleed. If the incision is not self-sealing, the gloved index finger should immediately be placed over the wound and pressure applied.[49]

Intravenous mannitol will shrink the vitreous volume and decrease a markedly elevated intraocular pressure, although there is some disagreement about its use since a dehydrated vitreous, in theory, promotes bleeding. When the wound is self-sealing, indirect ophthalmoscopy can be performed, provided the media are clear. Other viewing lenses have been developed, allowing the surgeon to view the fundus through the operating microscope.[50]

Further attempts of any anterior segment maneuvers (or release of the digital pressure if a finger secures the wound) should be delayed for at least fifteen minutes to give the hemorrhage a chance to clot. If inspection at that time reveals a lack of progression of a focal choroidal hemorrhage, one of us (RHO) has reported draining the hemorrhage through a sclerotomy performed 3.5-4.0 mm behind the limbus. Next, the cortex can be removed with a 27-gauge cannula through two paracenteses, then implanting a foldable lens through an unenlarged incision. Enlarging any incision in the face of a suprachoroidal hemorrhage is not recommended. Traditionally, if the anterior chamber is too shallow or the tension is too high, medical therapy should be initiated and completion of the surgery should be deferred to a later time.

CONCLUSIONS

Cataract surgery is a safe and elegant procedure, yet complications will be occasionally encountered by every cataract surgeon. We hope that the above discussions will help the reader in prevention, early identification, and successful management of intraoperative complications that may occur during cataract surgery.

REFERENCES

1. Gills JP: Ophthalmic anesthesia update: intracameral xylocaine. *Video J Cataract Refract Surg* 1996;12(4).
2. Osher R: Thermal Burns. *Video J Cataract Refract Surg* 1993; 9(3).
3. Osher R: New suturing techniques. *Audiovisual J Cataract Implant Surg* 1990; 6(3).
4. Mackool RJ, Holtz SJ: Descemet membrane detachment. *Arch Ophthalmol* 1977; 95(3):459-63.
5. Walland MJ, Stevens JD, Arther D: Repair of Descemet's membrane detachment after intraocular surgery. *J Cataract Refract Surg* 1995; 21(3):250.
6. Ellis DR, Cohen KL: Sulfur hexaflouride gas in the repair of

Descemet's membrane detachment. *Cornea* 1995; 14(4):436-7.
7. Assia EI, Levkovich-Verbin H, Blumenthal M: Management of Descemet's membrane detachment. *J Cataract Refract Surg* 1995; 21(6):714-7.
8. Minkovitz JB, Schrenck LC, Pepose JS: Spontaneous reattachment of an extensive Descemet's detachment. *Arch Ophthalmol* 1994; 112:551-52.
9. Wachler BB, Krueger RR: *American Journal of Ophthalmology* 1996; 122(1):109-10.
10. Kaufman SC, Insler MS: *Ophthalmic Surgery and Lasers* 1996; 27(11):963-6.
11. Brauweiler P: Bimanual irrigation/aspiration. *J Cataract Refract Surg* 1996; 22(8):1013-6.
12. Updegraff SA, Peyman GA, McDonald MB: Pupillary block during cataract surgery. *Am J Ophthalmol* 1994;117(3):328-32.
13. Davison JA: Capsular bag distension after endophacoemulsification and posterior chamber intraocular lens placement. *J Cataract Refract Surg* 1990; 16:99-108.
14. Holtz SJ: Post-operative capsular bag distension. *J Cataract Refract Surg* 1992; 18:310-17.
15. Nishi O, Nishi K: Intraocular lens encapsulation by shrinkage of the capsulorhexis opening. *J Cataract Refract Surg* 1993; 19(7):544-45.
16. Davison JA: Capsule contraction syndrome. *J Cataract Refract Surg* 1993;19(5):582-9.
17. Masket S: Postoperative complications of capsulorhexis. *J Cataract Refract Surg* 1993;19(6):721-4.
18. Hayashi K, Mayashi H, et al: Reduction in the area of the anterior capsular opening after polymethylmethacrylate, silicone, and soft acrylic intraocular lens implantation. *Am J Ophthalmol* 1997; 123(4):441-47.
19. Ota I, Miyake S, Miyake K: Dislocation of the lens nucleus into the vitreous cavity after standard hydrodissection. *Am J Ophthalmol* 1996; 121(6):706-8.
20. Drews R: Posterior capsular rupture: hydrodissection. *Video J Cataract Refract Surg* 1996; 12(2).
21. Osher R, Yu B, Koch D: Posterior polar cataracts: A predisposition to intraoperative posterior capsular rupture. *J Cataract Refract Surg* 1990; 16:157-162.
22. Shepard DM: The pupil stretch technique for miotic pupils in cataract surgery. *Ophthalmic Surgery* 1993; 24(12):851-2.
23. Miller KM, Keener GT Jr.: Stretch pupilloplasty for small pupil phacoemulsification *Am J Ophthalmol* 1994; 117(1):107-8.
24. McCuen BW 2d, Hickenbotham D, Tsai M, deJuan E Jr.: Temporary iris fixation with a micro-iris retractor. *Archives of Ophthalmology* 1989; 107(6):925-7.
25. Masket S: Avoiding complications associated with iris retractor use in small pupil cataract extraction. *J Cataract Refract Surg* 1996; 22(2):168-71.
26. Graether pupil expander for managing the small pupil during surgery. *J Cataract Refract Surg* 1996; 22(5):530-5.
27. Jaffe N: *Cataract Surgery and its Complications*, 3rd ed. St. Louis, CV Mosby, 1981, pp 368, 576-79.
28. Osher R, Cionni R: The torn posterior capsule: its intraoperative behavior, surgical management, and long term consequences. *J Cataract Refract Surg* 1990; 16(4):490-4.
29. Ross W: Management of dislocated lens fragments after pha-

coemulsification surgery. *Can J Ophthalmol* 1996; 31(5)234-40.

30. Kelman C: Posterior capsular rupture: PAL technique. *Video J Cataract Refract Surg* 1996; 12(2).

31. Castenada V, Tegler U, Tsai J, et al: Posterior curvilinear capsulorhexis. *Ophthalmology* 1992; 99(1):45.

32. Steinert RF, Wasson PJ: Neodymium:YAG laser anterior vitreolysis for Irvine-Gass cystoid macular edema. *J Cataract Refract Surg* 1989; 15(3):304-7.

33. Eller AW, Barad RF: Miyake analysis of anterior vitrectomy techniques. *J Cataract Refract Surg* 1996; 22(2):213-7.

34. Osher R: Dry vitrectomy. *Audiovisual J Cataract Refract Surg* 1992; 8(4).

35. Lambrow F, Stewart M: Management of dislocated lens fragments during phacoemulsification. *Ophthalmol* 1992; 99(8):1260-62.

36. Osher R, Corcoran K: presented at Cataract Congress, Houston, 1986.

37. Lane S, Lewis J, et al: New techniques for scleral fixation. *Video J Cataract Refract Surg* 1995; 11(2).

38. Panton RW, Salewski ME, Parker JS, et al: Surgical management of subluxed posterior-chamber intraocular lenses. *Arch Ophthalmol* 1993; 111(7):919-26.

39. Pfister DR: Stress fractures after folding an acrylic intraocular lens. *Am J Ophthalmol* 1996;121(5):572-4.

40. Koo EY, Lindsey PS, et al: Bisecting a foldable acrylic intraocular lens for explantation. *J Cataract Refract Surg* 1996; 22(suppl)2:1381-82.

41. Batlan SJ, Dodick JM: Explantation of a foldable silicone intraocular lens. *Am J Ophthalmol* 1996; 122(2):270-2.

42. Ernst P: Intraocular refolding. *Video J Cataract Refract Surg* 1996; 12(4).

43. McAuliffe K: Intraoperative IOL complications: Backwards. *Video J Cataract Refract Surg* 1993; 9(3).

44. Osher R: Pseudoexfoliation. *Audiovisual J Cataract Implant Surg* 1988; 4(4).

45. Cionni RJ, Osher RH: Endocapsular ring approach to the subluxed cataractous lens. *J Cataract Refract Surg* 1995; 21(3):245-9.

46. Arnold PN: Study of acute intraoperative suprachoroidal hemorrhage. *J Cataract Refract Surg* 1992; 18(5):489-99.

47. Price FW Jr., Whitson WE: Suprachoroidal hemorrhage in penetrating keratoplasty. *Ophthalmic Surg* 1994; 25(8):521-25.

48. Speaker M, Gueirleio P, Riet J, et al: A case controlled study of risk factors for intraoperative suprachoroidal expulsive hemorrhage. *Ophthalmol* 1991; 98:202-210.

49. Osher M: Emergency treatment of vitreous bulge and wound gaping complicating cataract surgery. *Am J Ophthalmol* 1957; 44:409-11.

50. Osher R: New Approaches to the management of threatened expulsive hemorrhage. Presented at the American Society of Cataract and Refractive Surgery Meeting, Seattle, WA, May, 1993.

CURRENT IOL MATERIALS AND TECHNOLOGY

Johnny L. Gayton, MD, Robert G. Martin, MD, Akef El-Maghraby, MD

Ocular surgical techniques and the technologies supporting them are enmeshed together in a movement toward efficacious, yet minimally disruptive, surgical interventions. Because intraocular lens development and cataract surgical techniques are inextricably bound together, surgeons have historically worked closely with the IOL industry.

In the past decade and a half, surgical advancements have led to a minimally invasive procedure involving very small, sutureless incisions at clear cornea. This type of surgical technique could only have been possible with the concurrent development of foldable lens technology. There are only two types of materials used in foldable lenses currently available in the United States, acrylic and silicone. In Europe, a hydrogel material is under testing, and a new material composed of a collagen copolymer, collamer, is being tested in the U.S.

The only acrylic lens now available in the U.S. is the Alcon AcrySof three-piece lens. It has a 6-mm optic composed of a random copolymer of phenylethyl acrylate and phenylethyl methacrylate that is cross-linked with butanediol diacrylate. A bondable benzotriazole derivative is incorporated for UV absorption. The high refractive index of 1.55 allows for a thin optic design.

The thermomechanical properties of the acrylic material result in a hard material at room temperature, and a soft, bendable material at somewhat higher temperatures. The IOL can be stored dry, heated in a warm BSS bath to fold, and then inserted with forceps. At the intraocular temperature of 37° C, the material behaves as a semi-elastic material. After insertion, the folded IOL will slowly unfold to its former shape.

Silicone lenses are available both as a three-piece IOL or as a single-piece plate-haptic IOL. Both are made of RMX-3 silicone elastomer, which has been in clinical use since mid-1986. The RMX-3 material has an index of refraction of 1.41. It can be cast molded, avoiding manufacturing residues, and is autoclavable.

STAAR Surgical's three-piece silicone lens is the Elastimide, available either in modified-J or modified-C loop configurations. The haptics are formed by photo-etching, and thus are not subject to haptic relaxation. The 12.5-mm Elastimide lens has a 6-mm biconvex optic.

The STAAR plate lens, the AA-4203, is 10.5-mm in length and can be implanted using an injector system. Newer, slimmer models of injectors allow this lens to be inserted through incisions as small as 2.6 mm. The AA-4203F has larger positioning holes for faster fibrosis within the capsule to quicken fixation. Both lenses are available with a UV filter.

The plate lens can only be implanted in the presence of an intact capsulorhexis, with no capsular tears. The bulky 6-mm optic fills the bag completely, and with the planar haptics fixates stably in the capsule. Because these lenses completely fill the bag, plate-haptic IOLs exhibit less posterior capsule opacification.

ACRYLIC AND SILICONE—SIDE BY SIDE COMPARISONS

Preference for acrylic versus silicone is largely surgeon dependent. There are many factors involved in choosing between the lenses, including cost, handling characteristics, ease of implantation, or marketing information. The only way to tell if there are actual clinical differences is to perform a side by side comparison in a comparative study.

Martin Study

We performed a randomized, prospective study of the AcrySof lens versus the STAAR AA-4203F silicone plate lens. Planned enrollment was 100 uncomplicated phacoemulsification cases. Patients were excluded if they experienced a ruptured or torn posterior capsule, or if surgical complications occurred.

Figure 12-1. Clinical assessment of inflammation in a randomized, prospective study comparing the Alcon Acrysof acrylic 3-piece lens with the Staar AA-4203F plate-haptic silicone lens (Martin). (A) Flare. (B) Cells.

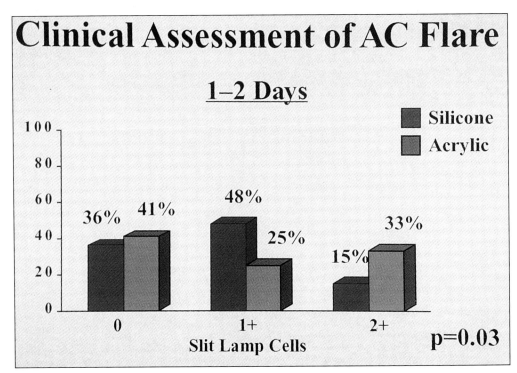

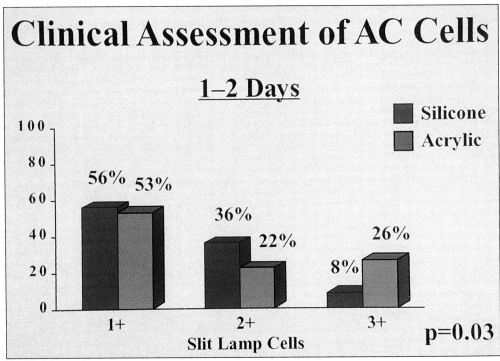

Actual enrollment was 103 patients, 52 receiving silicone and 51 receiving acrylic. Eighty-one percent of the silicone group and 69% of the acrylic group were female. Mean age in both groups was 70.5. Seventy percent of cases have been followed at least 5 weeks.

Figures 12-1 A&B show distribution of early postoperative inflammation. At one to two days after surgery, the acrylic group had a larger proportion of eyes graded as 3+ cells and a larger proportion with 2+ flare. The differences were 2-fold for flare and 3-fold for cells. These differences were statistically significant.

Differences in inflammation were probably due to the significantly ($p < 0.001$) longer operative time for acrylic cases. Silicone cases took an average 5.6 minutes of operative time while acrylic took an average 7.6 minutes, or 36% longer. The difference is attributable to the more difficult insertion of

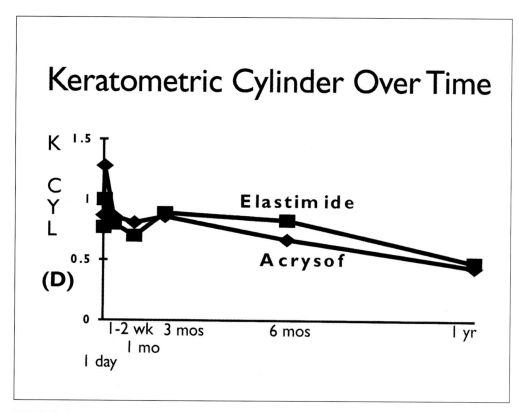

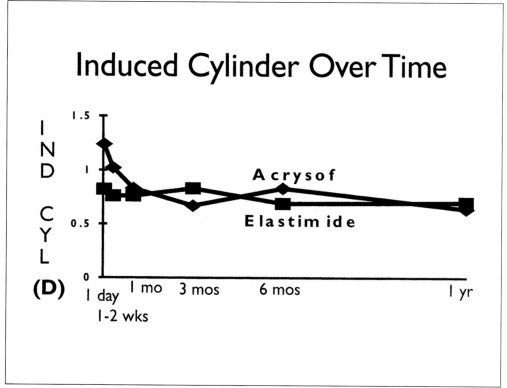

Figure 12-2. Astigmatism results in a bilateral, randomized, prospective study comparing the Alcon Acrysof acrylic 3-piece lens with the Staar Elastimide 3-piece silicone lens (Gayton). (A) Mean keratometric cylinder over time. (B) Induced cylinder over time.

AcrySof lenses compared to the STAAR plate-haptic lens. The incisions for the acrylic lenses were also a full millimeter longer at 3.75 mm compared to 2.65 mm for the silicone. This larger incision size could contribute to inflammation.

Table 12-1 shows the three to five week endothelial cell assessment. There were no significant differences in endothelial cell density, average cell size, or in other measures of endothelial health.

Figure 12-3. Best-corrected visual acuity results comparing the Elastimide eye with the Acrysof eye in each patient (Gayton). (A) One to two weeks postoperatively. (B) One month postoperatively.

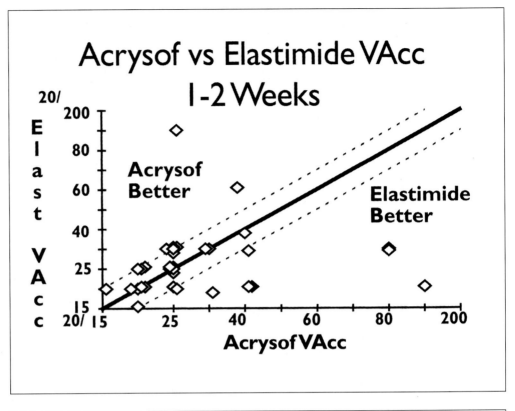

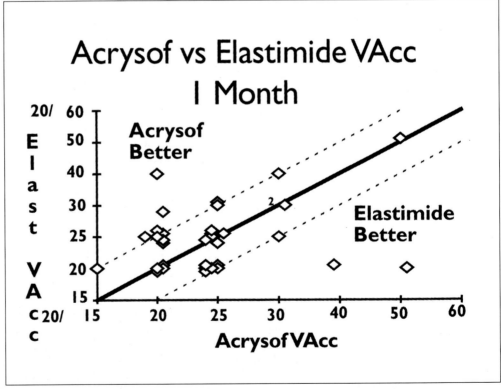

Gayton Study

We are conducting a randomized, bilateral comparison of the Alcon 3-piece Acrysof lens with the Staar 3-piece Elastimide lens. We intend to look at differences in astigmatism, visual performance, capsular opacity and YAG rates, and complications. One hundred bilateral patients will be enrolled. To ensure a fair comparison, patients with preoper-

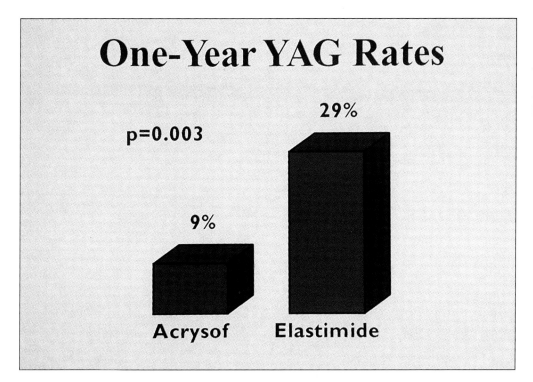

Figure 12-4. One-year results in a retrospective, matched study comparing YAG rates in Acrysof patients and Elastimide patients (Gayton).

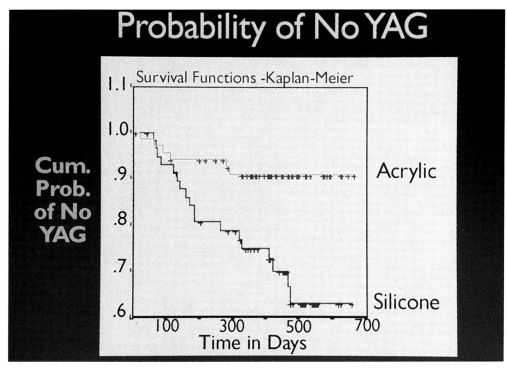

Figure 12-5. Life table survival curves in a retrospective, matched study comparing YAG rates in Acrysof patients and Elastimide patients. The curves demonstrate the cumulative probability of not having a YAG capsulotomy over time, and are statistically significantly different (p<0.005) between groups (Gayton).

ative pathology that could limit best-corrected acuity were not eligible. We currently have 38 patients with both eyes enrolled and at least 1 month data.

Figures 12-2 A&B show astigmatism results. We found no differences in either net astigmatism or surgically induced astigmatism between the two groups.

Figures 12-3 A&B show corrected acuity in the AcrySof

versus the Elastimide eyes. At one to two weeks, we found some patients with dramatically worse vision in one eye, usually the Acrysof eye. These differences were due to edema. There were four cases of edema in Acrysof eyes and one in Elastimide eyes. This difference in edema was most likely due to the more traumatic insertion of AcrySof lenses. By one month, the edema has resolved and almost all eyes are with-

TABLE 12-1

MEAN ENDOTHELIAL CELL DENSITY AT 3 TO 5 WEEKS POSTOPERATIVE

	Silicone Plate Mean (Standard Deviation)	Acrylic Three-Piece Mean (Standard Deviation)
Postoperative cell density	2081 (480)	2190 (357)
Postoperative cell size	492 (136)	467 (81)
Mean postoperative % hexagonal cells	54% (12.1%)	52% (11.1%)
Mean postoperative coefficient of variation	38 (7.1)	38 (9.0)

in one Snellen line of their fellow eye. The few cases with vision worse than 20/40 are due to macular changes not diagnosed preoperatively.

Although it is too early in this study to determine differential YAG rates, we are conducting a retrospective study to evaluate one-year rates. We collected a series of 100 consecutive Elastimide cases and matched them to 100 Acrysof cases by age, sex and date of surgery. Clinical data are being collected from charts, while the capsule status is determined from charts as well as phone interviews.

In the 132 cases already assessed (63 Elastimide and 69 Acrysof), the follow-up in the two groups was comparable, with a mean follow-up of 430 days in the Elastimide group and 436 in the AcrySof group. The one year YAG rates were highly statistically significantly different (p=0.003). The Elastimide group had a three-fold higher YAG rate, with 29% of cases receiving a YAG capsulotomy compared to 9% of AcrySof cases (Figure 12-4).

We used a life table statistical technique to verify this result. This method adjusts for individual differences in patient follow-up time. The probability of not having a YAG capsulotomy is plotted over time for each group in Figure 12-5. The probability of *not* having a YAG for the AcrySof group is 91% by a year and stays steady thereafter. For the Elastimide group the probability of not having a YAG decreases steadily and at a year is about 72%. The survival curves are significantly different between the groups (P<0.005). The groups also differ in the amount of time between surgery and YAG. The mean time to YAG is 141 days for the AcrySof group and 224 days for the Elastimide group.

COLLAMER™

The collamer material made by STAAR is a highly biocompatible and permeable collagen copolymer. The material is extremely hydrophilic, containing 30 to 35% water. The hydrophilic nature of a lens material is important because hydrophobic materials such as PMMA and silicone can increase the cellular response, or metaplasia, of lens epithelial cells at the capsular rim which can migrate from the anterior capsule to the posterior capsule. Proliferation of the cells can lead to Elschnig pearl clusters or fibrosis, leading to posterior capsule opacification.

The material has an excellent memory, allowing the lens to resume its original shape completely, making the lens very stable in the eye. The material has superb optical resolution capabilities, being clearer than silicone, and 98 to 99% transmissible. The resolving power of the material almost reaches theoretical limits.

The STAAR Surgical Collamer™ lens model CC-4203VF has completed Phase I of the FDA approval process, with 125 patients enrolled. Fifty-one of those patients have completed their 4 to 6 month evaluation. All 51 patients achieved 20/40 or better corrected visual acuity. Postoperative complications in this group were rare, with no corneal edema or macular reported at 4 to 6 months, and one case of iritis in a Fuch's dystrophy patient. Only three patients (5.9%) had a YAG capsulotomy performed.

SUMMARY

The Gayton study suggests that acrylic lenses have substantially lower YAG rates than silicone lenses of similar design, probably due to the more hydrophilic nature of acrylic. This advantage must be balanced against other concerns, such as ease of insertion and handling characteristics, which are often the deciding factor in choosing a lens.

NEW OPTICS

James P. Gills, MD, Harry Grabow, MD, Felix K. Jacobi, MD

After posterior chamber intraocular lenses were re-introduced as a viable technique in the late seventies, advances in IOL technology revolved around optimizing the overall design of the PMMA implants. Parameters evaluated and improved included better haptic material and configuration (toward flexible loop designs suited for bag fixation), sizing of the entire IOL (for better fixation and centration within the capsular bag), and optic configuration (biconvex vs. planoconvex which also impacts on posterior capsule opacification). The focus was to produce IOLs which were more safely and easily fixated entirely within the capsular bag with minimal risk of decentration, dislocation, or disruption of the posterior capsule.

By the early eighties, posterior-chamber IOLs were documented as very safe and efficacious. IOL removals were relatively rare and exchanges were mainly to remedy power errors or to reposition IOLs if surgical errors occurred.[1-3] Clinical studies during that time also helped clarify the role of IOL design in the etiology of posterior capsule opacification. One-piece IOLs are thought to produce lower rates of Nd:YAG capsulotomy.[1,2,4,5]

The next wave of advances in IOL technology was the introduction of compressible IOL materials discussed in Chapter 12. Current innovation in IOL technology revolves around the development of the IOL optic to increase the efficiency of the optic and to increase control over the final refraction. This chapter will summarize three innovations in optic design which have just been made available or which will soon be available: multifocal IOLs, minus-power IOLs, and toric IOLs.

MULTIFOCAL LENSES

Multifocal lenses have been under study for some time, but none has yet made it to the U.S. market. Currently one multifocal lens has made application to the U.S. FDA, and may be available soon.

The AMO® Array®

Allergan has developed a zonal progressive refractive multifocal intraocular lens called the AMO® Array®. The AMO Array is designed to provide functionally useful pseudo-accommodation, that is, to mimic a broad range of images at distance, intermediate and near.

The anterior surface curvature of the AMO Array is continual, and varies to refract light to distance, intermediate and near foci. The multifocal area within the central 4.7 mm diameter of the optic is comprised of alternated distance and near dominant zones. All zones are aspherized: the first zone, 2.1 mm diameter, is more distance dominant (i.e. more light is refracted to the distance focus and the rest to intermediate); the second zone, 2.1 - 3.4 mm, is more near dominant; the third zone, 3.4 - 3.9 mm, is primarily distance power; the fourth zone, 3.9 - 4.6 mm, is primarily near power; and the fifth narrow annular zone, 4.6 to 4.7 mm, is the transitional zone to a spherical periphery, and provides dioptric power for distance. Near zones provide 3.5 D add for near vision. Repeatable distribution of dioptric power for distance, intermediate and near foci is designed to maintain image quality and pseudoaccommodation in the presence of pupil size variation (Figure 13-1).

The surface aspherization of the AMO Array is such that approximately 50% of the available light is allocated to distance focus, which is similar to the transmittance of a normal crystalline lens of a 50+ year old person, for distance dominant performance. In this design, approximately 36% of light is allocated to near, and approximately 64% of the remaining light is allocated for the intermediate foci. Thus all available light is theoretically utilized. Distant dominant zones, particularly the first zone, are designed to provide adequate depth of focus around distance images.

Figure 13-1. Schematic drawing of the AMO® Array® multifocal optic.

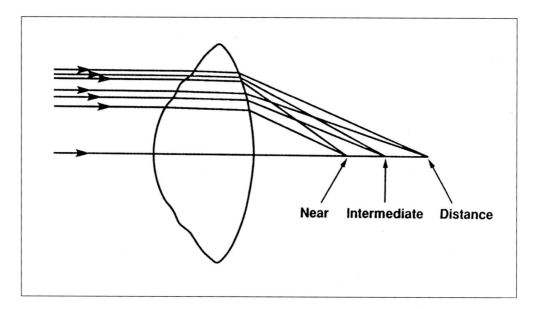

Figure 13-2. Picture of the three-piece second generation foldable silicone AMO® Array® model SA40N.

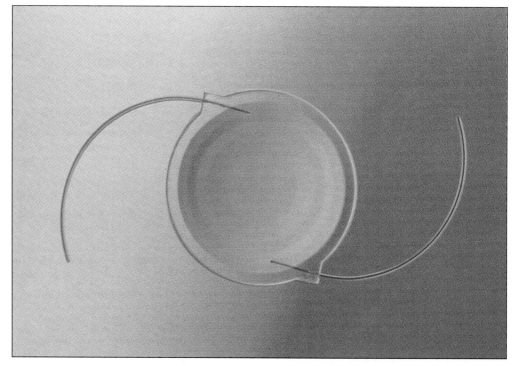

Lens Models

Four models of the AMO Array multifocal IOL have been studied; none of these models is approved for use in the United States at this time. Only the single-piece PMMA model PA154N and the three-piece second generation foldable silicone model SA40N (Figure 13-2) are marketed elsewhere.

Two single-piece models were developed: 1) the MPC25NB was a single-piece PMMA lens; 6.5 mm optic diameter with an overall diameter of 14.0 mm; J configuration, 10° angulated haptics, and 2) the PA154N is a single-piece PMMA lens; 6.0 mm optic diameter with an overall diameter of 12.5 mm; modified C configured, 5° angulated haptics.

Two three-piece silicone models were developed: 1) the SSM26NB was made from AMO SLM-1/UV® first generation silicone material; 6.0 mm optic diameter with an overall diameter of 13.0 mm; short C configured, 10° angulated polypropylene haptics; and center thickness from 1.32 mm for a 16 diopter lens up to 1.84 mm for a 24 D lens, and 2) the SA40N is made from AMO SLM2-UV® second generation silicone material; has a 6.0 mm optic diameter with an overall diameter of 13.0 mm; has short C configured, 10° angulated extruded PMMA monofilament haptics; and has a constant center thickness (0.9 mm for a 16 D lens to 1.0 mm for a 24 D lens) similar to that of the AMO PhacoFlex II® silicone monofocal IOLs model SI40NB.

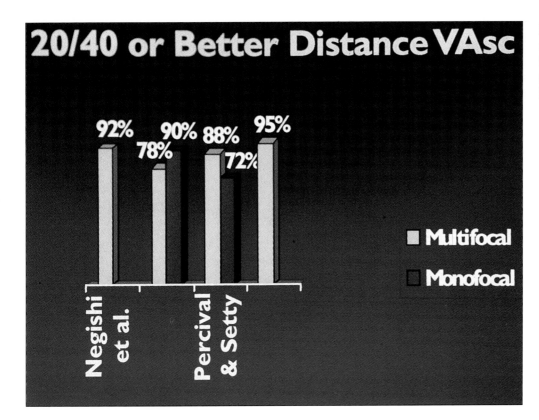

Figure 13-3. Various reported uncorrected distance acuities, percent of cases achieving 20/40 or better.

Results of the AMO Array

Unilateral Implantation

Distance Acuity

In a clinical evaluation of the MPC25NB, Negishi et al. reported that 91.9% of patients with less than 1.5 D of preoperative astigmatism achieved an uncorrected distance visual acuity of 20/40 or better three months after surgery.[6] In a previous study of the same lens, Negishi et al. reported that 69.2% of patients achieved an uncorrected distance visual acuity of 20/25 or better three months postoperatively.[7] Jacobi and Konen conducted a clinical evaluation using this lens and reported a mean uncorrected distance visual acuity of 20/32 twelve months postoperatively.[8]

In two comparative studies, Steinert et al. and Percival and Setty reported excellent postoperative results for patients implanted with this lens. Steinert et al. reported 78% of multifocal patients versus 90% of monofocal patients achieved 20/40 through three to six months.[9] Patients not achieving 20/40 had cylinder greater than 1 D and/or posterior capsular haze. Percival and Setty[10] reported that 88% of patients achieved an uncorrected distance visual acuity of 20/40 or better through four months postoperatively versus 72% for the monofocal control group.

Shoji and Shimizu reported that 95.2% of patients implanted with the SSM26NB achieved an uncorrected distance visual acuity of 20/40 or better ten months after surgery.[11] Schmidt et al.[12] reported a mean uncorrected distance visual acuity of 20/31 twelve months after surgery (Figure 13-3).

Several studies have demonstrated excellent corrected distance visual acuity. Negishi et al. reported that 97.8% of patients achieved a final best corrected distance visual acuity of 20/40 or better three months after surgery; 91.1% achieved 20/20 or better.[6] Negishi et al. also reported that 100% of patients achieved a final best corrected distance visual acuity of 20/20 of better through three months postoperative follow-up in an earlier study.[7] Jacobi and Konen reported that 75% of patients achieved a mean corrected distance visual acuity of 20/20 twelve months postoperatively.[8]

In a prospective randomized study of the MPC25NB versus a monofocal control group, Steinert et al. reported that 100% of both the multifocal and monofocal group achieved 20/40 or better corrected distance visual acuity at the three to six months postoperative follow-up visit.[9] Percival and Setty reported similar results; 100% of the multifocal and monofocal groups achieved a corrected distance visual acuity of 20/40 or better.[10]

Shoji and Shimizu[12] reported that 100% of patients achieved a corrected distance visual acuity of 20/40 or better at ten months; 88.1% 20/20 or better.[11] Schmidt et al. reported a mean corrected distance visual acuity of 20/20 twelve months after surgery (Figure 13-4).

Near Acuity

Negishi et al. reported that 62.2% of patients achieved an uncorrected near visual acuity of J3 or better through three months postoperative follow-up.[6] Jacobi and Konen reported a mean uncorrected near visual acuity of 20/40 twelve months postoperatively.[8]

Figure 13-4. Various reported best-corrected distance acuities, percent of cases achieving 20/20 or better.

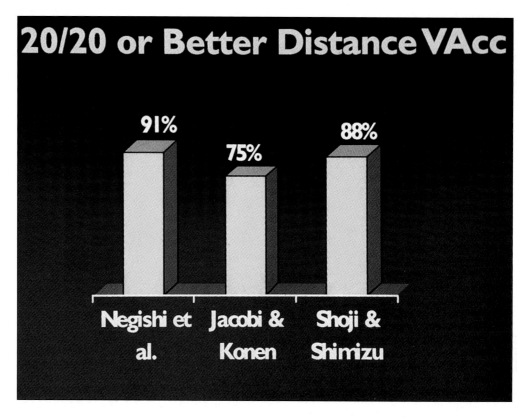

Steinert et al. reported a mean uncorrected near visual acuity of J3 for the multifocal patient group versus J7 for the monofocal control. This difference was statistically significant (p<0.0001).[9] Percival and Setty reported that 80% of the multifocal group versus 60% of the monofocal group achieved an uncorrected near visual acuity of J3 or better.[10]

Shoji and Shimizu[11] reported that 64.2% of patients achieved an uncorrected near visual acuity of J3 or better ten months after surgery (Figure 13-5).

Negishi et al. reported that 93.4% of patients achieved a distance corrected near visual acuity of J2 or better with additional add in place.[6] Jacobi and Konen reported a mean distance corrected near visual acuity of 20/25; the mean distance corrected near visual acuity with additional add was 20/22.[8] Steinert et al. reported a mean distance corrected near visual acuity with additional add of J1 for both the multifocal group and monofocal group; a mean distance corrected near visual acuity of J2 was achieved by multifocal patients compared to J5 for the monofocal patients.[9] This difference was statistically significant (p=0.0001). Patients in the multifocal group required significantly less additional add power for best near vision compared to patients in the monofocal group (1.36 D versus 2.37 D, respectively, p<0.0001).

Shoji and Shimizu[11] reported that 33.3% of patients achieved a distance corrected near visual acuity of J1 or better; 100% achieved J3 or better (Figure 13-6).

Functional Vision

Functional vision is defined as a patient's ability to see both 20/40 or better and J3 or better uncorrected. Percival and

Setty reported that 72% of patients achieved 20/40 or better and J3 or better unaided compared to 48% of patients in the monofocal control group.[10] Shoji and Shimizu reported that 64.3% of patients achieved 20/28 or better distance visual acuity and 20/50 or better near visual acuity unaided.

Optical/Visual Symptoms

Eisenmann et al. reported that patients with cataracts and the 3M multifocal IOL noticed larger halos (mean values: 22.2 sq.deg. and 19.2 sq.deg., respectively) than patients implanted with either the SSM26NB or a monofocal IOL (mean values: 13.7 sq.deg. and 12.6 sq.deg., respectively).[13] In a comparative study, Eisenmann and Jacobi were unable to demonstrate a statistically significant difference in the results of halo or glare measurements between groups of patients implanted with either the SSM26NB or a monofocal lens (mean values of halo blur circle size: 13.7 ± 4. 7 sq.deg. versus 12.6 ±5.2 sq.deg., respectively).[14] The difference between these measurements was not statistically significant. In an additional study, Eisenmann and Jacobi found that optical symptoms such as halos were much more frequently reported in patients implanted with the 3M diffractive multifocal IOL than in patients implanted with the MPC25NB.[15] Although the functional results of both lens groups were comparable, the AMO Array had fewer optical side effects than the 3M multifocal IOL.

Contrast Sensitivity

Steinert et al. reported a reduction in visual acuity at 11% contrast for patients implanted with the multifocal versus a monofocal IOL (mean Regan scores: 2.59 lines versus 4.37

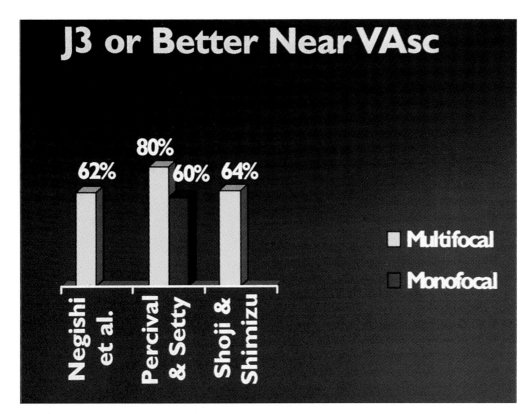

Figure 13-5. Various reported uncorrected near acuity, percent of cases achieving J3 or better.

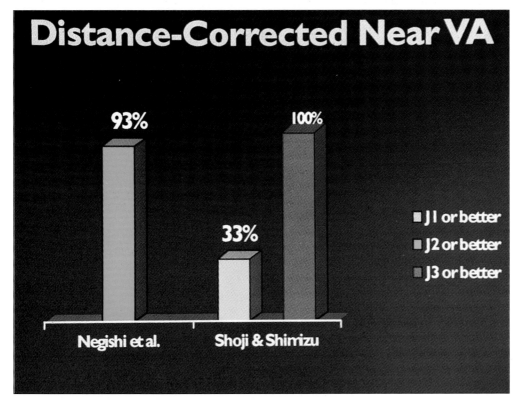

Figure 13-6. Various reported near acuity with distance correction in place, percent of cases achieving J1 or better, J2 or better, and J3 or better.

lines, respectively). This difference was statistically significant (p=0.0024).[9] However, results of a patient satisfaction survey did not demonstrate any perceived drawbacks that could be directly attributed to this reduction in contrast sensi-

tivity. Subjective scores for quality of vision at distance and near under different lighting conditions were similar for both groups. Percival and Setty reported a 2.1 line loss at 11% contrast for multifocal patients versus monofocal patients.[10]

Negishi et al. reported that mean contrast sensitivity and low contrast vision achieved by patients implanted with the MPC25NB were comparable to that achieved by monofocal patients.[7] Jacobi and Konen reported that contrast acuity was not affected clinically except at the low levels of illumination (11%) where there was a mean difference of 1.5 lines between multifocal patients versus monofocal patients.[8] These results were even more pronounced for multifocal patients under glare (2.5 line loss in poor lighting conditions).

Jacobi and Eisenmann reported that contrast acuity testing at high and medium contrast showed no difference between patients implanted with the multifocal versus a monofocal IOL.[16] However, at 11% contrast, the monofocal lens group performed significantly better than the multifocal lens group.

Negishi et al. reported that mean contrast sensitivity acuities were within normal ranges for all spatial frequencies.[6] Results for a comparable monofocal control group were not presented. Schmidt et al. reported a 13% reduction in visual acuity during contrast sensitivity testing with the 50% Regan chart versus the 96%, and in the presence of glare, a 90% reduction in visual acuity for the 11% chart.[12] Again, results for a comparable monofocal control group were not presented.

Bilateral Implantation of the AMO Array

In an optical measurement set-up, enabling the projection of images through an IOL in a physical eye into the eye of a "healthy" subject, Wagner et al. demonstrated that although contrast acuity was significantly reduced at the 11% contrast level in a unilateral set-up using the MPC25NB IOL, in the bilateral set-up binocular function was not impaired at the 11% contrast level.[17] In a study of bilaterally implanted SSM26NB patients versus unilateral patients, Liekfeld et al. reported that bilaterally implanted patients reported less disturbing optical phenomena.[18] The results of Wagner et al. demonstrate the need for prospective randomized studies testing contrast acuity between bilaterally implanted multifocal and monofocal patients.

In a study of the binocular function of patients, Javitt et al. conducted a retrospective quality of life analysis of 100 patients bilaterally implanted with the SSM26NB versus 103 patients bilaterally implanted with a three-piece foldable monofocal IOL.[19] Patients were interviewed over the telephone by an interviewer who was masked to the patients' implant status. Patients in both groups were asked to rate their degree of satisfaction and trouble with vision, and statistically significant differences were demonstrated for both categories. A higher proportion of multifocal patients versus monofocal patients were satisfied with their ability to see without glasses (rating scale of 0 to 4 where 3 equals "quite satisfied"—mean scores: 3.6 versus 2.9 daytime and 3.3 versus 2.8 at night, respectively, p<0.001). Patients with multifocal IOLs also reported less trouble with vision without spectacles (scale of 0 to 4 where 1 equals "some of the time"—mean scores: 0.4 versus 0.9 daytime, p<0.001 and 0.6 versus 0.9 at night p=0.014).

When asked about limitations while driving at night without spectacles, patients with multifocal IOLs showed a 51% increase in difficulty compared to patients with monofocal IOLs, which was not statistically significant (scale of 0 to 4 where 1 equals "slightly limited"—mean scores: 0.8 versus 0.5, p=0.164). The difference for limitations while driving at night decreased with spectacle wear (0.35 versus 0.08, p<0.05).

When patients were asked whether they were bothered by glare, halos or rings around lights, statistically significantly more patients with multifocal IOLs reported a greater degree of bother both with and without spectacles compared to monofocal patients (p<0.001). However, no correlation between overall ratings of trouble and satisfaction with vision with bother due to rings or halos was demonstrated, and patients with multifocal IOLs reported better overall health and happiness compared to those with monofocal IOLs (health, p<0.001 and happiness, p=0.018).

Overall results of the Javitt et al. study indicate that patients bilaterally implanted with the AMO Array achieved better patient outcomes for most variables versus bilaterally implanted monofocal patients. Additional studies using the questionnaire from this retrospective analysis are planned to determine if these results can be generalized to all patients implanted with the AMO Array.

Conclusion

Published data to date demonstrate excellent monocular and binocular results achieved by patients implanted with the AMO Array. The impact of optical/visual symptoms such as halos and glare, and the loss of acuity at low levels of contrast have not been demonstrated in the published literature to affect the performance of patients implanted with the AMO Array. The Premarket Approval Application for AMO Array model SA40N was submitted to the U.S. FDA in August of 1996.

Asymmetrical Bilateral Diffractive Multifocal IOLs

Asymmetrical bilateral multifocal IOL implantation combines the methods of multifocals and monovision, while minimizing their limitations. We (FKJ) bilaterally implant two types of a new diffractive multifocal IOL, which differ in the light distribution for the far and near focus. One eye receives a distant dominant multifocal lens, which has a light distribution of 70% for the far focus and 30% for the near. The fellow eye receives a near dominant multifocal lens with a light distribution of 30% for the far focus and 70% for the near (Figure 13-7).

The new multifocal is a diffractive silicone lens, which is currently produced as a prototype with a disc-haptic design by Chiron-Adatomed (Figure 13-8). The IOL has an optic diameter of 5.5 mm (>22 D) to 6 mm (≤22 D) and a total diameter of 10 mm. The lens optic is biconvex, aspheric, and has a diffractive zone of 4.5 mm in diameter on the posterior

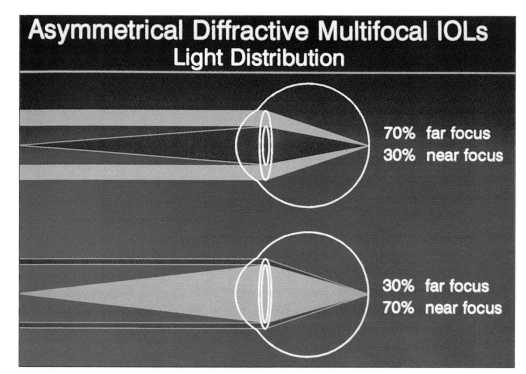

Figure 13-7. Light distribution for the far and near focus of the asymmetrical diffractive multifocal IOLs. One eye receives a distant dominant multifocal lens, which has a light distribution of 70% for the far focus and 30% for the near. The fellow eye receives a near dominant multifocal lens with a light distribution of 30% for the far focus and 70% for the near (Jacobi).

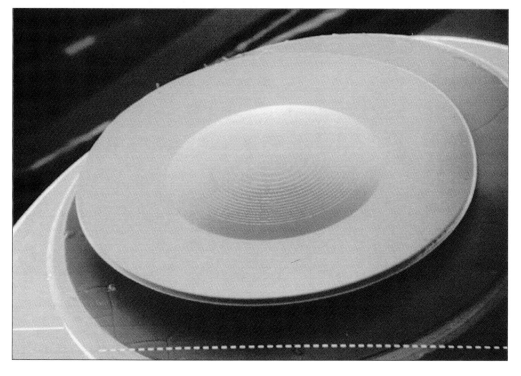

Figure 13-8. The diffractive silicone lens, currently produced as a prototype with a disc-haptic design by Chiron-Adatomed. The lens optic is biconvex, aspheric, and has a diffractive zone of 4.5 mm in diameter on the posterior surface (Jacobi).

surface. Due to its aspheric optic design, the lens shows a good modulation transfer function (MTF), which comes close to the MTF of a perfect diffraction-limited lens. Figures 13-9A&B show the MTF for a near dominant lens, measured through the near and far focus respectively.

Our current surgical technique involves a temporal clear-corneal incision, with phacoemulsification and lens implantation with an injector device. It is important to put the lens into the cartridge with the anterior surface showing upward, in order to have the diffractive pattern on the posterior surface after implantation (Figure 13-10).

Results of Asymmetrical Bilateral Multifocals

So far twelve patients have received bilateral implants in a prospective clinical trial. One subject was excluded because of significant posterior capsular opacification. The results

Figure 13-9. The modulation transfer functions for a near dominant lens (Jacobi). (A) Measured through the near focus. (B) Measured through the far focus.

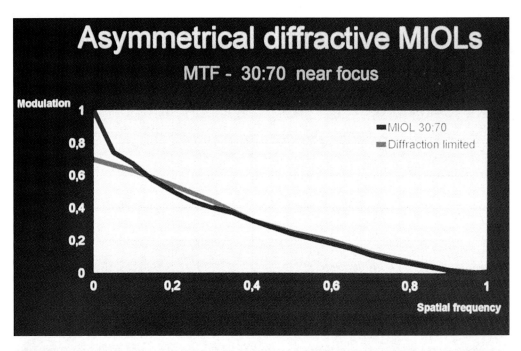

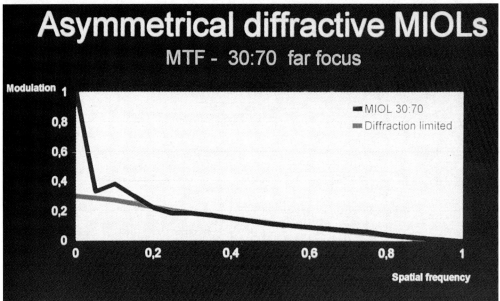

show that the asymmetrical light distribution has a pronounced effect on visual function.

Best-corrected visual acuity was significantly reduced in the near dominant IOL compared to the distant dominant lens. Only one subject achieved 20/20 with the near dominant lens. However, mean binocular visual acuity did not differ from monocular acuity with the distant dominant lens (Figure 13-11).

In distance-corrected near visual acuity, the near dominant IOLs performed better than distant dominant IOLs, but not significantly. Mean near visual acuity was slightly improved in binocular testing (Figure 13-12).

We compared binocular contrast acuity using the Regan contrast charts between our multifocal patients and an age- and visual acuity-matched group of monofocal pseudophakic patients. The binocular contrast acuity was significantly reduced in the multifocal subjects at the lowest contrast level (Figure 13-13).

In binocular visual function testing, no patient showed any clinical dysfunction. All patients showed stereoscopic acuity results in the Titmus and Randot test within the normal range.

Figure 13-14 demonstrates the clinical defocus curves of one of the bilaterally implanted patients. They show the typical bimodal curve which has the highest peak at the far focus for the distant-dominant lens and at near focus for the near-dominant lens. In binocular vision both curves add up

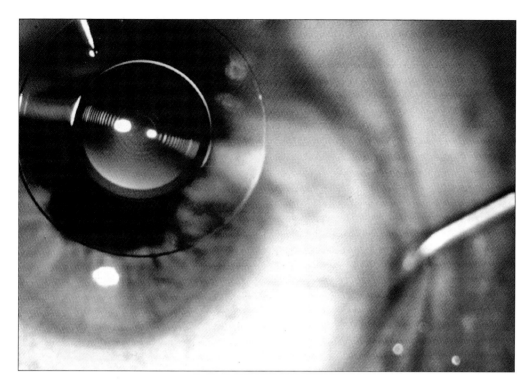

Figure 13-10. Implantation of the diffractive silicone IOL. It is important to put the lens into the cartridge with the anterior surface showing upward, in order to have the diffractive pattern on the posterior surface after implantation (Jacobi).

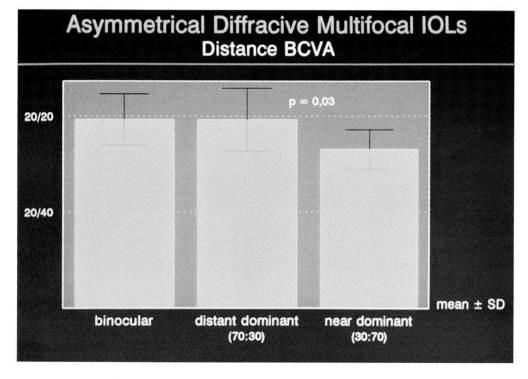

Figure 13-11. Best-corrected distance visual acuity measured OU, through the distant dominant lens, and through the near dominant lens (Jacobi).

to an improved visual acuity over the range of pseudoaccommodation.

Conclusions

Bilaterally implanted diffractive multifocal IOLs with an asymmetrical light distribution provide a good distance and near visual acuity with an improved function in the dominant focus. There is no reduction in mean binocular acuity compared to the monocular acuity with the distant-dominant lens alone, although binocular contrast acuity is reduced at the lowest contrast. This new multifocal lens can also be implanted in other combination, for example, bilateral distant-dominant lenses to further improve visual function in the far focus.

Figure 13-12. Near visual acuity with distance correction in place measured OU, through the distant dominant lens, and through the near dominant lens (Jacobi).

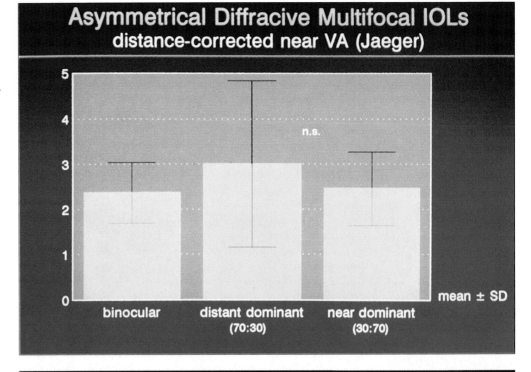

Figure 13-13. Binocular contrast acuity using the Regan contrast charts comparing multifocal patients and an age- and visual acuity-matched group of monofocal pseudophakic patients (Jacobi).

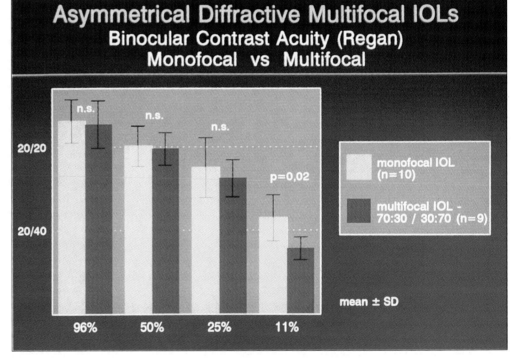

LOW AND MINUS POWER IOLS FOR HIGH MYOPES

Extreme myopes are often left with residual myopia after cataract extraction. Until now, the surgeon has had to settle for a zero power IOL or with leaving the patient aphakic. Allergan now makes low and minus power IOLs for extreme myopes, the AMO DuraLens® models PS-60 AMB and PS-

60AZB (Figure 13-15). The former lens is available in dioptric powers from +1 to +5, in 1 D steps, and the latter is available in powers ranging from –10 to 1 D, in 1 D steps. Both are single-piece PMMA lenses with a concave-convex shape.

Power calculation must be done with the Holladay IOL Consultants program (see Chapter 15). Third generation power calculation formulas do not accurately predict power in these very extreme cases, because they assume that the

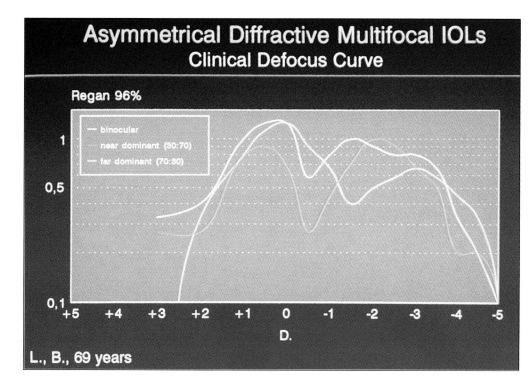

Figure 13-14. The clinical defocus curves of one of the bilaterally implanted patients, showing the typical bimodal curve which has the highest peak at the far focus for the distant-dominant lens and at near focus for the near-dominant lens (Jacobi).

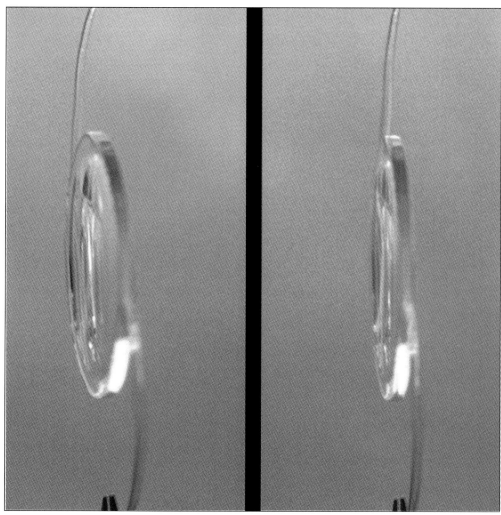

Figure 13-15. Stereo photo of the Allergan PS60AZB minus power IOL. Stereopsis can be appreciated with a stereo viewer (Gills).

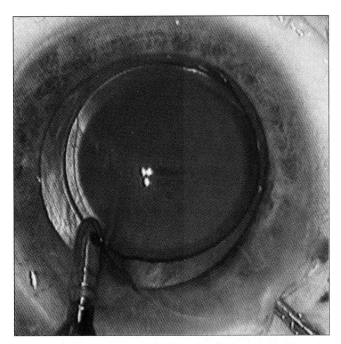

Figure 13-16. Insertion of minus IOL for high myope (Gills).

axial length is proportionate to other anatomical structures. Extreme myopes and extreme hyperopes have disproportionate axial lengths, and the Holladay formula adjusts for these differences to provide the most accurate power prediction currently available for the extreme case.

We have implanted minus power IOLs in two patients with extreme myopia (Figure 13-16). Refraction in the first was -13.00 -3.00 X 175 with best-corrected vision of 10/700. The patient was amblyopic and had Fuch's dystrophy. Axial length was 32.16 mm, anterior chamber depth was 3.3, and lens thickness was 4.3. Corneal diameter was 10.5 mm. An Allergan minus power IOL of –4 D was implanted through a 6-mm scleral incision at 9:30. Because of the Fuch's, Vitrax was given every 10 seconds to protect the endothelium.

At one day after surgery uncorrected vision was 20/50. At one week, uncorrected vision was also 20/50 and refraction was +1.00 –0.50 x 167 with 20/30 vision.

The second patient had a preoperative refraction of -17.50 -1.25 X 005. Preoperative best corrected vision was 20/200. Axial length was 30.81 mm, anterior chamber depth was 4.2 and lens thickness was 4.4. A –4.0 D Allergan lens was implanted through a 5.5 mm incision at 9:00. Postoperative refraction was plano -1.00 X 010, which was very close to the predicted postoperative refraction of -0.28 D computed using the Holladay IOL Consultant Software (see Chapter 15). The best-corrected acuity was 20/40.

These lenses can also benefit myopic pseudophakes who were overpowered at primary surgery. Implanting a second IOL of minus power reduces the total power while avoiding the disadvantages of IOL exchange. This application will be discussed more thoroughly in Chapter 14.

TORIC IOLS

The objective of a toric IOL is to incorporate astigmatism correction directly into the optic so as to avoid compromising corneal integrity by using relaxing incisions or an excimer laser. The STAAR toric IOL AA-4203 TF (Figure 13-17), based on STAAR's AA-4203 one-piece silicone IOL (see Chapter 12), is available with a 2 D or 3.5 D cylindrical correction in the IOL plane. The IOL provides approximately 1.4 D or 2.3 D of cylindrical correction at the corneal plane. Since the lens is identical to the plate-haptic silicone lens in all respects except the optic, small incision surgical techniques are used to minimize any surgically induced cylinder.

The steep meridian of the toric optic is 90° away from the long axis of the IOL. Once the lens is in the bag, the markings must be aligned with the steep corneal meridian as determined by keratometry.

At this time, enrollment in Phase I and Phase II FDA trials is complete, and follow-up is near complete. Anticipated submission of the PMA is July, 1997.

Results of Phase I and II

2.0 D Toric IOL

Phase I was a randomized, prospective, controlled evaluation of the 2.0 D toric IOL versus a non-toric optic IOL, and included 250 patients having 1.0 to 4.25 D of pre-existing keratometric astigmatism. Phase II was a prospective evaluation of both the 2.0 D and 3.5 D toric powers in 60 patients in the intended sub-populations, that is, lower astigmats received the 2.0 D toric while higher astigmats received the 3.5 D toric IOL.

In the studies of the 2.0 D toric, 95% of toric patients and 86% of control subjects had 4 or more months follow-up. Mean postoperative keratometric cylinder was virtually identical between the toric and control groups, 1.77 +/- 0.65 D and 1.67 +/- 0.58 D respectively. Similar keratometric cylinder means that any differences in refractive cylinder are directly attributable to the cylinder correction of the toric IOL.

Figure 13-18 demonstrates the distribution of postoperative refractive cylinder. One-third of toric patients had 0.5 D or less of refractive cylinder, and nearly two-thirds had 1 D or less. In contrast, 40% of control patients had more than 1.5 D, and nearly two-thirds had more than a diopter of refractive cylinder. Thus, the toric group demonstrates a clinically and statistically significant reduction in postoperative residual refractive cylinder (p=0.001).

Uncorrected distance acuity was slightly improved in the toric group, with 50% of the toric group versus only 36% in the control group seeing 20/40 or better. However, the difference is not statistically significant.

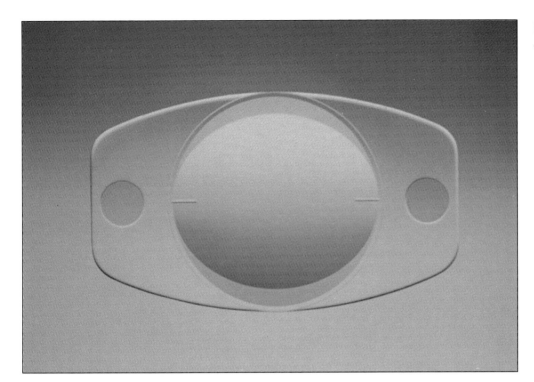

Figure 13-17. STAAR AA-4203TF toric optic IOL (Grabow).

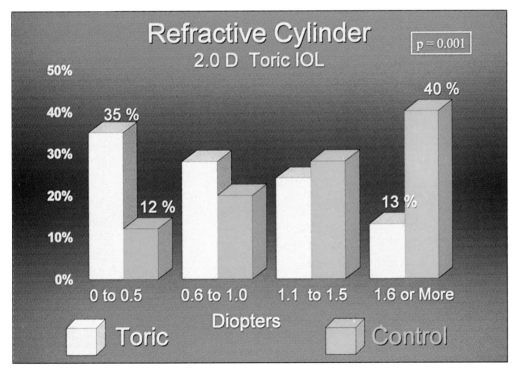

Figure 13-18. Distribution of postoperative refractive cylinder of the 2.0 D toric IOL group and control group (Grabow).

3.5 D Toric IOL

In the study of the 3.5 D toric lens, again the mean postoperative keratometric cylinder was virtually identical to the control group, 3.11 +/- 1.32 D for the toric and 2.93 +/- 0.83 D for the control, meaning that any differences in refractive cylinder are due to the toric correction.

Figure 13-19 demonstrates the dramatically reduced resid-ual refractive cylinder with the toric IOL. Toric subjects were 14 times as likely to achieve sub-clinical levels of cylinder than were control subjects (42% vs 3%). Further, 85% of control subjects had more than 1.5 D of cylinder versus only 25% of toric subjects.

The toric group did demonstrate a statistically significantly greater proportion of patients able to see 20/40 or better

Figure 13-19. Distribution of postoperative refractive cylinder of the 3.5 D toric IOL group and control group (Grabow).

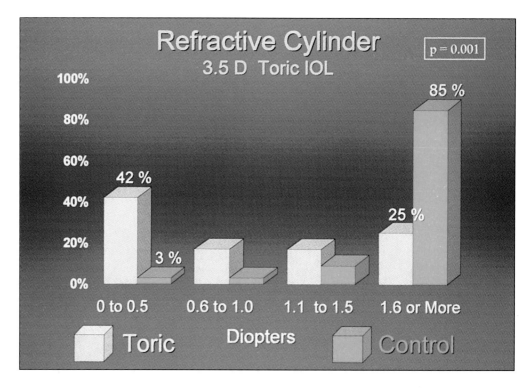

uncorrected compared to the control group, 76% vs 38%, respectively (p=0.04).

Conclusion

From a safety perspective, the STAAR 4203 silicone lens design has already been demonstrated to be safe before the FDA, and has been on the market for several years. In terms of effectiveness, the toric optic of the Model 4203TF dramatically reduces postoperative residual astigmatism.

REFERENCES

1. Apple DJ, Kincaid MC, Mamalis N, Olson RJ: *Intraocular Lenses: Evolution, Designs, Complications and Pathology.* Baltimore: Williams and Wilkins, 1989.

2. Apple DJ, Morgan RC, Tsai JC, Lim ES: Update on implantation of posterior chamber intraocular lenses. In: *Management and Care of the Cataract Patient.* Blackwell Scientific Publications Inc. Cambridge, Massachusetts, 1992.

3. Kraff MC, Sanders DR, Raanan MG: A survey of intraocular lens explantations. *J Cataract Refract Surg* 1986; 12:644-650.

4. Martin RG, Sanders DR, Souchek J, Raanan MG, DeLuca M: Effect of posterior chamber intraocular lens design and surgical placement on postoperative outcome. *J Cataract Refract Surg* 1992; 18:333-341.

5. Hansen SO, Solomon KD, McKnight GT, et al: Posterior capsular opacification and intraocular lens decentration. Part I: Comparison of various posterior chamber lens designs implanted in the rabbit model. *J Cataract Refract Surg* 1988; 14:605-613.

6. Negishi K, Nagamoto T, Hara E, et al: Clinical evaluation of a five-zone refractive multifocal intraocular lens. *J Cataract Refract Surg* 1996; 22:110-5.

7. Negishi K, Mori A, Hara E, et al: Clinical performance of a five-zone refractive multifocal IOL (AMO Array). *Journal of the Eye* 1994; 11:445-50.

8. Jacobi P, Konen W: Effect of age and astigmatism on the AMO Array multifocal intraocular lens. *J Cataract Refract Surg* 1995; 21:556:61.

9. Steinert RF, Post CT, Brint SF, et al: A prospective, randomized, double-masked comparison of a zonal-progressive multifocal intraocular lens and a monofocal intraocular lens. *Ophthalmology* 1992; 99:853-60.

10. Percival SPB, Setty SS: Prospectively randomized trial comparing the pseudoaccommodation of the AMO ARRAY multifocal lens and a monofocal lens. *J Cataract Refract Surg* 1993; 19:26-31.

11. Shoji N, Shimizu K: Clinical evaluation of the AMO silicone refractive multifocal intraocular lens. *IOL* 1994; 8:156-62.

12. Schmidt FU, Haring G, Eisenmann D, et al: Functionelle ergebnisse nach implantation von 138 refraktiven multifokalen intraocularlinsen vom typ AMO® ARRAY®. 9. Kongreß der DGII. Springer-Verlag Berlin Heidelberg 1995; 212-16.

13. Eisenmann E, Jacobi F, Dick B, Jacobi K: Computerisierte untersuchungen von blendempfindlichkeit und halos bei katarakt, mono- und multifokaler pseudophakie. *Spektrum Augen* 1996; 10:7-9.

14. Eisenmann D, Jacobi KW: Computerisiert untersuchung von blendempfindlichkeit und halos bei monofokaler und multifokaler pseudophakie 9. Kongreß der DGII. Springer-Verlag Berlin Heidelberg 1995; 204-207.

15. Eisenmann D, Jacobi KW: Die ARRAY-multifokallinse - funktionsprinzip und klinische ergebnisse. *Klin Monatsbl Augenheilkd* 1993; 203:189-194.

16. Jacobi FK, Eisenmann D: Klinische ergebnisse der AMO Array multifokallinse. *Spektrum Augen* 1996; 10:53-55.

17. Wagner R, Eisenmann D, Jacobi KW, Reiner J: Abbildungseigenschaften der AMO-Array-multifokallinse nach optischer implantation physikalischer augen. 9. Kongreß der DGII. Springer-Verlag Berlin Heidelberg 1995; 208-211.

18. Liekfeld A, Pham DT, Wollensak J: Funktionelle ergebnisse bei bilateraler implantation einer faltbaren refraktiven multi-fokalen hinterkammerlinse. *Klin Monats* Augen 1997; 207:283-286.

19. Javitt JC, Wang F, Trentacost DJ, et al: Outcomes of cataract extraction with multifocal intraocular lens implantation: functional status and quality of life. *Ophthalmology* 1997; 104:589-599.

MULTIPLE INTRAOCULAR LENS IMPLANTATION

James P. Gills, MD, Johnny L. Gayton, MD, Marsha Raanan, MS

In 1993, one of the authors (JLG) first presented a unique solution to the problem of providing adequate IOL power to a patient with microphthalmos and extreme hyperopia—two IOLs implanted back to back. Since then, many surgeons have taken up the technique, not only to treat high hyperopia, but also as a secondary technique to treat pseudophakic refractive errors to avoid the risks associated with lens exchange. With the advent of minus power IOLs, the technique can benefit even myopic pseudophakes. The technique is very helpful for patients who have had a corneal refractive procedure and are thus more likely to have post-cataract surgery refractive error. The technique also can be used to correct the often high refractive errors of pseudophakic PK patients, for whom lens exchange presents even greater levels of risk.

MULTIPLE IMPLANTS FOR HIGH HYPEROPES

The highly hyperopic patient presents the cataract surgeon with two potential problems. The first is the possibility of surgical complications that may arise from the structural nature of the hyperopic eye. The second is implanting adequate power while maintaining good optical quality and an accurate refraction.

Patients with short axial lengths often have very small anterior segments. About 20% of eyes with axial length less than 21 mm have disproportionately small anterior segment sizes.[1] In cases with shallow anterior chambers, we are less able to utilize clear corneal incisions (CCIs) because 2.5 mm takes up more area in a small cornea. Phacoemulsification is more challenging in a short eye. One of the challenges that may arise during phacoemulsification is pupillary block. Increased IOP from choroidal effusion or fluid misdirection is more common in hyperopic eyes and can cause a progressive shallowing of the anterior chamber as the eye hardens. Short eyes are at greater risk for expulsive hemorrhage. Another complication associated with a short eye is iris prolapse when the phaco tip is inserted. Patients with short eyes are at increased risk of angle closure glaucoma.

Predicting and fitting the correct IOL power in highly hyperopic patients is even more challenging due to IOL technology constraints and the limitations of current power formulas. Empirically derived power formulas were developed on "normal" eyes and by their nature are much less accurate for shorter and longer eyes. Current theoretical formulas have been improved enormously, providing fairly accurate power predictions for average and for moderately short and long eyes.[2-6] Nevertheless, these formulas still use empirically derived constants and estimates of optical relationships that remain more accurate for average or near-average length eyes, making power determination for high hyperopes much less predictable.

Furthermore, even when the surgeon is fairly confident of the calculated power, a lens of that power is often not commercially available. Highly hyperopic patients often require substantially higher power than 34 diopters, which is generally the upper limit of IOL power inventories. Microphthalmic eyes may require as much as 60 diopters of power in the IOL plane to provide a reasonable refraction. Even if the patient and surgeon are willing to tolerate delays, bureaucracy and added expense, custom making higher powered lenses poses tedious FDA-related problems concerning optical issues with high powered lenses. At high dioptric powers (over about 40 D), significant spherical aberrations occur. Such high powers require very steep radii, causing the lens to be shaped more like a sphere. The modulation transfer function is decreased. Thus resolution is compromised, with a severely distorted image quality.[7,8]

Because of these problems in predicting and providing adequate power for the high hyperope, severe undercorrection has often been the expected outcome. Better surgical technique, improved phacoemulsification technology, and better IOL designs have given us confidence in avoiding surgical complications in the hyperopic eye. The next step is to address the power issues. A practical solution to the problem of providing accurate power for the patient with a short eye is to implant two IOLs "piggyback" style, which together provide adequate power without any compromise in optical quality.

Dr. Johnny Gayton, M.D. first reported implantation of two IOLs in a case of extreme microphthalmos in 1993.[9] A number of surgeons have applied this strategy since 1993 to less extreme cases of hyperopia in which a single high power IOL would not have provided sufficient power and even to cases in which the required power was at or near the upper limit of power inventories.[10] Implanting two IOLs in these cases is preferable, because when the optical centers of the lenses are aligned, they provide better optical quality than a single high powered IOL. Good refractive and visual outcomes have been documented for hyperopes receiving double (and triple) implants.[10,11]

General Guidelines: Preoperative Measurements, Power Calculation and Patient Strategies

Axial Length Measurement

Accurate measurement of axial length and corneal curvature have always been the starting point for obtaining predictable refractive outcome. Used in conjunction with an appropriate power calculation formula and optimized constants (specific to both the IOL and the surgeon), accurate measurements result in good outcomes in the majority of cases.[2-4]

Accurate measurement of axial length in hyperopic eyes is especially important since any error is greatly magnified in proportion to the length of the eye. Yet it is in short eyes that accurate measurements are most difficult to obtain. Ultrasound axiometers are calibrated with average velocities for normal length eyes. These velocities are incorrect for short eyes, causing significant measurement errors.[7]

Performing applanation biometry is frequently difficult in short-eye cases with a shallow anterior chamber because it can be difficult to distinguish the initial "bang" echo from the iris and establish perpendicularity. Decreasing the ultrasound gain may be necessary when this occurs so each echo can be visualized but doing so can make the scan more difficult to perform. The most significant problem with applanation biometry is that the cornea is easily indented even in the hand of the most skilled ultrasound technician. Even the slightest indentation can cause significant measurement errors which are magnified when the eye is short.[2,7,12]

Immersion biometry can provide superior results in these cases.[13] First, it is impossible to applanate the cornea. Thus, by its very nature, immersion is more reliable. Second, it allows visualization of the corneal echoes. In order to obtain the most accurate measurement, the skilled ultrasound technician will watch for consistency of echo height, axial length, lens thickness, and anterior chamber depth readings.

Power Calculation

Optimizing axial length measurements does not guarantee the desired outcome. In a study one of the authors (JPG) performed with Dr. Jack Holladay,[7] several hyperopic patients were examined and more detailed anatomical measurements were taken. In most cases the short eye cases had normal anterior segment dimensions (corneal diameter, keratometry, and anterior segment length.) The "abnormality" was a foreshortened axial length due to a shortened posterior segment.

Based on these observations we can conclude that current third generation power formulas systematically generate hyperopic errors in power calculation among most short eye cases because they shorten the expected anterior chamber depth to the lens as a function of the axial length.[1] Thus they all predict the position of the lens to be too far anterior, resulting in a hyperopic error.

Dr. Holladay's recent multi-site study of power calculation in long and short eyes[1] has suggested that there are different "types" of eyes with respect to axial length and anterior segment size. About 80% of short eyes have normal anterior segment length while only 20% have short anterior segment sizes (see Figure 14-1). Examination of the relationship between predicted power (using current methods) and axial length for large, normal and small anterior segment sizes (Figure 14-2) shows that predicted emmetropia power is lower for short eyes.[1]

Holladay estimates that short axial length cases with normal anterior segment length and shortened posterior segment length may comprise about 80% of short eyes and 0.6% of all cataract cases (see Figure 14-1, Table 14-1),[1] or approximately 7200 cases per year (of about 1.2 million IOL cases) who would receive underestimated IOL power. A new Holladay power formula has been developed on almost 1000 eyes in this study (including 93 eyes with short axial length)[1]. It appears that white-to-white corneal diameter and lens thickness can be used along with anterior chamber depth to determine the size of the anterior segment and that all are important considerations for power calculation. These measurements help predict the exact location of the IOL in the short eye and increase prediction accuracy.

Holladay has reported that prediction accuracy in short eyes is significantly improved in the new Holladay-2 formula, which utilizes these extra measurements.[1] He reported a decrease in mean absolute error among short eye cases from about four and a half diopters when current formulas are used to a little less than 1 diopter when the new Holladay-2 formula is used. About 4% of eyes with average total axial lengths have anterior segment sizes which are large or small relative to the posterior segment (Figure 14-1) and may also benefit from the use of a power formula based on more measurements.

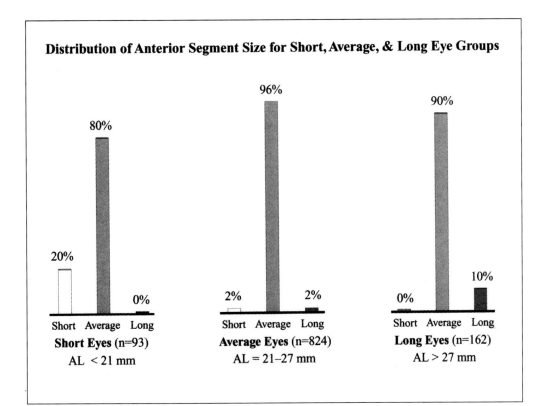

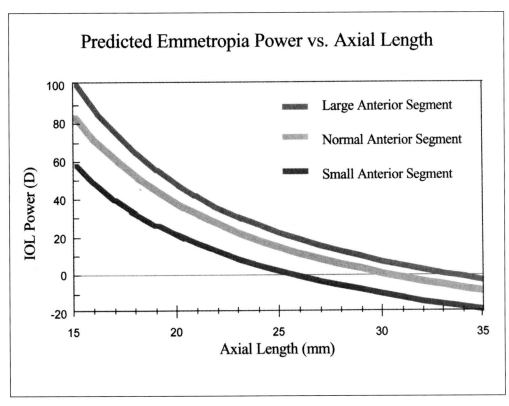

Figure 14-2. Schematic illustration of predicted emmetropia power (using current theoretic formulas) versus axial length for small, normal and large anterior segment sizes. Adapted from Holladay.[1]

Furthermore, when the "piggyback" technique is used in high hyperopes, power calculations must be adjusted again. By measuring the distance from the iris to the intraocular lens vertex, Holladay and Gills[12] determined that the anterior-most lens is in the usual position while the posterior-most lens is pushed back, causing additional hyperopic error. Apparently the anterior lens pushes the posterior lens further back due to the elastic nature of the capsular bag. Thus, additional power

TABLE 14-1

DISTRIBUTION OF AXIAL LENGTH VS. ANTERIOR SEGMENT SIZE IN GENERAL POPULATION

Anterior Segment Size	Axial Length		
	Short	**Normal**	**Long**
Large	0.0%	2.0%	0.1%
Normal	0.6%	94.1%	1.1%
Small	0.1%	2.0%	0.0%

Adapted from Holladay[1]

must be factored into the equation. The new Holladay-2 formula provides such adjustments.[1] For more discussion of the Holladay formulas, see Chapter 15.

Patient Selection and Strategies

When axial length is short, further measurements help us to make better predictions of the necessary IOL power. Classifying patients accordingly allows us to optimize refractive and visual outcome. We can better manage patient expectations regarding refractive outcome and, in fact, provide high hyperopes with better vision than they have ever had. Intraocular lens power becomes more predictable and thus less of a limiting factor in visual outcome. Benefits derived from surgical strategies to correct pre-existing astigmatism and providing fast visual recovery through the use of intraoperative anesthesia are no longer overshadowed by unpredictable power calculation. In short, the high hyperope can expect excellent refractive and visual outcome along with "average" axial length patients.

Patient and Surgeon Preparation

Anesthesia

All patients undergoing cataract surgery receive a thorough explanation of the type of anesthesia to be used, what to expect during surgery, and the risks involved with surgery. This is especially important with high hyperopes since compliance during surgery is critical. Topical anesthesia can be used for these patients, just as for cases with average axial lengths. However managing complications is certainly more difficult under topical anesthesia, and high hyperopes are at greater risk for certain complications such as shallow anterior chambers; iris prolapse; pupillary block while the pupil is dilated, which can result in a hard eye; and choroidal effusion or fluid misdirection which can increase the pressure in the eye. Beginning surgeons may prefer regional anesthesia for these cases.

Managing Expectations

It is important to manage patients' expectations. Frequently hyperopia is accompanied by amblyopia and the patient must be aware of the possibility of a limited improvement in vision. It is wise to test potential acuity in these cases. The amblyopic patient should be aware of the potential visual limitations. However, often amblyopic patients report that their vision after surgery is better than it ever has been.

If the patient is undergoing surgery for the first time, also explain the probability of a severe anisometropia problem. Rather than "balancing" the first eye for a less optimal result, suggest to the patient that both eyes be operated within several days to correct the anisometropia and avoid the need for full-time glasses.

If the patient is pseudophakic and underpowered in the contralateral eye, a second IOL can be implanted in the underpowered eye under topical anesthesia to provide the needed additional power. There is no need for a removal/exchange, which would be traumatic and increases the risk for retinal tears, cystoid macular edema, and cyclodialysis, and is associated with posterior or anterior capsule rupture, decreasing capsular support. The power of a secondary piggyback IOL is also more predictable than an IOL exchange for the following reasons:

1. The surgeon can never be 100% sure of the power of the original IOL
2. The surgeon can not be 100% confident that an exchanged IOL would be in the same plane as the old IOL
3. The secondary piggyback formula is calculated purely by the patient's refraction.

With current power formulas, there is still the possibility of underpowering the eye with a very short axial length even when double implants are used. The patient must be made aware of the possibility that an exchange of the anterior-most IOL may be necessary. One significant benefit of topical anesthesia is that the patient may be refracted immediately or on the next day to determine if an exchange is necessary. The early exchange of the IOL (sometimes on the same day) is uneventful without the risks of removal discussed earlier. Power "surprises", even among high hyperopes, are becoming less common as we learn more about power calculation in these cases.

Gills Method

IOL Selection and Surgical Procedure

All patients requiring 34 or more diopters of IOL power are given double implants. We had been using the original Holladay formula, but at this time we are using the Holladay-2 formula. Never use an empirical formula (regression-based) for short eye cases. They are much less accurate than theoretical formulas.[2,3,5,6] Even with current third generation theoretical formulas additional power will be needed. We added 2 to 3 diopters to the formula-predicted value before we switched to the new Holladay-2 formula.

The total required power is divided equally between the 2 IOLs. The surgeon should systematically monitor power

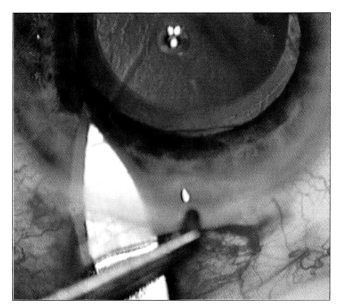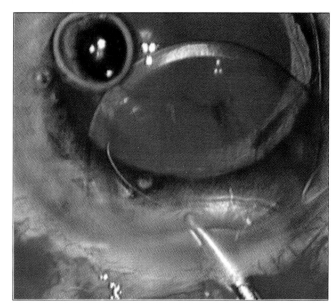

Figure 14-3. Insertion of secondary piggyback lens (Gills). (A) Enlargement of the SLiC incision to accommodate the PMMA lens. (B) Insertion of the lens, piggyback style, into the ciliary sulcus.

errors to arrive at an appropriate adjustment to the formula-predicted value, which will vary by formula, and by surgeon. Make sure that appropriate constants are used.

In secondary cases (underpowered pseudophakes), the necessary additional power is provided by implanting a second IOL of appropriate power with haptics fixated in the sulcus (Figure 14-3). In secondary cases the refraction is used to determine the power requirement. Our lens choices, strategies and power formulas for secondary cases are presented in Table 14-2.

We use PMMA single-piece biconvex IOLs with an optic size of 5.5 mm for primary piggyback cases (Figure 14-4A&B). The PMMA optic is thinner than a silicone optic making bag-fixation of two IOLs easier. The material is firmer so the IOL will hold position better. We generally use a self-sealing scleral-tunnel incision in these cases. The incision length must accommodate the 5.5-mm optic, and a 5.5-mm clear-corneal incision would have an increased risk of infection.

The incision is placed in the steep meridian to correct pre-existing astigmatism. In some cases limbal or corneal relaxing incisions are also performed to correct pre-existing astigmatism.[15] Both IOLs are bag-fixated with the haptics aligned.

We perform an immediate postoperative refraction to detect any power "surprises" which may then be corrected by an immediate exchange of the anterior lens.

Titrating the Postoperative Refraction

Following appropriate IOL power selection and good surgical technique, patients achieve excellent visual results. If the anterior-most IOL is misplaced, power errors can occur. For example, if it is completely in the sulcus there will be a 3

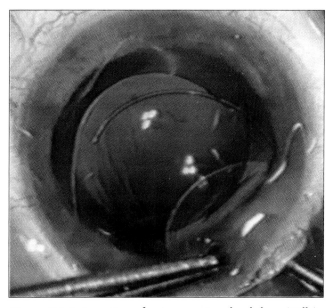

Figure 14-4. Insertion of primary piggyback lens (Gills).

to 6 D shift in the myopic direction. In one instance, a front IOL tilted, with one haptic in the bag and the other in the sulcus. This situation can result in both a shift in refraction in the myopic direction and induced refractive astigmatism.

Even if there is no misplacement of the IOL, with current formulas there are still power "surprises" in some cases. When topical anesthesia is used, the patient can actually be refracted on the same or next day to determine if there is a power error. An immediate exchange of the anterior-most IOL can be performed in a very low-risk, non-traumatic pro-

---

TABLE 14-2

RECOMMENDED IOL STYLES AND POWER CALCULATION METHODS WHEN USING "PIGGYBACK IOLS" FOR HIGH HYPEROPES AND RESIDUAL REFRACTIVE ERROR

I. Primary Piggybacks (High Hyperopes)

A. Formula: HOLLADAY 2

Total required power is divided in half between two lenses

Both IOLs are placed in the bag

Haptics are aligned

B. Lenses:

Ioptex UPB320GS

PMMA, biconvex, 5.5 mm optic, one-piece IOL

A Constant: 117.9

Diopter range: 16.0 to 24.0

Storz P359UV

PMMA, equiconvex, 5.5 mm optic, one-piece IOL

A Constant: 118.0

Diopter Range: 4.0 to 34.0

II. Secondary Piggybacks

A. Formula: Underpowered Pseudophake (hyperope)

1. Short eye (<21 mm):P=(1.5 x sph. equ.) +1

2. Avg. eye (22–26 mm):P=(1.4 x sph. equ.) +1

3. Long eye (>27 mm):P=(1.3 x sph. equ.) +1

B. Lenses:

Storz PO47UV

PMMA, equiconvex, 6.0 mm optic, sulcus, one-piece IOL

A Constant: 118.0

Diopter Range: 4.0 to 30.0

Allergan AMO PS60AMB

PMMA, concave/convex, 6.0 mm optic, sulcus, one-piece IOL

A Constant: 116.7

Diopter Range: 1.0 to 5.0

C. Formula: Overpowered Pseudophake (myope)

1. Short eye (<21 mm):P=(1.5 x sph. equ.) -1

2. Avg. eye (22–26 mm):P=(1.4 x sph. equ.) -1

3. Long eye (>27 mm):P=(1.3 x sph. equ.) -1

D. Lenses:

Allergan AMO PS60AZB

PMMA, Concave/convex, 6.0 mm optic, one-piece, post chamber IOL

A Constant 116.0

Diopter range: -1.0 to -10.0

NOTE: A Constants: Not necessary to consider for Secondary IOLs

Secondary IOLs are very low powers IOLs are always in the same position (sulcus)

---

cedure. In this way, the refraction may be titrated appropriately and all patients will enjoy good refractive outcome.

Results of Gills Piggyback IOLs in High Hyperopes

The results of a series of 51 highly hyperopic cataract patients are summarized in Figures 14-5 and 14-6. Mean preoperative hyperopia was 7.38 D (standard error = 0.34, range of 2.25 to 12 D). Total required power ranged from 30 to 55 diopters. Mean postoperative spherical equivalent was 0.56 D (standard error = 0.09, range of -2.25 to 0.87 D).

Figure 14-5 is a scatterplot of the change in spherical equivalent versus the preoperative refraction. Eighty-two percent of cases were within a diopter of emmetropia and 53% were within 0.5 D. Most of the cases had been targeted for a

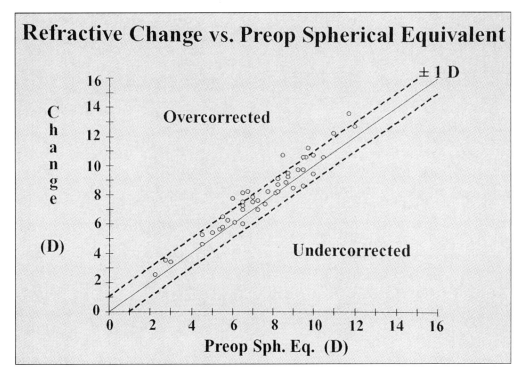

Figure 14-5. Scatterplot of achieved refractive change in spherical equivalent versus the preoperative spherical equivalent in 51 eyes with short axial lengths which received double implants. Most eyes were targeted for a residual refractive error of -0.5 D, although a few cases were targeted for 1.0-2.0 D of myopia for monovision. The targeted and achieved changes in spherical equivalent are highly correlated (Gills).

refraction of -0.5 D. A few were targeted for 1 to 1.5 diopters of myopia for monovision. Nine of the 51 cases (17%) were amblyopic or had conditions affecting visual outcome. In 16 of the 51 eyes, relaxing incisions were performed to correct pre-existing astigmatism. The reduction in cylinder for these cases averaged about a diopter.

We have clinically noted increased depth of focus (DOF) in many eyes receiving multiple implants. In a study comparing single-IOL cases with multiple-IOL cases, we performed defocus testing.[10] This procedure involves neutralizing the sphero-cylindrical refractive error with trial frames, adding plus and minus sphere in 0.25 diopter increments from +6 to -6 and measuring Snellen acuity at each step. The region between 0 and -3 diopters of defocus is of interest with respect to the patient's distance, intermediate and near vision. In a typical defocus pattern, the best distance vision occurs at 0 diopters defocus. Overminusing 1 to 2 diopters measures intermediate range vision. An overminus by as much as 2.5 to 3.5 diopters provides the near vision zone. The cutoff of functional uncorrected vision is 20/40. A typical monofocal IOL has a range of about 1.25 diopters of usable (20/40 or better) vision.

Overall, increased DOF was observed in 46% of eyes with a single IOL and 54% of eyes with double or triple implants. This difference was not statistically significant. However, in cases in which both eyes received primary surgery (i.e., the multiple IOL eye received both implants together, fixated in the capsular bag), 60% of multiple IOL eyes had increased DOF compared with 40% of single IOL eyes.

Shugar, et al. have presented data corroborating our clinical impression. In their study, eyes with multiple acrylic implants demonstrated a substantially greater depth of focus compared with eyes with single acrylic implants.[16]

Gayton Method

Multiple implant strategies are readily adaptable to individual surgery styles. Initially I used 2 plano-convex IOLs implanted with the plano sides together. However, when I began to correct underpowered pseudophakes by adding a second IOL, I found I could simply place a second biconvex optic on top of the biconvex lens already in place. Centration is excellent and the power is truly additive optically. There is some question as to whether a plano-convex IOL has a different effective power when placed with the plano surface anterior. Currently I use single-piece biconvex PMMA or Acrysof lenses. I prefer the Acrysof lens because it is the thinnest available, and allows me to use an incision as small as 3 to 3.5 mm. I use the technique on all cases requiring 30 D or more.

The posterior-most IOL is bag-fixated and the anterior-most IOL has the optic depressed into the bag. It is preferable to have the haptics of the anterior-most IOL in the bag, but they may be in the sulcus. Fixation strategies may vary from patient to patient and are certainly related to whether the implantation is a primary or secondary procedure, the style of IOL already in place, and the preferences of the surgeon. The insertion of the second IOL is generally easy.

Surgical Technique

I generally perform these cases under topical anesthesia. I construct a temporo-limbal wound of 3.0 mm in width, being careful to have a good anterior corneal lip, to help prevent iris chafing and prolapse. If limbal relaxing incisions are needed

Figure 14-6. Bar chart illustrating the deviation from emmetropia among the 51 eyes studied. Fifty-three percent were within 0.5 D of emmetropia and 82% were within a diopter of emmetropia (Gills).

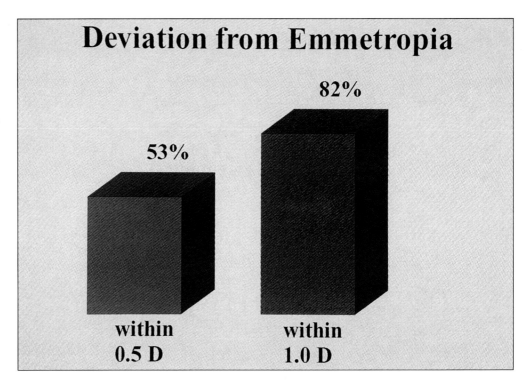

to correct preoperative astigmatism, they are made prior to entering the eye. I always deepen the chamber initially with Viscoat®. It maintains space well, protects the cornea, and helps prevent iris prolapse.

Following the capsulorhexis, I hydrodissect the nucleus with 1% lidocaine. Intraocular lidocaine has been the secret to painless surgery, especially in these short eyes. The nucleus is emulsified efficiently, trying to keep irrigation and operative time to a minimum, to lessen the likelihood of fluid misdirection and a hard eye. Following nuclear removal, I again hydrodissect with 1% lidocaine through a J-cannula, which provides additional anesthesia and eliminates struggling with subincisional cortex. Irrigation and aspiration then takes thirty seconds or less.

I then fill the bag with Provisc® due to its ease of removal, to lessen the likelihood of a postoperative IOP spike, which is more common in these short eyes. The wound is enlarged to 3.3 mm. The acrylic lens is placed in the bag using a longitudinal or moustache fold, depending on the surgeon's preference. Additional Provisc is added and the Provisc cannula is used to position the first lens. The second acrylic lens is then folded longitudinally and inserted in the bag. Frequently this lens has to be placed initially in the anterior chamber. The optic is then depressed into the bag. The haptics can be directly positioned, or dialed into the bag. I line up the haptics, evacuate the viscoelastic, and seal the wound with Gills mixture.

Power Calculation

As we have said above, power calculation is difficult in extremely short eyes and predictability is reduced. My guidelines are to: 1) implement good office systems for obtaining the most accurate measurements possible in these cases, 2) use a modern theoretical formula such as the Holladay or SRK/T, 3) continually individualize (optimize) the A-constant or ACD specifically for short eye patients in order to effectively adjust the calculation to avoid or lessen the hyperopic error discussed above. It helps, if possible, to use a single-style IOL (which may not be possible in secondary cases) in all short eye cases. I presently use the Holladay 2 formula for all primary cases and the Holladay R for all secondary cases. The following is a discussion of my power calculation techniques prior to having the Holladay IOL consultant software (see Chapter 15).

Analysis of my cases showed that for primary cases I needed to add 2.5 to 3 diopters of power to the total power predicted by the formula in use to achieve emmetropia. I have found that the most predictable method with the Holladay I formula system is to input a "desired" refraction of -1.5 D into the program and then add 1 D to the IOL power recommended, which gives an effective emmetropia power. If I am shooting for monovision, I will add another 2 or 3 D. I will of course add more if indicated by power results of a contralateral eye.

Even with this method, the predictability in short eye cases is less than can be expected with more normal axial lengths. I consider a final refraction of +0.5 to -2 D acceptable. With a larger power error, the anterior-most lens can be exchanged. For moderate myopic error, an RK procedure postoperatively may be preferable to disturbing the cataract wound (and risking induction of astigmatism) and more predictable than an IOL exchange.

The double implant strategy also can be used as a secondary procedure to reduce residual refractive error. Power calculation

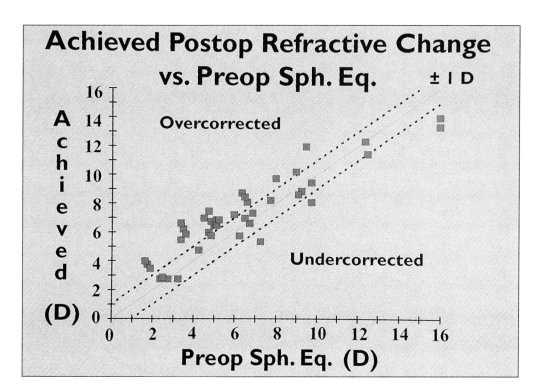

Figure 14-7. Achieved refractive change versus the preoperative spherical equivalent for the entire cohort of primary and secondary cases (Gayton).

for the second IOL is based on the refraction. For moderate to high hyperopia, add a second plus power IOL. For high myopia, add a minus power IOL. For underpowered pseudophakes, a good estimate of the needed power is the desired change in spherical x 1.5. For overpowered pseudophakes, it is simply the desired spherical equivalent change. That is, a +3.0 pseudophake who wants to be –1.0 postoperatively would need [+3 – (-1)] x 1.5 = 6 D IOL. A –3.5 pseudophake wanting to be -0.50 postoperatively would need a –4.0 D IOL.

Results of Gayton Method

We have collected a series of 41 patients over the last 3 years, with 49 eyes of these patients receiving double implants. Of these, 34 eyes were primary double implants and 15 were underpowered pseudophakes receiving secondary double implantation.

Among the primary cases, hyperopia ranged from 3.4 to 16 D, axial length from 15.5 to 21 mm, and calculated powers from 32 to 56 D. Three of the primary double implants were power "surprises" and required exchange of the anterior-most IOL. Among the secondary cases residual hyperopia ranged from 1.62 to 7.5 D.

Ninety-three percent of cases achieved acceptable results, defined as residual hyperopia <0.5 D or mild myopia. Figure 14-7 shows the achieved refractive change versus the preoperative spherical equivalent for the entire cohort. Most cases either were within 1 D of desired correction, or were mildly overcorrected, resulting in mild myopia. Figure 14-8 shows results for the secondary cases. Postoperatively, 76% were within the target range of refraction of 0 to –2 D, and all were within 1 D of this target range.

MINUS POWER LENSES FOR OVERPOWERED PSEUDOPHAKES

With minus power lenses, we can extend the piggyback technique to myopic pseudophakes. Implanting a second IOL of minus power avoids the disadvantages of IOL exchange, including capsular rupture, retinal tears, CME, and cyclodialysis. This technique has been used in penetrating keratoplasty cases, in a keratoconus case, and in a 32.5-mm length eye.

Using topical anesthesia in these cases allows the patient to be refracted immediately after implantation to verify if the power is correct. If there is still a residual error, the anterior lens can be exchanged immediately.

The necessary power reduction is determined based on the refraction. Table 14-2 shows the Gills' nomogram for power calculation. The level of power reduction is titrated based on axial length.

Results of Gills Minus Power Secondary Double Implant

Fourteen overpowered pseudophakes were given minus power IOLs to correct residual myopia. There were eight females and six males. Average age was 72.

Average axial length was 24.2 mm, ranging from 21.9 to 26.3. Mean preoperative spherical equivalent was -3.0 D, ranging from -1 to -5.25. Median implant power was -3.0 D. Target refraction was -0.5 D.

Postoperatively, the mean spherical equivalent of the cohort was reduced to -0.3 D, which was very close to target. Figure 14-9 is a scatterplot of the change in spherical equivalent versus the preoperative level of myopia. All cases are

Figure 14-8. Postoperative refraction versus residual refractive error (after primary surgery) in secondary multiple implant cases (Gayton).

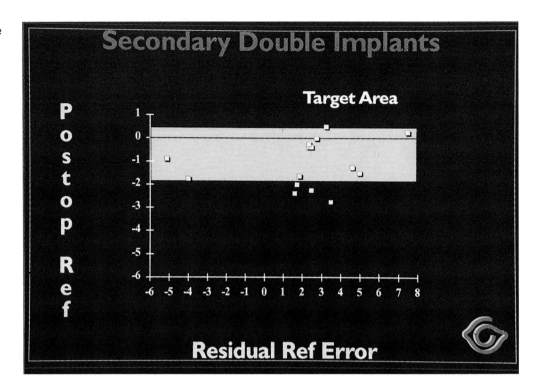

within a diopter of emmetropia. In fact, 82% of cases are within a half diopter of the target refraction of -0.5 D, and all were within one diopter of target.

Sixty percent of patients could see 20/40 or better uncorrected. All were 20/50 or better. Best corrected vision for the cohort was excellent, with 82% at 20/25 or better, and all at least 20/30. Figure 14-10 is a scatterplot of the postoperative versus preoperative best-corrected vision for each patient. Visions were either improved or within a line of the preoperative value in every case.

SECONDARY DOUBLE IMPLANTS IN PSEUDOPHAKIC PK PATIENTS

The management of refraction in post-PK patients is always problematic. Penetrating keratoplasty has an unpredictable effect on the refraction, and following refractive surgery on a donor cornea is less predictable than on virgin corneas.

Pseudophakia, however, presents an opportunity for the PK patient with high residual refractive error. While an IOL exchange may be too traumatic for a PK patient, refractive errors, both hyperopic and myopic, can be satisfactorily addressed with a secondary double implant. Power calculation for the secondary implant is the same as for other pseudophakes, but is slightly less predictable in PK patients. However, as in other secondary double implant cases, exchange of the secondary lens is easily performed if there is a power surprise. This technique may be the best hope for PK patients with visually disabling refractive errors.

Gayton Case Examples

Correcting Hyperopia

This case presented with anisometropia and asthenopia, with hyperopic astigmatism. Refraction was +0.5 +4.0 x 80 with visual acuity of 20/25. We implanted a secondary double implant with an inferior CRI to address the astigmatism. We targeted mild myopia, and implanted a 5 D IOL. Four months postoperatively, the refraction was -0.5 +0.25 x 74 with corrected acuity of 20/20 and uncorrected acuity of 20/30. More importantly, the visually disabling symptoms were alleviated.

Correcting Myopia

This case presented with myopic astigmatism, with a refraction of -6.50 +2.75 x 176. Uncorrected visual acuity was 20/200. We performed a secondary double implant with a minus power lens and a Troutman wedge. We again targeted mild myopia, and implanted a -4 D IOL. Two months postoperatively the refraction was -2.25 +2.75 x 90 with both corrected and uncorrected visual acuity of 20/40.

Results of Gayton PK Series

Figure 14-11 demonstrates the results of all 7 PK double implants performed. All but one case had a postoperative refraction within the targeted range of refraction of 0 to -2 D, and the remaining case was within 0.5 D of that target range. Thus this technique has been an effective and relatively predictable method of correcting refractive error in this population for whom other methods are often unpredictable or risky.

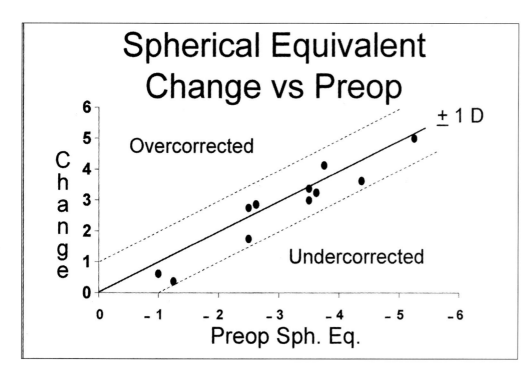

Figure 14-9. Change in spherical equivalent versus the residual myopia (after primary surgery) in cases receiving a minus power secondary implant (Gills).

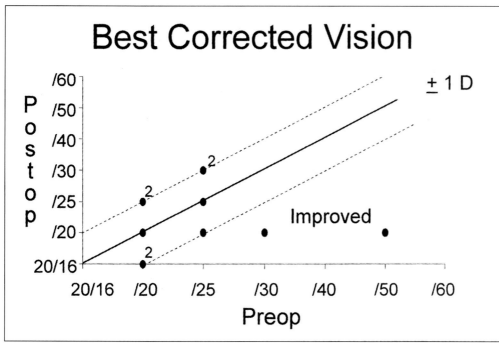

Figure 14-10. Postoperative versus pre-operative best-corrected vision for each patient in cases receiving a minus power secondary implant (Gills).

FUTURE CONCEPTS

For too long highly hyperopic patients have been at a disadvantage as they approached cataract surgery. They have had to settle for less than optimal visual and refractive outcomes. The innovative approach of implanting "piggyback" IOLs to provide adequate power has made a world of difference to the hyperopic patient. This strategy has been very successful and has provided a strong impetus to improve power calculation methods for short eyes. Now that we know we can *provide* enough power using double implants, we can no longer countenance less accurate power calculation methods for short axial lengths. In the near future we can expect power calculation to be much better. Indeed, we see greatly improved predictions in the early testing of the Holladay-2 formula, which uses more measurements to accurately determine power in short eyes and which factors in power adjustments when two IOLs are implanted.[1]

Another aid to providing better power prediction will be a better estimate of the exact position of the IOL in the eye. In

Figure 14-11.
Postoperative refraction versus residual refractive error (after primary surgery) in pseudophakic PK cases receiving a second implant (Gayton).

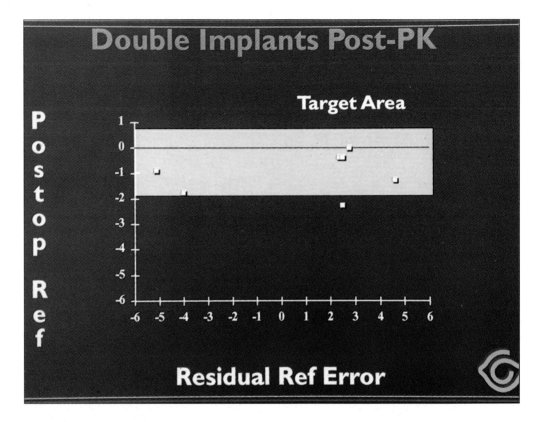

this regard, an important additional measurement to obtain would be the position of the ciliary sulcus. It is known that the IOL with flat loops centers about 0.2 mm behind the center of the sulcus. It has not been possible to measure the location of the ciliary sulcus in the past. With newer ultrasound units we can measure the distance from the front of the cornea to the ciliary sulcus. These units are generally used for other diagnostic work but will probably be adapted for use in measuring the sulcus location to provide an accurate measurement of the IOL location. When this occurs, we can look forward to even fewer power "surprises" in the high hyperope.

Also in the future will be the ability to "piggyback" toric and spherical IOLs to correct high levels of astigmatism along with high hyperopia, which will be an improvement in the management of astigmatism for patients with high cylinder.

REFERENCES

1. Holladay JR: Achieving emmetropia in extremely short eyes. Presented at the 1996 Annual Meeting of the American Academy of Ophthalmology, Chicago, IL.

2. Sanders, DR, Retzlaff JA, Kraff MC: A-scan biometry and IOL implant power calculations. In *Focal Points: Clinical Modules for Ophthalmologists.* San Francisco, CA, American Academy of Ophthalmology 1995; 13(10)1-14.

3. Holladay Jr, Prager TC, Chandler TY, et al: A three-part system for refining intraocular lens power calculation. 1988; 14:17-24.

4. Retzlaff JA, Sanders DR, Kraff MC: *Lens Implant Power Calculation: A Manual for Ophthalmologists and Biometrists,* 3rd ed. Thorofare, NJ: Slack Inc; 1990.

5. Sanders DR, Retzlaff JA, Kraff MC, et al: Comparison of the SRK/T formula and other theoretical and regression formulas. 1990; 16:341-346.

6. Hoffer KJ: The Hoffer Q formula: A comparison of theoretic and regression formulas. 1993; 19:700-712.

7. Holladay JR, Gills JP, Leidlein JL, Cherchio M: Achieving emmetropia in extremely short eyes with two piggyback posterior chamber intraocular lenses. *Ophthalmology* 1996; 103:1118-1123.

8. Smith WJ: *Modern Optical Emmetropia. The Design of Optical Systems.* New York, McGraw-Hill Book Co. 1966, pp. 50-52.

9. Gayton JL, Sanders VN: Implanting two posterior chamber intraocular lenses in a case of microphthalmos. 1993; 19:776-777.

10. Gills JP: The implantation of multiple intraocular lenses to optimize visual results in hyperopic cataract patients and under-powered pseudophakes. *Best Papers of Sessions, 1995 Symposium on Cataract IOL and Refractive Surgery Special Issue,* 1996.

11. Gayton JL, Raanan MG: Reducing refractive error in high hyperopes with double implants. In Gayton JL, *Maximizing Results.* Thorofare, NJ, Slack Inc., p. 139-148, 1996.

12. Holladay JT, Prager TC, Ruiz RS, Lewis JW: Improving the predictability of intraocular lens power calculations. *Arch Ophthalmol* 1986; 104:539-541.

13. Shammus HJF: A comparison of immersion and contact techniques for axial length measurement. *Am Intraocular Implant Soc J* 1984; 10:444.

14. Gills JP, Cherchio M, Raanan MG: The use of intraoperative unpreserved lidocaine to control discomfort during IOL surgery under topical anesthesia. *J Cataract Refract Surg*

1997 *in press*.

15. Gills JP, Cherchio M: Relaxing incisions for correcting astigmatism and optimizing near and distance vision. Presented at the 1995 annual meeting of the American Academy of Ophthalmology.

16. Shugar JK, Lee A, Shugar MC: Defocus curves for piggyback acrylic intraocular lenses in highly hyperopic eyes: Omniopia? Presented at the 1997 annual meeting of the American Society of Cataract and Refractive Surgery.

IOL POWER CALCULATION FOR THE UNUSUAL EYE

Jack T. Holladay, MD, FACS

INTRODUCTION

Several measurements of the eye are helpful in determining the appropriate intraocular lens power to achieve a desired refraction. These measurements include central corneal refractive power (k-readings), axial length (biometry), horizontal corneal diameter (horizontal white to white), anterior chamber depth, and lens thickness. The accuracy of predicting the necessary power of an intraocular lens is directly related to the accuracy of these measurements.[1,2]

Fyodorov first estimated the optical power of an intraocular lens using vergence formulas in 1967.[3] Between 1972 and 1975, when accurate ultrasonic A-scan units became commercially available, several investigators derived and published the theoretical vergence formulas.[4-9] All of these formulas were identical[10] except for the form in which they were written and the choice of various constants such as retinal thickness, optical plane of the cornea, and optical plane of the intraocular lens. These slightly different constants accounted for less than 0.50 diopters in the predicted refraction. The variation in these constants was a result of differences in lens styles, A-scan units, keratometers, and surgical techniques among the investigators.

IOL CALCULATIONS REQUIRING AXIAL LENGTH

Theoretical Formulas

The theoretical formula for intraocular lens power calculations has six variables. The six variables in the formula are: 1) corneal power (*K*), 2) axial length (*AL*), 3) intraocular lens (*IOL*) power, 4) effective lens position (*ELP*), 5) desired refraction (*DPostRx*), and 6) vertex distance (*V*). Normally, the intraocular lens power is chosen as the dependent variable

and solved for using the other five variables, where distances are given in millimeters and refractive powers given in diopters:

$$IOL = \frac{1336}{AL - ELP} - \frac{1336}{\dfrac{1336}{\dfrac{1000}{\dfrac{1000}{DPostRx} - V} + K} - ELP}$$

The only variable that cannot be chosen or measured preoperatively is the effective lens position (*ELP*). The improvements in intraocular lens power calculations over the past 30 years are a result of improving the predictability of the variable *ELP*. Figure 15-1 illustrates the physical locations of the variables.

The term "effective lens position" (*ELP*) was adopted by the FDA in 1995 to describe the position of the lens in the eye, since the term anterior chamber depth (ACD) is not anatomically accurate for lenses in the posterior chamber and can lead to confusion for the clinician. The *ELP* for intraocular lenses before 1980 was a constant of 4 mm for every lens in every patient (first generation theoretical formula). This value actually worked well in most patients because the majority of lenses implanted were iris clip fixation, in which the principal plane averages approximately 4 mm posterior to the corneal vertex.

In 1981, Binkhorst improved the prediction of *ELP* by using a single variable predictor, the axial length, as a scaling factor for *ELP* (second generation theoretical formula).[11] If the patient's axial length was 10% greater than normal (23.45 mm), he would increase the *ELP* by 10%. The average value of *ELP* was increased to 4.5 mm because the preferred location of an implant was in the ciliary sulcus, approximately 0.5

Figure 15-1. Physical locations of the variables used in formula.

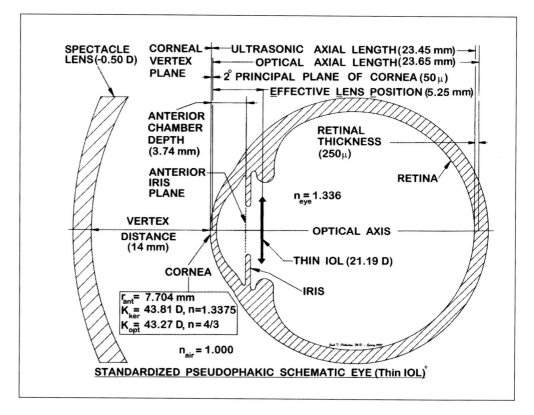

SPECTACLE LENS (-0.50 D)

CORNEAL VERTEX PLANE

ULTRASONIC AXIAL LENGTH (23.45 mm)

OPTICAL AXIAL LENGTH (23.65 mm)

2° PRINCIPAL PLANE OF CORNEA (50 μ)

EFFECTIVE LENS POSITION (5.25 mm)

ANTERIOR CHAMBER DEPTH (3.74 mm)

ANTERIOR IRIS PLANE

RETINAL THICKNESS (250 μ)

RETINA

$n_{eye} = 1.336$

VERTEX DISTANCE (14 mm)

OPTICAL AXIS

THIN IOL (21.19 D)

CORNEA

IRIS

$r_{ant} = 7.704$ mm
$K_{ker} = 43.81$ D, n=1.3375
$K_{opt} = 43.27$ D, n=4/3

$n_{air} = 1.000$

STANDARDIZED PSEUDOPHAKIC SCHEMATIC EYE (Thin IOL)®

mm deeper than the iris plane. Also, most lenses were convex-plano, similar to the shape of the iris-supported lenses.

The average *ELP* in 1996 has increased to 5.25 mm. This increased distance has occurred primarily for two reasons: the majority of implanted IOL's are biconvex, moving the principal plane of the lens even deeper into the eye, and the desired location for the lens is in the capsular bag, which is 0.25 mm deeper than the ciliary sulcus.

In 1988, we proved[4] that using a two-variable predictor, axial length and keratometry, could significantly improve the prediction of *ELP*, particularly in unusual eyes (third generation theoretical formula). The original Holladay 1 Formula was based on the geometrical relationships of the anterior segment. Although several investigators have modified the original Holladay two-variable prediction formula, no comprehensive studies have shown any significant improvement using only these two variables.

In 1995, Olsen published a four-variable predictor that used axial length, keratometry, preoperative anterior chamber depth and lens thickness.[12] His results did show improvement over the current two-variable prediction formulas. The explanation is very simple. The more information we have about the anterior segment, the better we can predict the *ELP*. This explanation is a well known theorem in prediction theory where the more variables that can be measured describing an event, the more precisely one can predict the outcome.

In a recent study,[13] we discovered that the anterior segment and posterior segment of the human eye are often not proportional in size, causing significant error in the prediction of the

ELP in extremely short eyes (< 20 mm). We found that even in eyes shorter than 20 mm, the anterior segment was completely normal in the majority of cases. Because the axial lengths were so short, the two-variable prediction formulas severely underestimated the *ELP*, explaining part of the large hyperopic prediction errors with current two-variable prediction formulas. After recognizing this problem, we began to take additional measurements on extremely short and extremely long eyes to determine if the prediction of *ELP* could be improved by knowing more about the anterior segment. Table 15-1 shows the clinical conditions that illustrate the independence of the anterior segment and the axial length.

For the past year, we have been gathering data from 35 investigators around the world. Several additional measurements of the eye have been taken, but only 7 preoperative variables (axial length, corneal power, horizontal corneal diameter, anterior chamber depth, lens thickness, preoperative refraction, and age) have been found to be useful for significantly improving the prediction of *ELP* in eyes ranging from 15 to 35 mm.

The improved prediction of ELP is not totally due to the formula, but is also a function of the technical skills of the surgeons who are consistently implanting the lenses in the capsular bag. A 20 D IOL that is 0.5 mm axially displaced from the predicted *ELP* will result in approximately a 1.0 D error in the stabilized postoperative refraction. However, when using piggyback lenses totaling 60 D, the same axial displacement of 0.5 mm will cause a 3 D refractive surprise; the error is directly proportional to the implanted lens power.

TABLE 15-1

CLINICAL CONDITIONS DEMONSTRATING THE INDEPENDENCE OF THE ANTERIOR SEGMENT AND AXIAL LENGTH

Anterior Segment Size	Axial Length		
	Short	Normal	Long
Small	Small eye Nanophthalmos	Microcornea	Microcornea + Axial myopia
Normal	Axial hyperopia	Normal	Axial myopia
Large	Megalocornea + Axial hyperopia	Megalocornea	Large eye Buphthalmos + Axial myopia

This direct relationship to the lens power is why the problem is much less evident in extremely long eyes, since the implanted IOL is either low plus or minus to achieve emmetropia following cataract extraction.

The Holladay 2 Formula and the interim results of the 35 investigators were presented at the June, 1997 ASCRS meeting. Software programs that implement the new formula were available in 1996. Once these additional measurements become routine among clinicians, a new flurry of prediction formulas using 7 or more variables will emerge, similar to the activity following our two-variable prediction formula in 1988.[4] The standard of care will reach a new level of prediction accuracy for extremely unusual eyes, just as it has for normal eyes. Calculations on patients with axial lengths between 22 and 25 mm with corneal powers between 42 and 46 D will do well with current third generation formulas (Holladay 1[4], SRK/T[14] and Hoffer Q[15]). In cases outside this range, the Holladay 2 should be used to assure accuracy.

Normal Cornea with No Previous Keratorefractive Surgery

Clear Lensectomy for High Myopia and Hyperopia

The intraocular power calculations for clear lensectomy are no different than the calculations when a cataract is present. The patients are usually much younger, however, and the loss of accommodation should be discussed thoroughly. The actual desired postoperative refraction should also be discussed, since a small degree of myopia (-0.50 D) may be desirable to someone with no accommodation to reduce dependence on spectacles.

This procedure is usually reserved for patients who are outside the range of other forms of refractive surgery. Consequently, the measurements of axial length, keratometry, etc., are usually quite different from typical cataract patients because of their degree of refractive error. In most of the cases with high myopia, the axial lengths are extremely long (> 26 mm). In cases of high hyperopia, the axial lengths are very short (< 21 mm).

In patients with myopia exceeding 20 D, removing the clear lens often results in postoperative refractions near emmetropia with no implant. The exact result depends on the power of the cornea and the axial length. The recommended lens powers usually range from -10 D to +10 D in the majority of these cases. The correct axial length measurement is very difficult to obtain in these cases because of the abnormal anatomy of the posterior pole. Staphylomas are often present in these eyes, and the macula is often not at the location in the posterior pole where the A-scan measures the axial length. In these cases it is recommended that a B-scan be performed to locate the macula (fovea) and recheck the measurement determined by A-scan. I have personally seen 3 to 4 D surprises because the macula was on the edge of the staphyloma, and the A-scan measured to the deepest part of the staphyloma. Such an error results in a hyperopic surprise because the distance to the macula is much shorter than the distance to the center of the staphyloma. The third generation theoretical formulas yield excellent results if the axial length measurement is accurate and stable.

In patients with hyperopia exceeding +8 D, the axial lengths are often less than 21 mm and require lens powers that exceed the normal range (> 34 D). In these cases piggyback lenses are necessary to achieve emmetropia.[15] The only formula available at this time in these eyes is the Holladay 2. If the required lens power is less than or equal to 34 D, then the piggyback lenses are not required and third generation theoretical formulas may be used.

PiggyBack IOLs to Achieve Powers above 34 D

Patients with axial lengths shorter than 21 mm should be calculated using the Holladay 2 Formula. In these cases, the size of the anterior segment has been shown to be unrelated to the axial length.[15] In many of these cases the anterior segment size is normal and only the posterior segment is abnormally short. In a few cases, however, the anterior segment is proportionately small to the axial length (nanophthalmos). The differences in the size of the anterior segment in these cases can cause an average of 5 D hyperopic error with third generation formulas because they predict the depth of the anterior chamber to be very shallow. Using the newer formula can reduce the prediction error in these eyes to less than 1 D.

Accurate measurements of axial length and corneal power are especially important in these cases because any error is magnified by the extreme dioptric powers of the IOLs. Placement of both lenses in the bag with the haptics aligned is essential. Inadvertently placing one lens in the bag and the other in the sulcus can cause a 4 diopter refractive surprise.

Patients with Previous Keratorefractive Surgery (RK, PRK, and LASIK)

The number of patients who have had keratorefractive surgery (radial keratotomy—RK, photorefractive keratectomy—PRK, or laser-assisted in-situ keratomileusis—LASIK) has been steadily increasing over the past 20 years. With the advent of the excimer laser, these numbers are predicted to increase dramatically. Determining their corneal power accurately is difficult and usually is the determining factor in the accuracy of the predicted refraction following cataract surgery. Providing this group of patients the same accuracy with intraocular lens power calculations as we have provided our standard cataract patients presents an especially difficult challenge for the clinician.

Methods of Determining Corneal Power

Accurately determining the central corneal refractive power is the most important and difficult part of the entire intraocular lens calculation process. Our current instruments for measuring corneal power make too many incorrect assumptions with corneas that have irregular astigmatism. The cornea can no longer be compared to a sphere centrally, the posterior radius of the cornea is no longer 1.2 mm steeper than the anterior corneal radius, etc. Because of these limitations, the calculated method and the trial hard contact lens method are most accurate, followed by corneal topography, automated keratometry, and finally manual keratometry.

Calculation Method

For the calculation method, three parameters must be known: the K-readings and refraction before the keratorefractive procedure, and the stabilized refraction after the keratorefractive procedure. It is important that the stabilized postoperative refraction be measured before any myopic shifts from nuclear sclerotic cataracts occur. It is also possible for posterior subcapsular cataracts to cause an apparent myopic shift, similar to capsular opacification, where the patient wants more minus in the refraction to make the letters appear smaller and darker. The concept which we described in 1989 subtracts the change in refraction due to the keratorefractive procedure at the corneal plane from the original K-readings before the procedure, to arrive at a calculated postoperative K-reading.[16] This method is usually the most accurate because the preoperative Ks and refraction are usually accurate to ± 0.25 D. An example calculation to illustrate the calculation method is given.

Example:

Mean Preoperative K = 42.50 @ 90° and 41.50 @ 180° = 42.00 D

Preoperative Refraction = -10.00 + 1.00 X 90°, Vertex = 14 mm Postoperative Refraction = -0.25 + 1.00 X 90°, Vertex = 14 mm

Step 1. Calculate the spheroequivalent refraction for refractions at the corneal plane (SEQ(sbc)) from the spheroequivalent refractions at the spectacle plane (SEQ(sbs)) at a given vertex, where

    a. SEQ = sphere + 0.5 (cylinder)

    b.

$$SEQ_c = \frac{1000}{\dfrac{1000}{SEQ_s} - Vertex(mm)}$$

Calculation for *preoperative* spheroequivalent refraction at corneal plane

    a. SEQ(sbR) = -10.00 + 0.5 * (1.00) = -9.50 D

$$SEQ_c = \frac{1000}{\dfrac{1000}{-9.50} - 14} = -8.38\,D$$

Calculation for *postoperative* spheroequivalent refraction at corneal plane

    a. SEQ(sbR) = -0.25 + 0.5 * (1.00) = +0.25 D

$$SEQ_c = \frac{1000}{\dfrac{1000}{+0.25} - 14} = +0.25\,D$$

Step 2. Calculate the change in refraction at the corneal plane.

Change in refraction = Preoperative SEQ(sbc) - Postoperative SEQ(sbc)

Change in refraction = -8.38 - (+.025) = -8.68 D

Step 3. Determine calculated postoperative corneal refractive power.

Mean Postoperative K = Mean Preoperative K - Change in refraction at corneal plane

Mean Postoperative K = 42.00 - 8.68 = 33.32 D

This value is the calculated central power of the cornea following the keratorefractive procedure. For IOL programs requiring two K-readings, this value would be entered twice.

Trial Hard Contact Lens Method

The trial hard contact lens method requires a plano hard contact lens with a known base curve and patients whose cataract does not prevent them from being refracted to approximately ±0.50 D. This tolerance usually requires a visual acuity of better than 20/80. The patient's spheroequivalent refraction is determined by normal refraction. The refraction is then repeated with the hard contact lens in place. If the spheroequivalent refraction does not change with the contact lens, then the patient's cornea must have the same power as the base curve of the plano contact lens. If the patient has a *myopic shift* in the refraction with the contact lens, then the base curve of the contact lens is *stronger* than the cornea by the amount of the shift. If there is a *hyperopic shift* in the refraction with the contact lens, then the base curve of the contact lens is *weaker* than the cornea by the amount of the shift.

Example:

The patient has a current spheroequivalent refraction of +0.25 D. With a plano hard contact lens with a base curve of 35.00 D placed on the cornea, the spherical refraction changes to -2.00 D. Since the patient had a myopic shift with the contact lens, the cornea must be weaker than the base curve of the contact by 2.25 D. Therefore, the cornea must be 32.75 D (35.00 - 2.25), which is slightly different than the value obtained by the calculation method. In equation form, we have

SEQ Refraction *without* hard contact lens = +0.25 D

Base Curve of Plano hard contact lens = 35.00 D

SEQ Refraction *with* hard contact lens = -2.00 D

Change in Refraction = -2.00 - (+0.25) = -2.25 D (myopic shift)

Mean Corneal Power = Base Curve of Plano HCL + Change in Refraction

Mean Corneal Power = 35.00 + -2.25

Mean Corneal Power = 32.75 D

This method is limited by the accuracy of the refractions which may be limited by the cataract.

Corneal Topography

Current corneal topography units measure more than 5000 points over the entire cornea and more than 1000 points within the central 3 mm. This additional information provides greater accuracy in determining the power of corneas with irregular astigmatism compared to keratometers. The computer in topography units allows the measurement to account for the Stiles-Crawford effect, actual pupil size, etc. These algorithms allow a very accurate determination of the anterior surface of the cornea. They provide no information, however, about the posterior surface of the cornea. In order to accurately determine the total power of the cornea, the power of both surfaces must be known.

In normal corneas that have not undergone keratorefractive surgery, the posterior radius of curvature of the cornea averages 1.2 mm less than the anterior surface.[17] In a person with an anterior corneal radius of 7.5 mm using the Standardized Keratometric Index of Refraction of 1.3375, the corneal power would be 45.00 D. Several studies have shown that this power overestimates the total power of the cornea by approximately 0.56 D. Hence, most IOL calculations today used a net index of refraction of 1.3333 (4/3) and the anterior radius of the cornea to calculate the net power of the cornea.

Using this lower value, the total power of a cornea with an anterior radius of 7.5 mm would be 44.44 D. This index of refraction has provided excellent results in normal corneas for IOL calculations.

Following keratorefractive surgery, the assumptions that the central cornea can be approximated by a sphere (no significant irregular astigmatism or asphericity) and that the posterior corneal radius of curvature is 1.2 mm less than the anterior radius are no longer true. Corneal topography instruments can account for the changes in the anterior surface, but are unable to account for any differences in the relationship to the posterior radius of curvature. In RK, the mechanism of having a peripheral bulge and central flattening apparently causes similar changes in both the anterior and posterior radius of curvature so that using the net index of refraction for the cornea (4/3) usually gives fairly accurate results, particularly for optical zones larger than 4 to 5 mm. In RKs with optical zones of 3 mm or less, the accuracy of the predicted corneal power diminishes. Whether this inaccuracy is due to the additional central irregularity with small optical zones or the difference in the relationship between the front and back radius of the cornea is unknown at this time. Studies measuring the posterior radius of the cornea in these patients will be necessary to answer this question.

In PRK and LASIK, the inaccuracies of these instruments to measure the net corneal power is almost entirely due to the change in the relationship of the radii of the front and back of the cornea, since the irregular astigmatism in the central 3 mm zone is usually minimal. In these two procedures, the anterior surface of the cornea is flattened with little or no effect on the posterior radius. Using a net index of refraction (4/3) will overestimate the power of cornea by 14% of the change induced by the PRK or LASIK, i.e. if patient had a 7 D change in the refraction at the corneal plane from a PRK or LASIK with spherical preoperative Ks of 44 D, the actual power of the cornea is 37 D and the topography units will give 38 D. If a 14 D change in the refraction has occurred at the corneal plane, the topography units will overestimate the power of the cornea by 2 diopters.

In summary, the corneal topography units do not provide accurate central corneal power following PRK, LASIK and in RKs with optical zones of 3 mm or less. In RKs with larger optical zones the topography units become more reliable. The calculation method and hard contact lens trial are always more reliable.

Automated Keratometry

Automated keratometers are usually more accurate than manual keratometers in corneas with small optical zone (≤ 3 mm) RKs because they sample a smaller central area of the cornea (nominally 2.6 mm). In addition, the automated instruments often have additional eccentric fixation targets that provide more information about the paracentral cornea. When a measurement error on an RK cornea is made, the instrument almost always gives a central corneal power that is greater than the true refractive power of the cornea. This error occurs because the samples at 2.6 mm are very close to the paracentral knee of the RK. The smaller the optical zone and the greater the number of the RK incisions, the greater the probability and magnitude of the error. Most of the automated instruments have reliability factors that are given for each measurement helping the clinician decide on the reliability in the measurement.

Automated keratometry measurements following LASIK or PRK yield accurate measurements of the front radius of the cornea because the transition areas are far outside the 2.6 mm zone that is measured. The measurements are still not accurate, however, because the assumed net index of refraction (4/3) is no longer appropriate for the new relationship of the front and back radius of the cornea after PRK or LASIK, just as with the topographic instruments. The change in central corneal power as measured by the keratometer from PRK or LASIK must be increased by 14% to determine the actual refractive change at the plane of the cornea. Hence, the automated keratometer will overestimate the power of the cornea proportional to the amount of PRK or LASIK performed.

Manual Keratometry

Manual keratometers are the least accurate in measuring central corneal power following keratorefractive procedures, because the area that they measure is usually larger than automated at 3.2 mm in diameter. Therefore, measurements in this area are extremely unreliable for RK corneas with optical zones ≤ 4 mm. The one advantage with the manual keratometer is that the examiner is actually able to see the reflected mires and the amount of irregularity present. Seeing the mires does not help get a better measurement, but does allow the observer to discount the measurement as unreliable.

The manual keratometer has the same problem with PRK and LASIK as topographers and automated keratometers, and is therefore no less accurate. The manual keratometer will overestimate the change in the central refractive power of the cornea by 14% following PRK and LASIK.

Choosing the Desired Postoperative Refraction Target

Determining the desired postoperative refractive target is no different than in other patients with cataracts in which the refractive status and the presence of a cataract in the other eye are the major determining factors. A complete discussion of avoiding refractive problems with cataract surgery is beyond the scope of this text, and is thoroughly discussed in the reference given.[18] A short discussion of the major factors will follow.

If the patient has binocular cataracts, the decision is much easier because the refractive status of both eyes can be changed. The most important decision is whether the patient prefers to be myopic and read without glasses, or near emmetropic and drive without glasses. In some cases the surgeon and patient may choose the intermediate distance (-1.00 D) for the best compromise. Targeting for monovision is certainly acceptable, provided the patient has successfully utilized monovision in the past. Trying to produce monovision in a patient who has never experienced this condition may cause intolerable anisometropia and require further surgery.

Monocular cataracts allow fewer choices for the desired postoperative refraction, because the refractive status of the other eye is fixed. The general rule is that the operative eye must be within 2 D of the non-operative eye in order to avoid intolerable anisometropia. In most cases this means matching the other eye or targeting for up to 2 D nearer emmetropia, i.e. if the unoperative eye is -5.00 D, then the target would be -3.00 D for the operative eye. If the patient is successfully wearing a contact in the unoperative eye or has already demonstrated his ability to accept monovision, then an exception can be made to the general rule. However, should the patient be unable to continue wearing a contact, the necessary glasses for binocular correction may be intolerable and additional refractive surgery may be required.

Special Limitations of Intraocular Lens Power Calculation Formulas

As discussed previously, the third generation formulas (Holladay 1, Hoffer Q and the SRK/T) and the new Holladay 2 are much more accurate than previous formulas for the more unusual the eye. Older formulas such as the SRK1, SRK2 and Binkhorst 1 should not be used in these cases. None of these formulas will give the desired result if the central corneal power is measured incorrectly. The resulting errors are almost always in the hyperopic direction following keratorefractive surgery, because the measured corneal powers are usually greater than the true refractive power of the cornea.

To further complicate matters, the newer formulas often use keratometry as one of the predictors to estimate the effective lens position (*ELP*) of the intraocular lens. In patients who have had keratorefractive surgery, the corneal power is usually much flatter than normal and certainly flatter than before the keratorefractive procedure. In short, a patient with a 38 D cornea without keratorefractive surgery would not be expected to be similar to a patient with a 38 D cornea with keratorefractive surgery. Newer IOL calculation programs are now being developed to handle these situations and will improve our predictability in these cases.

Intraoperative Visualization and Corneal Protection

Intraoperative visualization is usually more difficult in patients with previous RK than in the normal cataract patient and is somewhat similar to severe arcus senilis or other conditions that cause peripheral corneal haze. The surgeon should be prepared for this additional difficulty by making sure that the patient is lined up to visualize the cataract through the optical zone. This usually means lining the microscope perpendicular to the center of the cornea, so that the surgeon is looking directly through the optical zone at the center of the cataract. When removing the peripheral cortex, the eye can be rotated so that visualization of the periphery is through the central optical zone. It is also prudent to coat the endothelium with viscoelastic to minimize any endothelial cell loss, since the keratorefractive procedure may have caused some prior loss.

Intraoperative Autorefractor/Retinoscopy

Large refractive surprises can be avoided by intraoperative retinoscopy or hand-held autorefractors. These refractions should not be relied upon, however, for fine-tuning the intraocular lens power since there are many factors at surgery that may change in the postoperative period. Factors such as the pressure from the lid speculum, axial position of the intraocular lens, intraocular pressure, etc. may cause the intraoperative refraction to be different than the final stabilized postoperative refraction. If the intraoperative refraction is within 2 D of the target refraction, no lens exchanges should be considered unless intraoperative keratometry can also be performed.

Postoperative Evaluation

Refraction on the First Postoperative Day

On the first postoperative day following cataract surgery, patients who previously have had RK usually have a hyperopic shift, similar to the first postoperative day following their RK. This phenomenon is primarily due to the transient corneal edema that usually exaggerates the RK effect. These patients also exhibit the same daily fluctuations during the early postoperative period after their cataract surgery as they did after the RK. Usually this daily shift is in a myopic direction during the day due to the regression of corneal edema after awakening in the morning.[19] Because the refractive changes are expected and vary significantly among patients, no lens exchange should be contemplated until after the first postoperative week or until after the refraction has stabilized, whichever is longer.

Very few results of cataract surgery following PRK and LASIK are available. In the few cases that have been performed, the hyperopic shift on the first day and daily fluctuations appear to be much less, similar to the early postoperative period following these procedures. In most cases the stability of the cornea makes these cases no different than patients who have not had keratorefractive surgery.

Long-term Results

Long-term results of cataract surgery following RK are very good. The long-term hyperopic shifts and development of against-the-rule astigmatism over time following cataract surgery should be the same as in the long-term studies following RK. The problems with glare and starburst patterns are usually minimal because the patients have had to adjust to these unwanted optical images following the initial RK. If the patient's primary complaint before cataract surgery is glare and starbursts, it should be made clear to the patient that only the glare due to the cataract will be removed by surgery, and the symptoms that are due to the RK will remain unchanged.

Long-term results following PRK and LASIK are nonex-

istent. Since there are no signs of hyperopic drifts or development of against-the-rule astigmatism in the 5 year studies following PRK, one would not expect to see these changes. However, the early studies following RK did not suggest any of these long-term changes either. Only time will tell whether central haze, irregular astigmatism, etc. will be problems that develop in the future.

IOL CALCULATIONS USING KS AND PREOPERATIVE REFRACTION

Formula and Rationale for Using Preoperative Refraction vs. Axial Length

In a standard cataract removal with IOL implantation, the preoperative refraction is not very helpful in calculating the power of the implant because the crystalline lens will be removed so dioptric power is being removed and then replaced. In cases where no power is being removed from the eye, such as secondary implant in aphakia, piggyback IOL in pseudophakia, or a minus IOL in the anterior chamber of a phakic patient, the necessary IOL power for a desired postoperative refraction can be calculated from the corneal power and preoperative refraction—the axial length is not necessary. The formula for calculating the necessary IOL power is given below[20]:

$$IOL = \cfrac{1336}{\cfrac{1336}{\cfrac{1000}{\cfrac{1000}{PreRx} - V} + K} - ELP} - \cfrac{1336}{\cfrac{1336}{\cfrac{1000}{\cfrac{1000}{DPostRx} - V} + K} - ELP}$$

where ELP = expected lens position in mm (distance from corneal vertex to principal plane of intraocular lens), IOL = intraocular lens power in diopters, K = net corneal power in diopters, PreRx = preoperative refraction in diopters, DPostRx = desired postoperative refraction in diopters, and V = vertex distance in mm of refraction.

Calculation From Preoperative Refraction

As mentioned above, the appropriate cases for using the preoperative refraction and corneal power include 1) secondary implant in aphakia, 2) secondary piggyback IOL in pseudophakia and 3) a minus anterior chamber IOL in a high myopic phakic patient. In each of these cases no dioptric power is being removed from the eye, so the problem is simply to find the intraocular lens at a given distance behind the cornea ELP that is equivalent to the spectacle lens at a given vertex distance in front of the cornea. If emmetropia is not desired, then an additional term, the desired postoperative refraction (DPostRx), must be included. The formulas for calculating the predicted refraction and the back-calculation of the effective lens position ELP are given in the reference and will not be repeated here.[20]

Example: Secondary Implant for Aphakia

The patient is 72 years old and is aphakic in the right eye and pseudophakic in the left eye. The right eye can no longer tolerate an aphakic contact lens. The capsule in the right eye is intact and a posterior chamber intraocular lens is desired. The patient is -0.50 D in the left eye and would like to be the same in the right eye.

Mean Keratometric K = 45.00 D
Aphakic Refraction = +12.00 sphere @ vertex of 14 mm
Manufacturers ACD Lens Constant = 5.25 mm
Desired Postoperative Refraction = -0.50 D

Each of the values above can be substituted in the refraction formula above except for the Manufacturers ACD and the measured K-reading. The labeled values on intraocular lens boxes are primarily for lenses implanted in the bag. Since this lens is intended for the sulcus, 0.25 mm should be subtracted from 5.25 mm to arrive at the equivalent constant for the sulcus. The *ELP* is therefore 5.00 mm. The K-reading must be converted from the measured keratometric K-reading (n = 1.3375) to the net K-reading (n = 4/3), for the reasons described previously under corneal topography. The conversion is performed by multiplying the measured K-reading by the following fraction:

$$Fraction = \frac{(4/3)-1}{1.3375-1} = \frac{1/3}{0.3375} = 0.98765$$

Mean Refractive K = Mean Keratometric K * Fraction
Mean Refractive K = 45.00 * 0.98765 = 44.44 D

Using the Mean Refractive K, aphakic refraction, vertex distance, *ELP* for the sulcus, and the desired postoperative refraction, the patient needs a 22.90 D IOL. A 23 D intraocular lens would yield a predicted refraction of -0.57 D.[20]

Example: Secondary PiggyBack IOL for Pseudophakia

In patients with a significant residual refractive error following the primary intraocular lens implant, it is often easier surgically and more predictable optically to leave the primary implant in place and calculate the secondary piggyback intraocular lens power to achieve the desired refraction. This method does not require knowledge of the power of the primary implant nor the axial length. This method is particularly important in cases where the primary implant is thought to be mislabeled. The formula works for plus or minus lenses, but negative lenses are just becoming available at this time.

The patient is 55 years old and had a refractive surprise after the primary cataract surgery and was left with a +5.00 D spherical refraction in the right eye. There is no cataract in the left eye and he is plano. The surgeon and the patient both desire him to be -0.50 D, which was the target for the primary implant. The refractive surprise is felt to be from a mislabeled intraocular lens, which is centered in-the-bag and would be very difficult to remove. The secondary piggyback intraocular lens will be placed in the sulcus, since trying to place the second lens in-the-bag several weeks after the primary surgery is very difficult. More importantly, it may displace the primary lens posteriorly, reducing its effective power and leaving the patient with a hyperopic error. Placing the lens in the sulcus minimizes this posterior displacement.

Mean Keratometric K = 45.00 D
Pseudophakic Refraction = +5.00 sphere @ vertex of 14 mm
Manufacturers ACD Lens Constant = 5.25 mm
Desired Postoperative Refraction = -0.50 D

Using the same style lens and constant as the previous example and modifying the K-reading to net power, the formula yields a +8.64 D intraocular lens for a -0.50 D target. The nearest available lens is +9.0 D which would result in -0.76 D. In these cases extreme care should be taken to assure that the two lenses are well centered with respect to one another. Decentration of either lens can result in poor image quality and can be the limiting factor in the patient's vision.

Example: Primary Minus Anterior Chamber IOL in a High Myopic Phakic Patient

The calculation of a minus intraocular lens in the anterior chamber is no different than the aphakic calculation of an anterior chamber lens, except the power of the lens is negative. In the past these lenses have been reserved for high myopia that could not be corrected by RK or PRK. Since most of these lenses fixate in the anterior chamber angle, concerns of iritis and glaucoma have been raised. Nevertheless, several successful cases have been performed with good refractive results. Because successful LASIK procedures have been performed in myopias up to -20.00 D, these lenses may be reserved for myopia exceeding this power in the future. Interestingly, the power of the negative anterior chamber implant is very close to the spectacle refraction for normal vertex distances.

Mean Keratometric K = 45.00 D
Phakic Refraction = -20.00 sphere @ vertex of 14 mm
Manufacturers ACD Lens Constant = 3.50 mm
Desired Postoperative Refraction = -0.50 D

Using an *ELP* of 3.50 and modifying the K-reading to net corneal power yields -18.49 D for a desired refraction of -0.50 D. If a -19.00 D lens is used, the patient would have a predicted postoperative refraction of -0.10 D.

REFERENCES

1. Holladay JT, Prager TC, Ruiz RS, Lewis JW. Improving the predictability of intraocular lens calculations. *Archives of Ophthalmology* 1986; 104:539-541.
2. Holladay JT, Prager TC, Chandler TY, Musgrove KH, Lewis JW, Ruiz RS. A three-part system for refining intraocular lens power calculations. *J Cataract and Refract Surg* 1988; 13:17-24.
3. Fedorov SN, Kolinko AI, Kolinko AI: Estimation of optical power of the intraocular lens. *Vestnk Oftalmol* 1967; 80:27-31.

4. Fyodorov SN, Galin MA, Linksz A. A calculation of the optical power of intraocular lenses. *Invest Ophthalmol* 1975; 14:625-628.

5. Binkhorst CD. Power of the prepupillary pseudophakos. *Br J Ophthalmol* 1972; 56:332-337.

6. Colenbrander MC. Calculation of the power of an iris clip lens for distant vision. *Br J Ophthalmol* 1973;57:735-740.

7. Binkhorst RD. The optical design of intraocular lens implants. *Ophthalmic Surg* 1975; 6:17-31.

8. van der Heijde GL. The optical correction of unilateral aphakia. *Trans Am Acad Ophthalmol Otolaryngol* 1976; 81:80-88.

9. Thijssen JM. The emmetropic and the iseikonic implant lens: computer calculation of the refractive power and its accuracy. *Ophthalmologica* 1975; 171:467-486.

10. Fritz KJ. Intraocular lens power formulas. *Am J Ophthalmol* 1981; 91:414-415.

11. Binkhorst RD. *Intraocular lens power calculation manual. A guide to the author's TI 58/59 IOL Power Module.* 2nd ed, New York, Richard D Binkhorst, 1981.

12. Olsen T, Corydon L, Gimbel H. Intraocular lens power calculation with an improved anterior chamber depth prediction algorithm. *J Cataract Refract Surg* 1995, 21:313-319.

13. Holladay JT, Gills JP, Leidlein J, Cherchio M: Achieving emmetropia in extremely short eyes with two piggy-back posterior chamber intraocular lenses. *Ophthalmology* 103:1118-1123, July, 1996.

14. Retzlaff JA, Sanders DR, Kraff MC. Development of the SRK/T intraocular lens implant power calculation formula. *J Cataract Refract Surg* 1990; 16:333-340.

15. Hoffer KJ. The Hoffer Q formula: A comparison of theoretic and regression formulas. *J Cataract Refract Surg* 1993, 19:700-712.

16. Holladay JT. IOL Calculations following RK. *Refractive and Corneal Surgery Journal* 1989, 5(3):203.

17. Lowe RF, Clark BA: Posterior Corneal Curvature. *Br J Ophthal* 1973, 57:464-470.

18. Holladay JT, Rubin ML: Avoiding refractive problems in cataract surgery. *Survey of Ophthalmology* 1988, 32(5):357-360.

19. Holladay JT. Management of hyperopic shift after RK. *Refractive and Corneal Surgery Journal* 1992, 8:325.

20. Holladay JT. Refractive power calculations for intraocular lenses in the phakic eye. *Am J Ophthalmol* 1993, 116:63-66.

Nd:YAG Laser Capsulotomy

CHAPTER 16

Robert G. Martin, MD, Manus C. Kraff, MD, Marsha Raanan, MS

Opacification of the posterior capsule (PCO) following extracapsular cataract surgery remains the single most frequent postoperative sequelae among pseudophakic patients. The consequent visual loss necessitates subsequent Nd:YAG capsulotomy. Despite the recognized efficacy and safety of YAG laser capsulotomy, it is nonetheless a secondary procedure with added costs and additional risks to the patient. Risks include IOL damage, IOL subluxation, retinal detachment, glaucoma and CME. Most current risk assessments focus on retinal detachment.

Current discussions of the use of newer IOL materials and their relative YAG rates indicate the high degree of concern over the rate of YAG capsulotomy. Furthermore, managed care environments put pressure on surgeons to lower and/or "justify" the need for subsequent surgical procedures. The purpose of this chapter is to provide a general overview of the current rate estimates of YAG capsulotomy among the newer IOL materials and styles compared with PMMA and to review the efficacy and safety of the YAG procedure in the current surgical environment.

The etiology of posterior capsule opacification following extracapsular cataract extraction is not fully understood. However, it is generally described as a cellular response of lens epithelial cells to various stimuli associated with the surgical procedure: contact with the IOL, surgical trauma, and the dynamics of the capsular bag surrounding the IOL following surgery. The cells migrate to the posterior capsule, where they may form Elschnig pearl clusters or fibrosis leading to opacification of the capsule. The development of posterior capsular opacity is affected by IOL design, IOL fixation within the eye, and the IOL material.[1-8] One-piece biconvex IOLs have been shown to result in lower YAG rates. Bag-fixation of the IOL decreases the YAG rate as well. This effect of design and placement results from the IOL having maxi-

mal contact with the capsule, creating a barrier to the proliferation and migration of cells.

Since the lens epithelial cell response to contact with the IOL causes cell proliferation, increasing biocompatibility of the IOL should be beneficial. However, the relative effects of IOL design and material on incidence of capsular opacity are not yet well documented. There are few published long-term studies of silicone IOLs, and acrylic IOLs have only recently been approved in the U.S.

ESTIMATED RATES OF ND:YAG CAPSULOTOMY

PMMA

Reported rates of Nd:YAG capsulotomy among PMMA IOL cases range from about 15% to 40% depending on the length of follow-up.[1-4,9,10] One of the authors (RGM) previously reported a study of the clinical outcomes of 600 various PMMA IOL styles.[5] The 3-year rate of YAG capsulotomy for one-piece biconvex lenses was 25%. This rate agrees with the 3-year YAG rate of other large scale studies.[9,10]

Silicone

One of the authors (RGM) is conducting a long-term follow-up study of plate-haptic silicone IOLs (STAAR models AA4203 and AA4203F). YAG capsulotomy had been performed in 25% of the overall group of cases at the time of this evaluation (1-year follow-up). Survival analysis methods were used to adjust for case-to-case differences in length of follow-up. The rates were 24.3% of F-series cases and 25.1% of non-F IOLs (Figure 16-1). In a previously reported series (presented at the 1996 annual meeting of the ASCRS), Martin and Mincie also found the YAG rate of silicone plate-haptic IOLs to be in this range (26%).

Figure 16-1. Survival plot of the cumulative probability over time of not requiring YAG capsulotomy. The red curve represents probabilities for Staar model AA4203F IOLs which have larger positioning holes to enhance fixation of the IOL. The green curve represents probabilities among the model AA4203 IOL with smaller positioning holes (Martin).

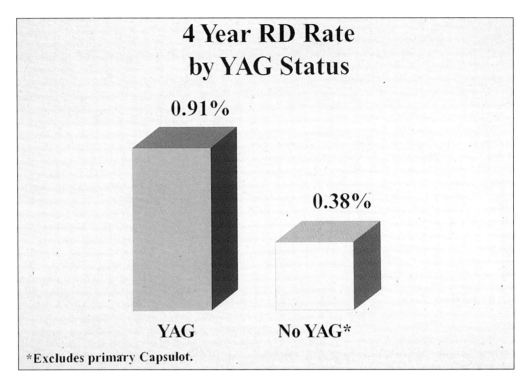

There have not been many studies reporting direct comparisons of YAG rates among PMMA, silicone, and acrylic IOLs. Comparative studies are important because YAG rates are influenced not just by the IOL material, design and placement, but by the decision criteria used to schedule the procedure. Presumably YAG capsulotomy is performed based on significant decrease in vision or presence of visual disturbances. However, these criteria can differ somewhat by practice due to demographic factors and access to the laser, etc.

In the current IOL surgical environment we operate on cataracts sooner due to the decreasing risk-to-benefit ratio. In an outcomes analysis of cases submitted under the American Board of Eye Surgery IOL Certification program (presented at the 1995 annual meeting of the American College of Eye Surgeons, Fort Lauderdale, FL), preoperative visions were worse among cases having surgery prior to 1988 compared with cases operated on subsequently. Expectations of good vision have increased as the efficacy and predictability of good outcome has improved. Patients and surgeons want visual loss due to PCO corrected.

Mammalis and coauthors[1] reported the results of a comparative study of one-piece plate-haptic silicone IOLs and three-piece silicone IOLs. The rate of YAG capsulotomy was 39% for the three-piece silicone IOL (AMO modified c-loop silicone lens) and 30% for the plate-haptic silicone IOL (STAAR AA4203). Average follow-up was 18 months. The YAG procedures were performed significantly longer after IOL implantation in the three-piece group.

One of the authors (MCK) evaluated the rate of YAG capsulotomy in his initial series of 200 plate haptic silicone (STAAR AA4203) IOLs 1 year after FDA approval of the lens.

He compared the rate with a series of 400 PMMA cases performed just prior to initiating the silicone series. One-year YAG rates were compared to adjust for the longer follow-up among the PMMA cases. The overall rate of YAG capsulotomy was greater among PMMA cases. The time between IOL surgery and the YAG procedure was significantly longer among the silicone cases (only 1 case prior to a year), compared with PMMA cases (over half performed by 8 months).

Acrylic IOLs

Oshika and co-authors reported YAG rates of acrylic IOLs to be 11.1 percent at 2 years of follow-up.[11] They reported less aqueous flare among acrylic IOL cases than among PMMA or silicone lenses. One of the authors (RGM) is conducting a randomized prospective study of acrylic and plate-haptic silicone IOLs (see Chapter 12) and has not observed early postoperative differences in aqueous flare or cells between acrylic and silicone IOLs.

Gayton has reported the results of a retrospective comparison[12] of 100 three-piece acrylic IOLs (Alcon AcrySof®) with 100 three-piece silicone (STAAR Elastimide) matched on age, sex, and date of surgery. All patients were examined at 1 year or contacted to determine the status of the capsule. The 1-year YAG rate was 29% in the Elastimide group and 9% in the acrylic group. Life-Table methods were used to adjust for individual differences in follow-up. The difference in YAG rates was statistically significant. Gayton also observed that the time between IOL surgery and YAG capsulotomy was longer for Elastimide cases.

While the study showed a reduction in YAG rate for acrylic versus silicone, no conclusions can be drawn regarding

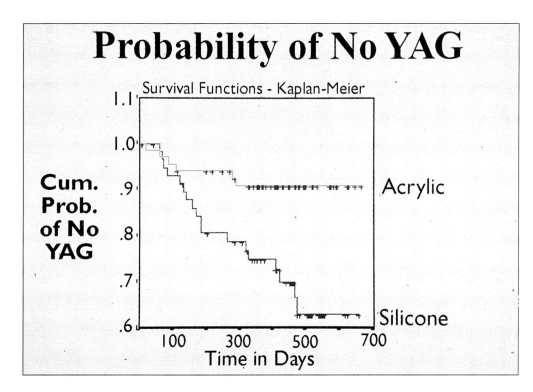

Probability of No YAG

Survival Functions - Kaplan-Meier

Cum. Prob. of No YAG

Acrylic

Silicone

Time in Days

Figure 16-2. Survival plot of the cumulative probability over time of not requiring YAG capsulotomy. The pink curve represents probabilities for the 3-piece Staar Elastimide model IOL. The green curve represents probabilities among the Alcon Acrysof three-piece IOL (courtesy of Johnny Gayton, MD).

acrylic versus all silicone lenses, because design factors into the rate as well. In the Gayton study, the groups were equivalent in terms of design, as both were three-piece lenses. However, it appears that the three-piece Elastimide lens has a higher YAG rate than the plate-haptic silicone IOL. As there are no studies comparing AcrySof with the plate-haptic silicone lens, it is not known which factor, lens design or material, impacts more on the YAG rate.

EFFICACY OF YAG CAPSULOTOMY

The expected rates of PCO and subsequent YAG capsulotomy are not yet clear as we move more and more to foldable IOLs and more biocompatible materials. Nevertheless even if the rate of PCO is significantly decreased to 10%-15%, there will still be significant numbers of these procedures each year.

In debates over YAG rates and the rates of post-YAG complications, we must remember to reassess the risk-to-benefit ratio of this procedure. The fact that YAG capsulotomy is very safe and has an extremely beneficial effect on final postoperative outcome is often overlooked.

One of the authors (RGM) conducted a study of the outcomes of YAG capsulotomy. The study was undertaken to document the benefits to the patient of the YAG capsulotomy in a broad sense.

Subjects and Methods

The study was carried out in an outpatient ambulatory surgical center. A sequential cohort of 200 post-cataract surgery patients who were scheduled for Nd:YAG capsulotomy were enrolled into the study with no exclusions based on patholo-

gy. Patients were of either sex and were between 55 and 85 years of age. Only one eye from each patient (the first eye to be scheduled for the YAG procedure) was used in the study. The only exclusion criterion was previous ocular surgery in the study eye other than the earlier cataract procedure.

Prior to the YAG procedure, each patient was given a comprehensive baseline visual examination. Included in the exam were uncorrected visual acuity, refraction, best-corrected visual acuity, contrast sensitivity evaluation (Multicontrast Vision Tester), and glare testing (BAT). Each patient also completed a questionnaire at that time to evaluate the patient's personal impression of visual function indoors and outdoors, visual disturbance, satisfaction level, and impact of vision on lifestyle. The questionnaire was designed to elicit information concerning visual function at near and far distances, in dim and bright settings, and for daily living and recreational activities. Some items required a "yes or no" response but most asked for responses chosen from a four-point scale (none, mild, moderate, severe). Patients were also directly asked about specific visual symptoms such as glare, halos, and decreased color brightness.

At the time of the pre-YAG examination, the level of posterior capsule opacification was graded as clear, mild, moderate, or severe. The uncorrected and best-corrected visual acuity achieved following the original cataract procedure was collected from the medical chart. These visions served as the baseline for measuring visual impairment due to the opacity prior to the YAG procedure.

Within a 1- to 2-month period following Nd:YAG capsulotomy, visual acuity, refraction, BAT glare, and Multicontrast Vision Tester vision were evaluated again. The

Figure 16-3. Scatterplot of best-achieved post-IOL corrected visual acuity versus pre-YAG corrected visual acuity. The numbers next to points indicate multiple observations (Martin).

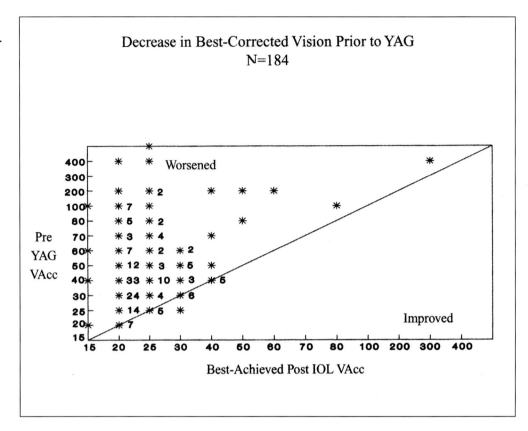

Figure 16-4. Percent of patients with perceived improvement in various visual symptoms following YAG capsulotomy (Martin).

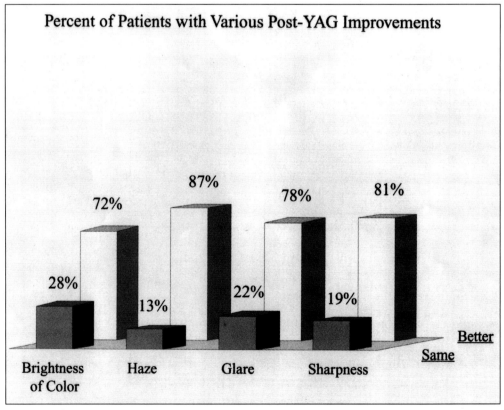

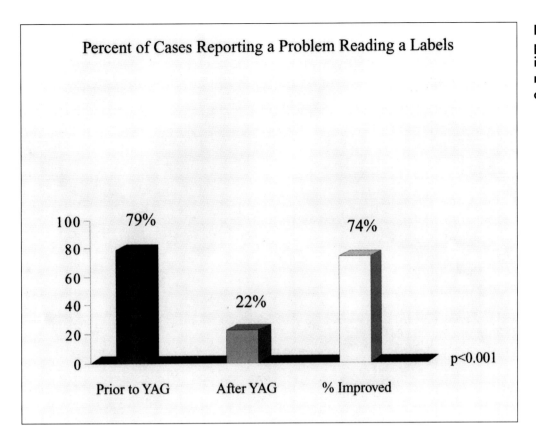

Figure 16-5. Percent of patients reporting improvement in ability to read labels following YAG capsulotomy (Martin).

patient was re-interviewed at that time using the original questionnaire but without reference to the original interview. In addition, patients were asked to assess the benefit of the YAG procedure.

Items on the questionnaire were tabulated to determine the percent of respondents choosing each level of function (0=none, 1=mild, 2=moderate, or 3=severe; or 0=never, 1=sometimes, 2=often, or 4=always) for a given item. In addition, pre-YAG scores were subtracted from post-YAG scores, item-by-item, to determine the percent of patients who reported improvement for a given item regardless of baseline level. Pre-YAG versus post-YAG results (percent improved versus percent not improved) were tested for significance using chi-square analysis with continuity correction.

Results

Completed questionnaires were obtained for 191 of the 200 patients enrolled in the study. Of these cases the majority (78%) were graded as having moderate opacity prior to the YAG procedure, 11% had severe opacity and 11% were graded as mild but were considered candidates for the procedure based on visual function and other criteria. Pre-YAG pathology other than the opacity included age-related macular degeneration (14.7%), diabetic retinopathy (3.7%), and cystoid macular edema (0.5%).

The decrease in best-corrected visual acuity as a result of the opacification in this cohort of patients is shown in Figure 16-3. In this figure, optimal best-corrected acuity just prior to

the YAG procedure is plotted against the best-corrected acuity achieved following the IOL surgery. With few exceptions, these patients experienced substantially diminished best-corrected vision. The points on the diagonal equivalency line represent those few patients whose lane-test vision did not worsen prior to the YAG procedure. However, all of these patients, in addition to the one patient with higher lane-measured vision, complained of glare, halos, haze, visual distortion, etc., and all had capsular opacities graded as moderate to severe.

On the questionnaire administered prior to the YAG procedure, patients were asked about the perceived changes in the quality of their vision. Almost 80% reported that their vision had worsened. Although some indicated that their vision had improved, all of these patients had lost more than a line of best-corrected visual acuity on examination and all reported other visual problems on their questionnaires.

Figure 16-4 summarizes how patients perceived changes in their vision following the YAG procedure. In all categories (brightness of color, haze, glare, and image sharpness), a substantial majority of patients reported improvements. To further refine these subjective appraisals of vision by patients, we evaluated their responses to a number of questions related to some practical aspects of daily living. The "percent improvement" was determined, which represents the proportion of patients who reported improvement for a given visual function item regardless of the baseline level of function. The perceived quality of post-YAG vision was substantially improved among these patients for many items, including label reading (Figure

Figure 16-6. Percent of patients reporting improvement in ability to read the newspaper following YAG capsulotomy (Martin).

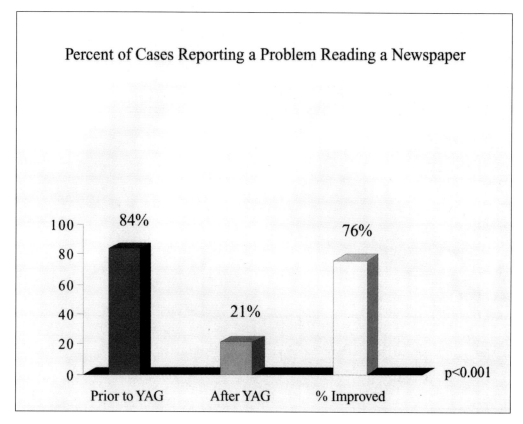

Percent of Cases Reporting a Problem Reading a Newspaper

Prior to YAG: 84%
After YAG: 21%
% Improved: 76%
p<0.001

Figure 16-7. Percent of patients able to see clearly across the street at dusk and during the day before and after YAG capsulotomy (Martin).

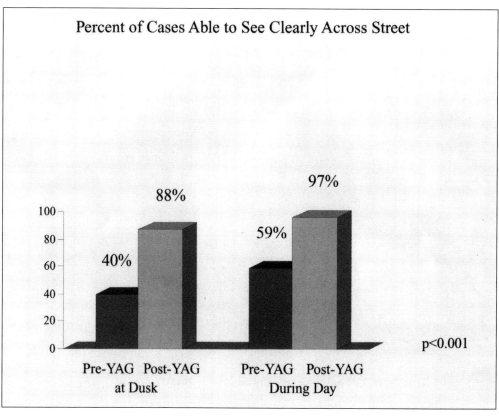

Percent of Cases Able to See Clearly Across Street

Pre-YAG at Dusk: 40%
Post-YAG at Dusk: 88%
Pre-YAG During Day: 59%
Post-YAG During Day: 97%
p<0.001

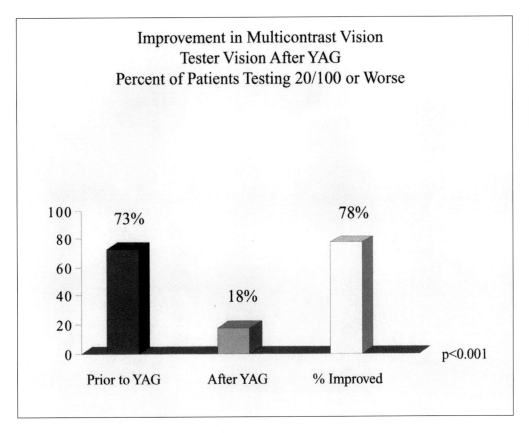

16-5), reading newspapers (Figure 16-6), and seeing across the street at daylight and at dusk (Figure 16-7). Patients also showed improvements in contrast sensitivity testing (Figure 16-8). Pre-YAG visual clarity problems were sharply reduced (Figure 16-9), and there was a dramatic improvement in comfort level for night driving (Figure 16-10).

The lane-measured best-corrected vision probably demonstrates efficacy most dramatically. In Figure 16-11 the post-YAG best-corrected visions are plotted versus the pre-YAG corrected vision. With few exceptions the patients showed marked improvement, many by very large amounts. Those few patients whose lane-tested vision did not improve still increased in functional vision as measured by glare testing, contrast sensitivity testing, or by subjective perception.

Summary of Study

This study demonstrated the magnitude of the benefits achieved by YAG capsulotomy for patients developing PCO following surgery. In our experience, the 4-year rate of opacity requiring YAG capsulotomy is about 25% among cases with one-piece PMMA IOLs and may be nearly as high among silicone IOLs. Thus roughly a quarter of patients will experience the level of decreased vision shown in Figure 16-3 within 2 to 4 years after cataract surgery. To restore and maintain the improved vision gained through cataract extraction to this large number of patients is a benefit that surpasses by far the very small rates of post-YAG complications.

RISK OF RETINAL DETACHMENT FOLLOWING ND:YAG CAPSULOTOMY

The most significant reported risk following YAG capsulotomy is retinal detachment (RD). However, our own work and other studies suggest that this risk remains small and to a large degree is associated with other factors; namely long axial length, younger age at the time of cataract surgery and, to a lesser extent, male sex. Even among these higher-risk patients such as long-eye patients, the risk of RD is certainly at or under 3% by all accounts even among older studies.

One of the authors (MCK) conducted a retrospective study of 3608 PMMA cases, determining the status of the capsule and rate of RD throughout a 4-year follow-up period. When the RD rate was compared between cases that had undergone YAG capsulotomy, and cases with intact capsules (Figure 16-12), the rate was found to be over twice as high (0.91% vs 0.38%). However, when these groups were stratified by axial length, the rate differences between open and intact cases was much reduced (Figure 16-13). Significantly higher risk of RD was associated with cases with very long axial lengths.

One of the authors (RGM) conducted a retro-prospective study of 500 cases which had undergone YAG capsulotomy comparing them with 500 matched controls (cases with intact capsules but matched by axial length (within 3 ordinal levels) and week of surgery). Each case was followed forward by medical chart. If the patient had not been seen within a month of the study initiation, the information on YAG status and

Figure 16-9. Improvement in visual clarity following YAG capsulotomy (Martin).

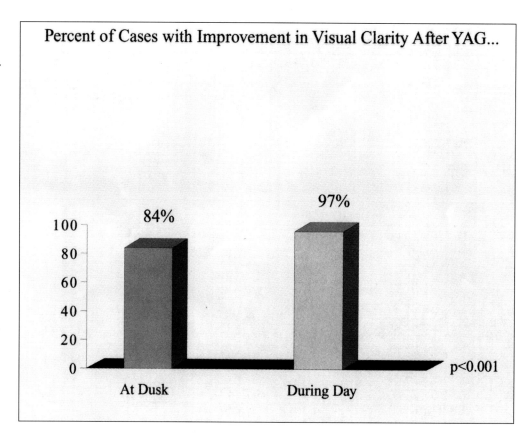

Figure 16-10. Improvement in night driving comfort level following YAG capsulotomy (Martin).

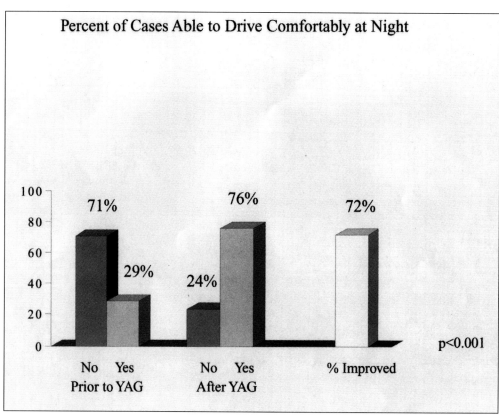

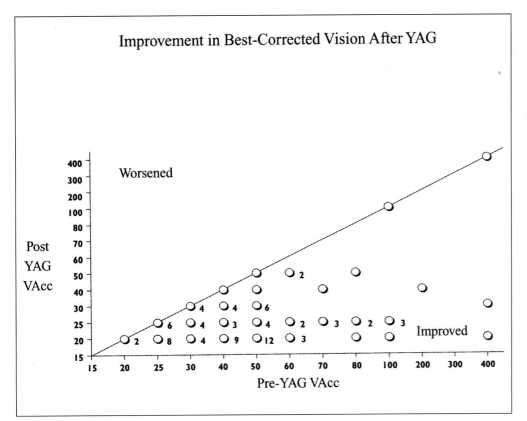

Figure 16-11. Scatterplot of pre-YAG best-corrected visual acuity versus post-YAG corrected acuity. The numbers next to points indicate multiple observations (Martin).

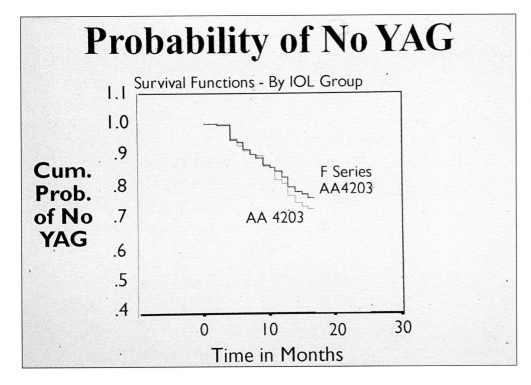

Figure 16-12. Four-year retinal detachment rate among PMMA cases that did (blue bar) and did not (yellow bar) receive YAG capsulotomy (Kraff).

Figure 16-13. Four-year retinal detachment rate among PMMA cases that did (blue bar) and did not (yellow bar) receive YAG capsulotomy, stratified by axial length. Front bars represent average axial length (below 24 mm), middle bars represent longer axial lengths (24-26 mm), and back bars represent very long axial lengths (>= 27 mm) (Kraff).

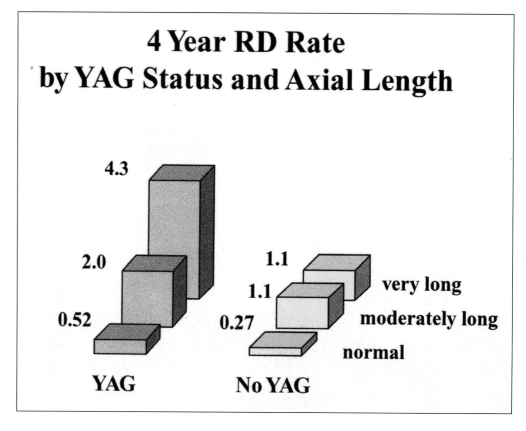

4 Year RD Rate by YAG Status and Axial Length

TABLE 16-1

REPORTED RATES OF RETINAL DETACHMENT FOLLOWING ND:YAG CAPSULOTOMY

Author	Number of Cases	Rate of RD
Coonan et al1[3]	95	3.2%
Flicker et al1[4]	582	2.0%
Dardenne et al1[5]	1000	1.6%
Javitt et al[9]	13,709	1.6%
Rickman-Barger et al[16]	397	1.6%
Van Westenbrugge, Gimbel, et al[17]	218	0.9%
Kraff (reported herein)	774	0.9%
Nielson, Naeser, et al[10]	345	0.29%
Martin (reported herein)	500	0.2%

occurrence of RD, retinal tears, or holes was determined by phone interview with the patient, a referring caregiver, or a family surrogate. The cohorts were chosen such that the potential post-surgical follow-up time was 3 years.

Of the 1,000 cases in the study, 6 experienced retinal detachment; 1 from the YAG group and 5 from the control group. The overall rate (unadjusted for differing follow-up) was 0.60% overall, 0.20% among YAG cases, and 1.0% among the controls. The number of events was too small to statistically compare the RD rates by life table analysis. However, among the cases of RD, mean age was lower and mean axial length was higher than in the overall group, reflecting the risk factors of younger age and higher axial length reported in other studies.

Various reported rates of RD following YAG capsulotomy are presented in Table 16-1. The rates in the Martin study are similar to other studies reported in the last 10 years. Retinal detachment, while serious, is a rare event for the average patient.

Newer IOL materials may effect a decrease in posterior capsular opacity rates. Nevertheless, YAG capsulotomy remains a safe and highly effective procedure to restore good vision among patients with posterior capsular opacity.

REFERENCES

1. Mammalis N, Phillips B, Kopp CH, et al. Neodymium:YAG capsulotomy rates after phacoemulsification with silicone posterior chamber intraocular lenses. *J Cataract Refract Surg* 1996; 22:1296-1302.
2. Miyake K. The significance of inflammatory reactions following cataract extraction and intraocular lens implantation. *J Cataract Refract Surg* 1996; 22:759-763.
3. Miyake K, Ota I, Miyake S, et al. Correlation between intraocular lens hydrophylicity and anterior capsule opacification and aqueous flare. *J Cataract Refract Surg* 1996; 22:764-769.
4. Born CP, Ryan DK. Effect of intraocular lens optic design on

posterior capsular opacification. *J Cataract Refract Surg* 1990; 16:188-192.

5. Martin RG, Sanders DR, Souchek J, Raanan MG, et al. Effect of posterior chamber intraocular lens design and surgical placement on postoperative outcome. *J Cataract Refract Surg* 1992; 18:333-341.

6. Frezzotti R, Caporossi A. Pathogenesis of posterior capsule opacification. Part I: epidemiological and clinical statistical data. *J Cataract Refract Surg* 1990; 16:347-352.

7. Frezzotti R, Caporossi A, Mastrangelo D, et al. Pathogenesis of posterior capsule opacification. Part II: histopathological and in-vitro culture findings. *J Cataract Refract Surg* 1990; 16:353-360.

8. Obstbaum SA. The posterior capsule. *Implants Ophthalmol* 1988; 2:110-116.

9. Javitt JC, Tielsch JM, Canner JK, Kolb MM, et al. National outcomes of cataract extraction-increased risk of retinal complications associated with Nd:YAG laser capsulotomy. *Ophthalmology* 1992; 99:1487-1498.

10. Nielsen NE, Naeser K. Epidemiology of retinal detachment following extracapsular cataract extraction: A follow-up study with an analysis of risk factors. *J Cataract Refract Surg* 1993; 19:675-680.

11. Oshiku T, Suzuki Y, Kizaki H, Yaguchi S. Two year clinical study of a soft acrylic intraocular lens. *J Cataract Refract Surg* 1996; 22:104-109.

12. Gayton J. A comparison of Alcon AcrySof with STAAR Elastimide IOLs. Presented at the 1997 annual meeting of the ASCRS, Boston, MA.

13. Coonan P, Fung WE, Webster RG, Allen AW, Abbott RL. The incidence of retinal detachment following extracapsular cataract extraction. *Ophthalmology* 1985; 92:1096-1101.

14. Flicker LA, Vickers S, Capon MR, Mellerio J, et al. Retinal detachment following Nd:YAG posterior capsulotomy. *Eye* 1987; 1:86-89.

15. Dardenne M-U, Gerten G-J, Kokkas K, Kermani O. Retrospective study of retinal detachment following Neodymium:YAG laser posterior capsulotomy. *J Cataract Refract Surg* 1989; 15:676-680.

16. Rickman-Barger L, Florine CW, Larson RS, Lindstrom RL. Retinal detachment after Neodymium:YAG laser posterior capsulotomy. *Am J Ophthalmol* 1989; 107:531-536.

17. Van Westenbrugge JA, Gimbel HV, Souchek J, Chow D. Incidence of retinal detachment following Nd:YAG laser capsulotomy after cataract surgery. *J Cataract Refract Surg* 1992; 18:352-355.

EXTENDING THE BENEFITS OF MODERN SURGICAL TECHNIQUE

Johnny L. Gayton, MD, Robert G. Martin, MD,
James P. Gills, MD, Michelle Van Der Karr

Although the majority of cataract patients today benefit from modern surgical technique, there are some patients who, due to some pre-existing pathology or need for combined surgery, do not receive the most advanced, minimally invasive cataract procedure. However, advances in technology and new combined procedures make micro-incision cataract surgery available to a growing range of patients who previously could not receive sutureless small incision surgery, or even phacoemulsification.

MANAGING THE PATIENT WITH FUCH'S DYSTROPHY

Protecting the Compromised Cornea with Viscoelastic

In the past Fuch's dystrophy has been considered a relative contraindication for phacoemulsification. Cataract patients with corneal decompensation, edema, and bullae were usually referred to a corneal specialist for transplants before proceeding with the cataract extraction. This group of patients received little or no benefit from the ever-improving small incision procedures because most had corneas which could not withstand the phacoemulsification.

For the last two or three years this author (JPG) has found that patients with Fuch's dystrophy actually tolerate the phacoemulsification procedure quite well if the technique is modified to provide maximum protection of the cornea with viscoelastic. When endothelial cell count is 1500 cells per mm^2 or less the following technique is used.

Technique

A scleral-tunnel incision is preferred for these patients and is definitely used if cell count is less than 1300 cells per mm^2. Reduced phaco power and lower flow are necessary to minimize trauma to the endothelium. Viscoelastic is added through the paracentesis port during the *earliest* stage of the phaco. The viscoelastic is added very frequently with frequency dependent upon the preoperative cell count (Table 17-1) and the presence of corneal edema. The viscoelastic I prefer is Vitrax®, which is one of the shorter-chain, lower molecular weight dispersive agents with high viscosity and longer retention. I believe it lasts longer in the eye than all other agents. However there are other viscoelastics with these characteristics (Table 17-2). While it is important to use a shorter-chain dispersive viscoelastic, the frequency of application is more important. With frequent injection the anterior chamber can be kept sufficiently deepened at all times to protect the endothelium.

When the cell count is 700 cells per mm^2, viscoelastic is injected so frequently (every 2-3 seconds) that it is helpful to use the viscoelastic cannula as the secondary instrument during the phacoemulsification (Figure 17-1).

Postoperative Management

Because a short-chain viscoelastic agent with high retention is used it is difficult to remove, and the patient must be carefully monitored during the perioperative period. Most will experience an IOP spike to some degree. If necessary a paracentesis through the sideport incision may be performed to immediately lower the IOP.

Pred Forte® and sodium chloride ointments are administered (10 times) immediately after surgery. By saturating the cornea in this manner immediately postoperatively, early corneal edema is minimized. On the first postoperative day the medications are administered every hour. Subsequent medication is based on the appearance of the cornea

Clinical Results

I first used this technique in 50 cases who had Fuch's dystrophy and severe enough endothelial deficiency to have war-

TABLE 17-1
INJECTION FREQUENCY OF VISCOELASTIC

Cells Visualized Preoperatively	Injection Frequency During Phaco
<500 cells	Every 2 seconds
500-700 cells	Every 3 seconds
700-800 cells	Every 5 seconds
1000 cells	Every 8-10 seconds

ranted a corneal transplant. Of these 50 cases only 5 required a graft after cataract surgery.

Currently we enroll all Fuch's dystrophy patients into an ongoing study to monitor the clinical outcomes. Diagnosis criteria for the study are made on the basis of clinical appearance of the cornea, endothelial cell density, and central pachymetry. Surgical parameters collected include incision type, anesthesia, phaco time and power setting. The type of viscoelastic, volume and frequency of viscoelastic injection is recorded. The major clinical outcome parameters are the need for subsequent corneal transplant and serially measured postoperative endothelial cell counts. In Fuch's patients it is difficult to determine how much postoperative cell loss there is due to the uneven density of cells. Secondary measures include pachymetry and postoperative vision.

During the six month period between July 1, 1995 and December 31, 1995 106 cataractous eyes with Fuch's dystrophy and/or endothelial cell density of 1500 cells per mm² or less received phacoemulsification using the technique described above.

There were no serious complications in the early postoperative period. There were no uncontrollable IOP spikes. Mean IOP following surgery was 16.8 mmHg (standard deviation=7.8). The range of pressures was from 5 to 42 with only 2 cases above 30 mm Hg and 25% between 20 and 30 mmHg.

On the first postoperative day only 5% of eyes exhibited 1+ (trace) edema. Similarly, 95% patients had no anterior chamber reaction and 5% had only trace levels of flare or cells.

For the present analysis an attempt was made to contact patients who had not been examined recently by the author (JPG), to determine if a corneal graft had been performed elsewhere. Eighty percent of patients were contacted. Minimum follow-up of these cases to date has been 1.4 years and ranges to 2 years. Mean follow-up is 1.7 years. To date there have been no corneal transplants necessary during the average 1.7-year follow-up. Specular microscopy was available at 3 months or later (mean time of final endothelial cell count = 8.1 months) for half the patients. Mean preoperative cell density by specular microscopy was 1176 cells per mm² (range=500-1500, standard deviation=242) and mean postoperative cell density was 1128 cells per mm² (range=400-1500, standard deviation=268). Mean percent cell loss was 4.0%.

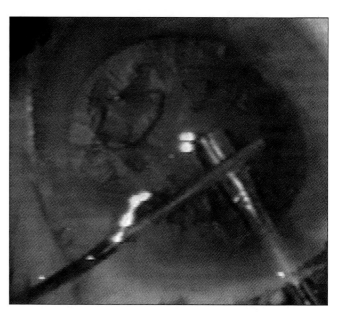

Figure 17-1. Injection of viscoelastic during phaco to protect the cornea (Gills).

Preoperative pachymetry was 0.55 (standard deviation=0.03) preoperatively and 0.58 postoperatively (standard deviation=0.04). At an average of 1.7 months postoperatively, 95.5% of cases had best corrected vision of 20/40 or better and 62% were 20/25 or better.

There was no statistically significant correlation between phacoemulsification time and endothelial cell loss. The same power and vacuum were used in all cases.

Reducing the Need for Combined Cataract/Corneal Transplant Procedures

The 106 patients in the series reported above have been able to avoid grafts and maintained good corrected vision for up to 2 years. All but 5 of our original group have not needed transplants. As we have optimized the cataract/IOL procedure for the majority of our patients we have been able to rethink some of our traditional practice patterns and extend the benefits of modern technique to groups of patients previously excluded due to complicated preoperative pathology. By reducing the risk to benefit ratio, we have been quite successful in this group.

COMBINED CATARACT AND GLAUCOMA PROCEDURES

Alternatives to Trabeculectomy

Patients with both glaucoma and cataract face the possibility of undergoing two separate invasive procedures, a cataract extraction and trabeculectomy. Performing both procedures at the same time is one way to reduce the morbidity. However, the patient must still undergo an invasive procedure

TABLE 17-2
A PARTIAL LIST OF SHORT-CHAIN VISCOELASTICS WITH HIGH RETENTION

Viscoelastic	Manufacturer	Properties
Vitrax® 3.0% sodium hyaluronate	Allergan Medical Optics	Short chain, lower molecular weight with high viscosity
Viscoat® 3% sodium hyaluronate and 4% chondroitin sulfate	Alcon Laboratories Inc.	Very short chain, low molecular weight, most dispersive
Ocucoat®	Storz Ophthalmics Inc.	Short Chain, low molecular weight, dispersive
Amvisc Plus® 1.6% sodium Hyaluronate	Chiron Vision	Still highly retentive but easier to remove

to treat the glaucoma in addition to the cataract extraction, which increases the possibility of complication.

Complications of a trabeculectomy include hyphema, cells in the anterior chamber, a shallow anterior chamber possibly with choroidal detachments, endophthalmitis, or suprachoroidal hemorrhage. Trabeculectomies often fail at some point as the eye heals itself, and have been known to be less successful in young eyes and those who produce large amounts of fibrous tissue.

Less invasive methods of surgically treating glaucoma that can be performed at the time of cataract surgery are now being explored. These procedures promise to simplify combined procedures, and further reduce morbidity and complications.

Cataract Surgery with Endoscopic Laser Cycloablation — Gayton Technique

A new endoscopic diode laser, the Microprobe, developed by Dr. Martin Uram and manufactured by Endo Optiks, Inc., may allow the surgeon to provide good control of glaucoma with less postoperative inflammation. The technique combines a self-sealing cataract incision and extraction procedure with cyclodestruction of the ciliary processes with the laser. The laser can be inserted within the phaco incision, which reduces the invasiveness of the combined procedure. The instrument permits extremely precise ablation and may avoid the complications associated with filtration procedures.

The endoscope laser has two basic components, the laser endoscope and the equipment console. The console contains the light source, video camera, video monitor, video recorder, and the diode laser, which is tuned to the 810-nm wavelength. Three fiber groupings, the image guide, the light guide, and the laser guide, are packaged into the endo-probe. The reusable 20-gauge probe with 0.89 cannula allows a 70-degree field of view with a depth of focus from 0.5 to 15 mm. This style is particularly helpful in phakic patients because of its small size. The 18-gauge probe allows a 110-degree field of view with a depth of focus from 1.0 to 30 mm. This probe permits greater image clarity and visualization. Both probes work equally well.

When performing endoscopic laser cycloablation, the surgeon must adjust to viewing the video monitor rather than the operating microscope. The surgical approach can be limbal or through the pars plana. The limbal approach is preferable unless an AC lens is present, because of the ease of construction of the limbal incision. Also, the limbal wound is easily decompressed should the patient experience a postoperative pressure rise.

Due to an early problem with immediate postoperative IOP spikes, we now use antiglaucoma medications preoperatively and immediately postoperatively. The preoperative medical regimen includes: Alcaine, Maxitrol, Neosyn, Voltaren, Ciloxan, and Mydriasyl. Intraoperatively we use 10 mg of Decadron IV and 1 amp Mannitol IV.

The procedure begins with a self-sealing cataract incision. This incision can be placed temporally for an astigmatically neutral procedure, or at the steepest axis for a small amount of astigmatism correction. Following a peribulbar block, the conjunctiva is disinserted from the limbus with a 0.12 forceps and Westcott scissors. A 3.2-mm keratome is then used to fashion the self-sealing wound starting at the limbus and going 1.5 mm into clear cornea. The anterior chamber is then entered with the same keratome. Healon GV is used to fill the anterior chamber. A 360 degree capsular tear is fashioned with capsulorhexis forceps. One percent unpreserved lidocaine is injected into the nucleus. Following phacoemulsification, hydrodissection, and cortical removal, the wound is enlarged to accommodate the appropriate implant which is inserted into the capsular bag.

Following lens implantation, viscoelastic is injected between the posterior surface of the iris and the anterior capsule. Healon GV is chosen for several reasons: 1) it does not absorb the 810 nm wavelength of the laser, 2) it is more easily cleared from the fragile probe than other viscoelastics, 3) it maintains space well, and 3) it provides excellent visibility.

The probe is then inserted through the cataract incision and advanced under the iris until the ciliary processes come into view (Figure 17-2). The light intensity is controlled by moving the foot pedal from side to side. Orientation is achieved by turning the probe until the iris is superior and the lens is inferior. The processes are treated until they shrink and

Figure 17-2. The endoscopic laser probe is placed under the iris (Gayton).

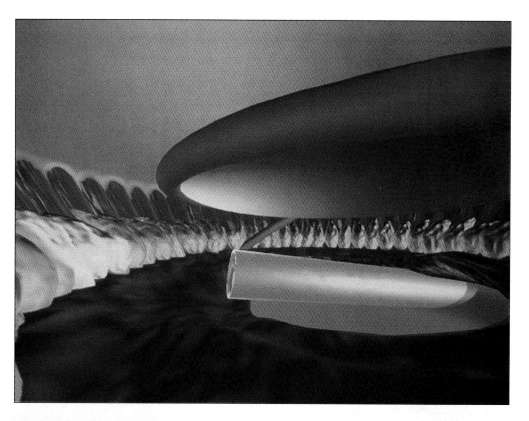

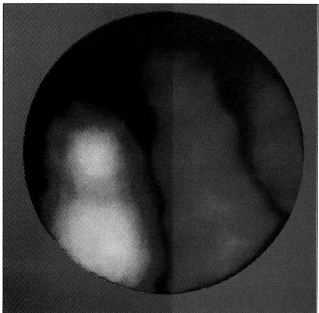

Figure 17-3. The ciliary processes are treated until they become chalky white. The ciliary process on the left has been treated (Gayton).

the initial procedure, and if the patient needs additional treatment I add another 120° of treatment. If a patient has severe glaucoma, consider starting with 360° of treatment

Following the procedure the Healon is removed and the wound sealed with BSS. One drop of Iopidine is instilled, and Tobradex and Atropine ointments are applied. The eye is patched shut. Postoperatively, the patient uses beta blocker or Iopidine, and Diamox tid. Antibiotic steroids are instilled every hour.

Results of Endoscopic Laser Cyclodestruction Combined with Cataract Surgery

A randomized study was conducted comparing combined cataract/endo laser with combined cataract/trabeculectomy. Twenty-nine endo cases have been randomized against 28 trabeculectomy cases.

Figures 17-3A&B show the mean IOP in the early and late postoperative periods. The endo cases do not achieve an immediate reduction in IOP as do the trabeculectomy cases. However, by one month, both groups stabilize at about 16 mmHg.

Thirty-eight percent (11) of endo cases versus 43% (12) of trabeculectomy cases achieved IOP control at the final available postoperative visit without medication. Pressure control was defined as IOP < 19 mmHg with no worsening of symptoms. Another 41% (12) of endo cases and 36% (10) of trabeculectomy cases were controlled with medication. Twenty-one percent (6) of endo cases and 25% (7) of trabeculectomy cases were not controlled at the last available visit. Uncontrolled IOP was defined as 19 mmHg or above or worsening glaucoma symptoms.

become chalky white (Figure 17-3). They can be treated singly or by a continuous painting technique. Start at 0.5 mW and adjust the power up or down as needed. Coagulation bubbles should be avoided. Treat 240° of ciliary processes at

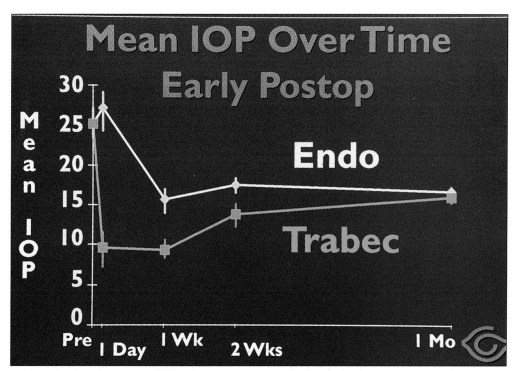

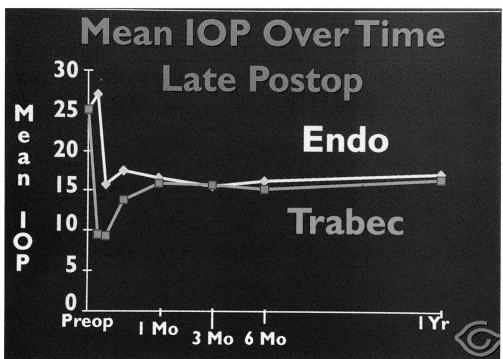

Figure 17-4. Mean IOP over time in a randomized study comparing cataract surgery combined with endoscopic laser treatment versus cataract surgery combined with trabeculectomy. Yellow lines represents the endo group, while the blue lines represent the trabeculectomy group (Gayton). (A) Mean IOP between preoperative and 1 month postoperative visits. (B) Mean IOP between preoperative and 1 year postoperative visits.

The endo group had much quieter eyes than the trabeculectomy group. Figure 17-5 shows the percent of cases with 4+ cells and flare over time. The endo group had significantly fewer cases of maximally rated edema at one day and one week. Moreover, 59% of the trabeculectomy group had hyphema versus none in the endo group (Figure 17-5).

Pressure spiking in the first 24 hours is always a concern with combined cataract/glaucoma patients, and was seen in both groups. There were two pressure spikes in the trabeculectomy group and six in the endo group. Two patients in each group had high inflammation that persisted past one month, but it eventually resolved. There were seven cases in the trabeculectomy group experiencing early hypotension and shallow chambers.

Only one endo case was a treatment failure, that is, requiring further surgical intervention. However, eight trabeculectomy cases, or 28% of the cohort, were treatment failures.

Figure 17-5. Percent of cases presenting with 4+ cells and flare in a randomized study comparing cataract surgery combined with endoscopic laser treatment versus cataract surgery combined with trabeculectomy. The yellow blocks represent the endo group while the pink blocks represent the trabeculectomy group (Gayton).

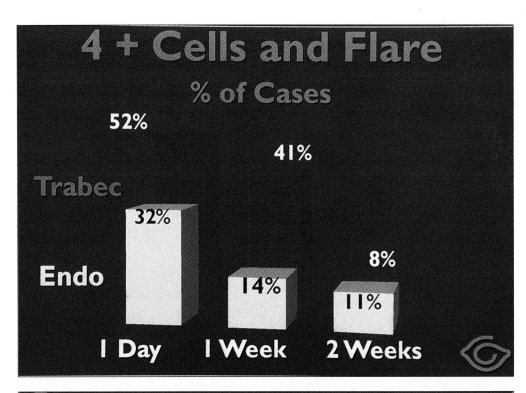

Figure 17-6. Percent of cases presenting with hyphema in a randomized study comparing cataract surgery combined with endoscopic laser treatment versus cataract surgery combined with trabeculectomy (Gayton).

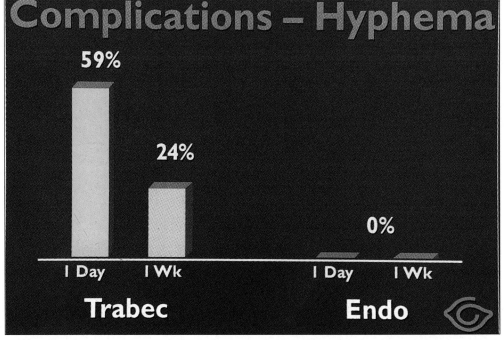

Because there is no bleb to fail with the endo procedure, we consider it the technique of choice when dealing with intractable cases that have proved refractory to both medication and other surgical options.

Cataract Surgery and Deep Sclerectomy with Collagen Implant

One alternative to trabeculectomy has been the placement of glaucoma drainage devices that act as shunts to relieve pressure by diverting intraocular fluid into a bleb. Examples of such setons are the Molteno, Baerveldt, Krupin and White shunts, which all work by the placement of a tube directly into the anterior chamber with a space-maintaining plate secured in a sub-scleral space.

Unfortunately, these devices have demonstrated a relatively low rate of success due to wound healing factors, and expose the patient to the risk of serious complications such as hyphema, hypotony, shallow chambers, suprachoroidal hemorrhage, or corneal decompensation.

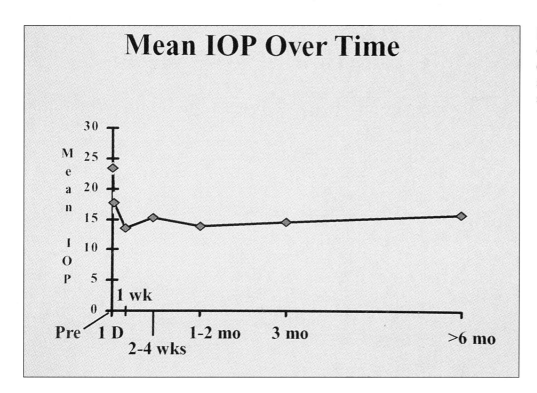

Figure 17-7. Mean IOP over time in a series of cases receiving cataract surgery and a scleral tissue implant (Martin).

The effect of these devices can be temporary, as well, as the implant becomes clogged with inflammatory or pigmentary debris. The collagen meshwork that generates around the plate can become increasingly dense over time, reducing the aqueous flow. Antimetabolites, such as 5-fluorouracil (5-FU) and mitomycin-C (MMC), can be administered to inhibit fibroblast production and external scarring of the bleb. However, injecting these drugs further exposes the patient to complications.

New glaucoma devices have been developed that are extraocular devices which act primarily as space maintainers. These devices do not require penetration into the anterior chamber, and thus are less invasive and carry less risk of complications than previous glaucoma devices.

The glaucoma wick, developed at the Fyodorov Institute for Staar AG is a collagen-based absorbable implant made from porcine scleral tissue. This biocompatible material has no known systemic immunologic reaction.

The device is placed in a non-penetrating sclerectomy site adjacent to Schlemm's canal. Upon placement in the eye, the device swells up to six times its size as it absorbs the ocular fluids to facilitate drainage. Approximately one week after placement, the implant begins to dissolve and is replaced by a new collagen fibril meshwork, which sustains the exit pathway. The intraocular pressure is reduced by additional release of fluid at the limbal edge of Descemet's membrane. The aqueous fluid is absorbed through the walls of the ciliary processes, into the blood stream, into the suprachoroidal space, and the subconjunctiva.

The advantages of this procedure is that drainage is constant and immediate. There is no penetration of globe, a decreased risk of hypotony, no need for 5-FU or mitomycin, and a low complication rate.

Experience With Device

In a randomized, prospective comparison to trabeculectomy in Europe, patients receiving the glaucoma wick had significantly less inflammation, flat chambers, hyphema, choroidal detachments, or hypotony.

Case Examples

Although the device has not yet been approved for study in the United States, one of the authors (RGM) has implanted 2 cases outside the U.S.

The first of these patients presented preoperatively with an IOP of 24 mmHg and moderate nerve damage. The patient was on Iopidine 1 gtt TID. After receiving the implant, the patient had cataract surgery 2 months postoperatively. Six weeks post-cataract surgery, the IOP was 19 mmHg, and the patient was well controlled without meds.

The second patient had an IOP preoperatively of 25 mmHg, with severe nerve damage and loss of rim. The patient was taking Timoptic 1 gtt BID and Betagan 1 gtt QD. The patient then had cataract surgery combined with placement of the wick device. One month postoperatively, the IOP was 12 mmHg and the patient was well controlled without meds.

Scleral Tissue Implant

Although the glaucoma wick device is not yet available, one of the authors (RGM) has devised a similar procedure using the patient's own scleral tissue for implantation. A superior fornix-based flap is made superiorly with Westcott scissors and Colibri forceps. A 4x4 mm one-third depth flap is made with a diamond knife to the anterior limbus. Next, a

Figure 17-8. Distribution of high IOP in a series of cases receiving cataract surgery and a scleral tissue implant (Martin).

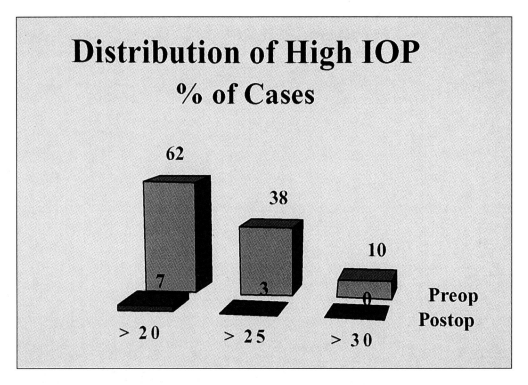

Figure 17-9. Distribution of cases in a series of cases receiving cataract surgery and a scleral tissue implant requiring various number of glaucoma medications (Martin).

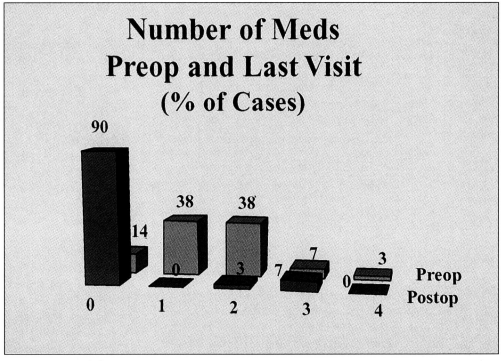

5-sided second scleral incision is begun with the apex of the incision ending at the central posterior incision. This incision is shelved forward with a diamond knife so that Schlemm's canal is unroofed. This flap is then cut off with Vannas scissors. A piece is fashioned measuring about 3 mm by 1.5 mm and sutured with 20/20 10-0 nylon in a radial fashion to the central bed, so that the head of it abuts Schlemm's canal. Next a rectangular flap is sutured using two interrupted 10-0 nylon

sutures to the apex of the posterior incision creating a tunnel. Conjunctiva is closed by a combination of wetfield cautery and an interrupted 10-0 nylon suture. The cataract is then approached temporally with a clear-corneal incision.

Results

Thirty cases have been performed with at least 1-2 month follow-up. Figure 17-7 shows the mean IOP over time for the cohort. There was a statistically significant drop in IOP from

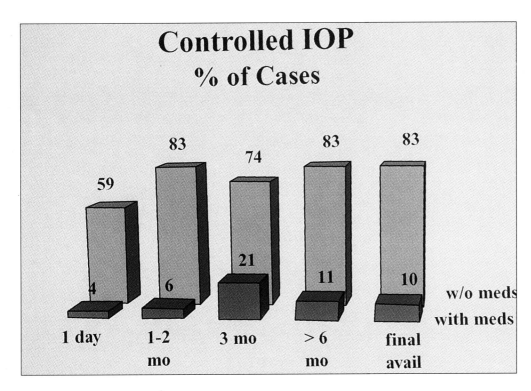

preoperative at every time period. The mean preoperative IOP of 24 mmHg was reduced to a mean of 15 mmHg at the final available visit. Figure 17-8 demonstrates the distribution of high IOP pre- and postoperatively. While preoperatively 38% of cases had IOP > 25 mmHg, postoperatively no cases had IOP that high.

Figure 17-9 shows the reduction of medication required by the cohort. Although preoperatively almost half the cases required two or more glaucoma medications, postoperatively 90% were not on any glaucoma medications. There was a statistically significant drop in number of meds at every time period.

Figure 17-10 shows the percent of cases achieving IOP control, either with or without medications, across time. At the final available visit, 83% of cases achieved control without medication. Only 7%, or two cases, remain uncontrolled at the final available visit.

Discussion

The glaucoma wick procedure appears to be effective in managing glaucoma, with results comparable or better than trabeculectomy. The technique is less invasive and safer. Although the procedure using the patient's sclera is a reasonable facsimile of the wick procedure, the availability of the STAAR glaucoma wick will make the procedure easier and less invasive.

SUMMARY

The cataract patient frequently presents with other ophthalmologic pathologies that in the past have precluded phacoemulsification or advanced incisional techniques. However, with advanced in phacoemulsification technique, and new, less invasive methods of surgically treating glaucoma, more patients are able to enjoy the benefits of state-of-the-art technique.

STRATEGIES FOR APPLYING STATE OF THE ART TECHNIQUES

CHAPTER 18

James P. Gills, MD

The previous chapters in this book have presented the most recent developments and techniques in cataract surgery. However, the purpose of this book is not simply to provide up-to-date techniques, but to offer strategies for improving outcomes for our patients. The privilege of performing cataract surgery on a patient provides us with an opportunity to offer that patient the best outcome possible, which often means performing extra procedures to correct other problems such as strabismus or astigmatism. Even many of the little "extras" we can add to our routine surgery, such as checking the IOP one hour postoperatively, can dramatically improve the safety and efficacy of our procedures.

STRATEGIES FOR ANESTHESIA

Avoiding Bupivicaine in Retrobulbar Blocks

David Guyton, M.D. has pointed out that many of the post-surgical patients presenting with double vision had received bupivicaine in their retrobulbar block. It is possible that bupivicaine causes muscle toxicity, resulting in double vision. Since I was the one to introduce the drug into this country in September, 1968, it is my responsibility to alert the ophthalmic community and suggest other alternatives, such as Citanest, which is a short-acting anesthetic usually used for dental work, but applicable to cataract surgery. The drug is extremely effective and to date we have noticed no cases of muscle toxicity.

Preparing the Patient for Topical Anesthesia

Patients should understand all their options for anesthesia. Topical anesthesia should be explained in great detail and the patients thoroughly evaluated to be sure they are good candidates. It has been extremely helpful in my practice for my postoperative patients who are leaving the OR explain their experience to other patients waiting for surgery. In counseling patients, I avoid words such as "anesthesia" or "medication", and instead explain that "special solutions" will be used to bathe the eye and eliminate sensation.

Topical anesthesia requires a partnership with the patient. In the patient prep area, the staff explains to the patient in detail how to fixate and be most cooperative during surgery. We must move beyond the old mentality of putting the patient on the OR table, inserting an IV line, and the surgeon working in solitude while the anesthetist writes in the chart. Instead, the nurse anesthetist must talk to the patient throughout the procedure, offering reassurance and helping the patient to keep the eye positioned correctly. Cataract surgery with topical anesthesia is very demanding and requires a great deal of communication between the patient, surgeon, and staff.

INSTRUMENTATION

The right tool for the job is a maxim that applies well to modern cataract surgery. Not only choosing appropriate instrumentation, but also knowing how and when to use the instruments at our disposal, can make the cataract surgery safer and easier.

Dripper

I have used a dripper during cataract surgery for years. Robert Drews, M.D. developed the Drews Dripper, made by Katena (Figure 18-1). I modified the design slightly because our microscopes were slightly different. More recently, Thomas Hedges, M.D. developed the Hedges Corneal Wetting Pack, which also works very well. The flow rate of a dripper can be adjusted, which reduces dryness and improves visualization for the surgeon.

Figure 18-1. Katena's Drews Dripper.

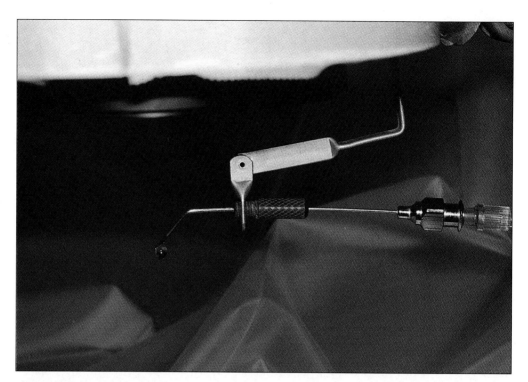

Figure 18-2. Anterior chamber maintainer.

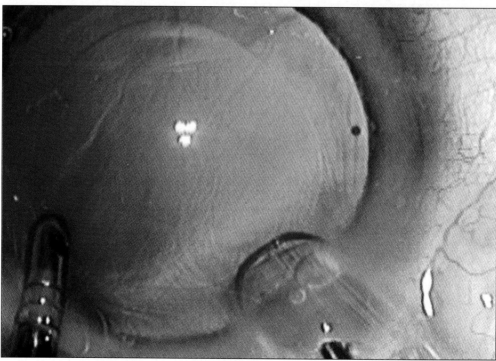

It is important not to have the flow rate set too high, because the oil and mucous layers of the tear film can be washed from the cornea, which causes tremendous discomfort and a diffuse keratitis postoperatively. Usually a flow setting of one drop every 3 to 4 seconds is adequate. Cases where the oil layer is almost nonexistent may require a higher setting to wet the cornea sufficiently.

Anterior Chamber Maintainer

Viscoelastic is used at the beginning of the case to fill the anterior chamber, but the anterior chamber maintainer (Figure 18-2) is used from the point of polishing the capsule to the end of the case to ensure that there is no viscoelastic left in the eye at the end of surgery. The A/C maintainer markedly reduces the incidence of elevated IOP that occurs

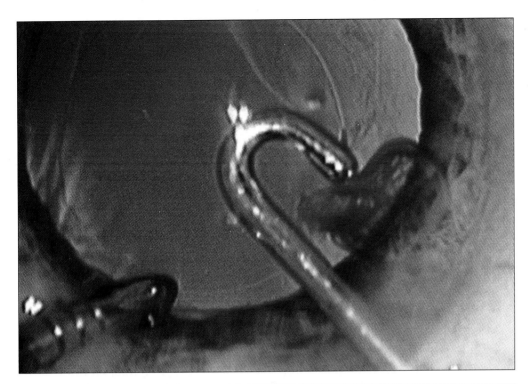

Figure 18-3. Retrieving cortex with a U cannula.

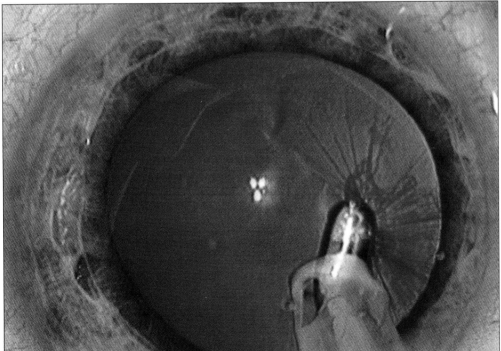

postoperatively from viscoelastic that remains in the anterior chamber.

Irrigation and Aspiration Tip

It is important to keep the I&A tip up during irrigation and aspiration. If the tip is turned to the side, it is easy to tear the capsule. This point is especially important when working at 12 o'clock, as it is the most common area to have a posterior capsular tear, and it usually occurs during I&A. When in doubt, leave any cortex in that area and retrieve with a U cannula (Figure 18-3).

Some surgeons prefer to remove all the peripheral cortex with phacoemulsification because it is faster. They feel that speed makes the procedure safer. However, if a capsule is inadvertently opened, usually it happens during phaco. It is more dangerous to remove peripheral cortex with phaco, and

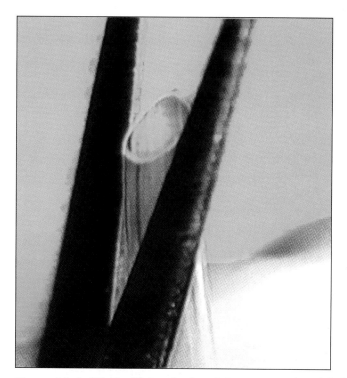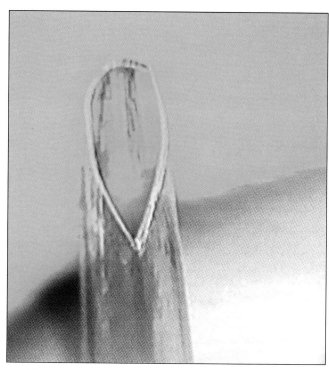

Figure 18-4. (A) Modifying the lens injector cartridge. (B) The modified injector.

it is safer with I&A. What is gained in speed could be lost in complications such as rupture of the posterior capsule. Therefore, I use I&A to remove peripheral cortex.

STRATEGIES FOR IMPLANTING FOLDABLE LENSES WITH THE INJECTOR

Injector Modification

Current injectors can cause inadvertent wound stretching and tearing while inserting IOLs through small clear-corneal incisions. We make the bevel larger by cutting the tip of the STAAR AA-4203 injection cannula at a greater angle (Figures 18-4A&B). This modification allows the inserter to be compressed, reducing stretching and distortion of the wound. Less trauma to the original incision preserves the self-sealing quality of the wound and decreases the likelihood of endophthalmitis. This modification also allows the wound itself to act as an extension of the injector, allowing the injector to be partially inserted, thus permitting the use of incisions as small as 2.1 mm (see Chapter 4).

Partial Insertion

When inserting a foldable lens, the injector should be only partially introduced into the incision. However, the injector tip must be inserted past the endothelium. If the tip is not inserted far enough into the incision, Descemet's membrane could be stripped. I hold the instrument with my right hand and brace my elbow against my side. Bracing the elbow

allows fine, precise movements. The person who screws in the IOL should use both hands. Pressure must be applied to the posterior sclera with the injector cartridge. Otherwise, the lens may be forced backwards out of the incision.

As the lens clears the mouth of the incision, slowly pull the injector back so that as the optic is introduced, the injector is just at the inner orifice. This technique of slowly removing the injector as the IOL unfolds creates pressure on the incision. Creating pressure on the incision as the lens is introduced into the anterior chamber results in a slower, more controlled unfolding of the IOL and less tissue stretch. The pressure should be at its greatest when the lens has emerged halfway from the injector (Figure 18-5).

After inserting the IOL, a common mistake is to neglect to check that the lens is completely in the bag. While the lens may appear to be in the bag, looks can be deceiving. I place a collar button over the top of the lens and grab the edge to make sure that it is indented all the way around, which indicates it is in the bag (Figure 18-6). This simple step can avoid problems such as residual myopia or reflections from the edge of the IOL due to lens shift. These problems could result in a dissatisfied patient who requires a lens repositioning or exchange.

STRATEGIES FOR THE DIFFICULT CASE

Fixed Pupils

Frequently, fixed pupils are associated with pseudoexfoliation or trauma. These pupils are handled most often by sim-

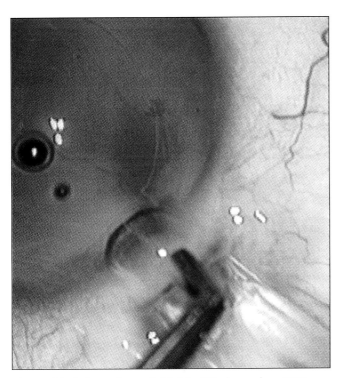

Figure 18-5. Inserting a foldable IOL through a SLiC incision with a modified injector cartridge.

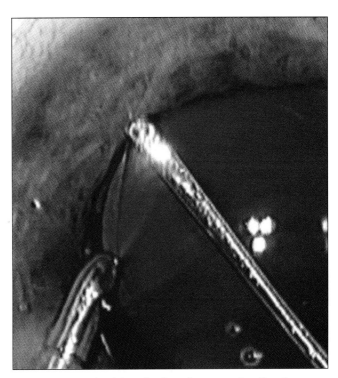

Figure 18-6. Checking the lens for capsular fixation.

ple stretching. There have been many techniques described to stretch the pupil. We have found the simplest method is to open the pupil slightly to 4 or 5 mm with a cyclodialysis spatula and a Graether collar button (Figure 18-7). Only if absolutely necessary do we open larger, because the more a pupil is stretched the less likely it will return to a functional size, which can result in significant symptoms. Stretching the pupil larger than 9 mm may result in a fixed and dilated pupil after surgery. To reduce this risk, I instill Eserine ung or some similar miotic after surgery to constrict the pupil.

At one time I felt a pupil up to 6, 7, or even 8 mm added extra safety and made the surgery easier to complete. However, I find I can now easily operate through a 2 or 3 mm pupil. In glaucoma cases, very hard lenses, and frequently short eyes, I stretch the pupil to at least 3 to 4 mm. I would rather phaco through a moderately sized pupil than one that is miotic. Although I have operated through 1 to 2.5 mm pupils of glaucomatous eyes, the pseudoexfoliation and density of the cataract that is so frequently present in these cases increases the difficulty of the procedure. Stretching the pupil slightly to a more moderate size provides more "relaxation room" and added security, making phacoemulsification easier.

Many other methods can be used to enlarge the pupil. We have used iris hooks on several occasions and found them very effective in holding a torn iris out of the way of the phaco tip. There are various lens stretchers made for the purpose, although I see no benefit to them over a collar button and a cyclodialysis spatula, which seem to be less cumber-

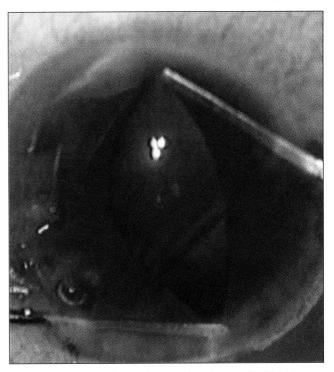

Figure 18-7. Stretching the pupil with a cyclodialysis spatula and Graether collar button.

some in the anterior chamber. In fact, most of the instruments I have seen could potentially cause complications such as capsular rupture.

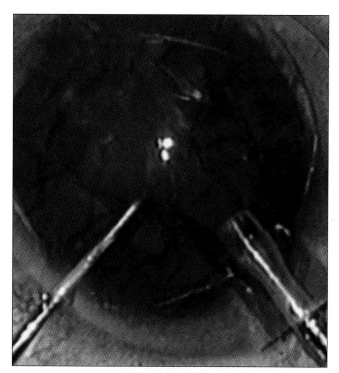

Figure 18-8. Phacoemulsification outside of the capsular bag.

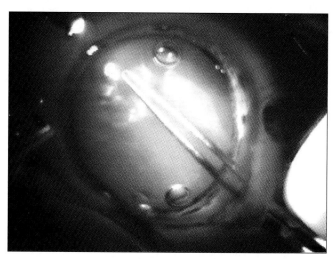

Figure 18-9. Capsulorhexis using a light pipe to improve visualization of the capsule.

When operating on a patient with a fixed pupil, always expect a dislocated lens or loose zonules. When the zonules are loose, the supracapsular phacoemulsification technique of Dr. Maloney (see Chapter 9), in which the cataract is removed from the bag, may be safer (Figure 18-8).

The Hypermature Cataract

Continuous curvilinear capsulotomies are difficult to perform on mature cataracts. In some cases, the cataract can be so mature that scissors are needed to open the capsule because it is so scarred and dense. If the cataract is totally white or brunescent, it can be difficult to visualize the capsule to perform capsulorhexis. My solution to this problem is to use a light pipe to follow at the edges of the tear with the microscope light off, which illuminates the edges of the capsule that otherwise would not be visible (Figure 18-9).

Occasionally I operate on patients with cataracts that are so hypermature they are actually morgagnion. These cases are best handled by entering the anterior chamber with a cannulat to find the nucleus. It is important to localize this area so that the cannula does not penetrate both layers of the capsule and through into the vitreous.

I then make a small capsulotomy in the capsule with the forceps, using a light pipe for illumination. If I can not visualize anything because of the white, oozing cataract, I will use a small gauge cannula, 25 or 27, and irrigate out the anterior cortical white milky material. After that material is almost completely irrigated out, I will frequently fill out the capsular bag and the anterior segment with viscoelastic to create a cushion between the anterior and posterior capsule. Because of the absence of nucleus in some areas of these cataracts, a posterior capsular tear could occur if there is no space between the two capsules.

I learned the importance of using viscoelastic to prevent penetration of the posterior capsule from a single case of inadvertent capsular rupture requiring a vitrectomy, which occurred after a series of over 2,000 cases with no vitreous loss. This particular patient was 37-years old. The cortex had been mostly absorbed and just a thin bit of white nucleus remained. The lesson from this cases is that although a cataract appears white, it may actually be very thin, so without viscoelastic a needle can easily penetrate both layers of the capsule.

Because the hypermature lens frequently has few zonules and the capsules are very loose, it can be helpful to use another instrument to steady the capsule while pulling the tear. When starting the capsular tear, I frequently use an iris hook, or a notched instrument like a collar button, to pull the capsule in the opposite direction from the tear to avoid stress on the zonules. As the tear approaches the area of the zonules, I may again use a hook through a second port to hold the capsule intact as I pull away from it. It is probably best at this time to grasp small sections of the capsule at a time to avoid excessive traction on the zonules.

Extremely Hard Cataracts

In about 1 in every 5,000 cases, I find I need to perform a planned extracapsular extraction for an extremely hard nucleus. However, usually I am able to phacoemulsify the hard nucleus, but proceed slowly, and frequently refill the anterior chamber with viscoelastic to reduce the incidence of postoperative corneal edema.

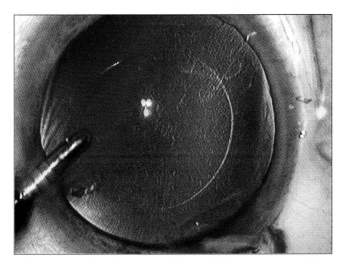

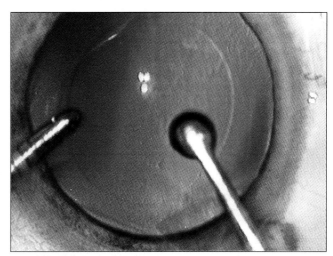

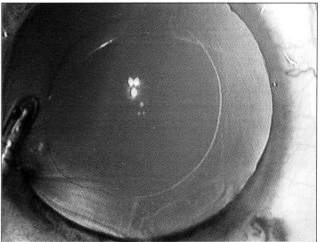

Figure 18-10. The importance of polishing the capsule. (A) Note the cells on the posterior capsule before polishing (top, left). (B) Polishing the posterior capsule with a chalazion curette (top, right). (C) Note clarity of the posterior capsule after polishing (bottom).

There is a great deal of energy required to phaco a dense cataract. Even a perfectly executed case may result in corneal edema. I frequently try to crack these cataracts because I find that the most effective technique. However, a decision must be made for each surgery which would be the most advantageous method: divide and conquer, chopping, or cracking. I use a low power setting and use pulse so that: the sclera or cornea doesn't burn (depending on the type of incision), and less energy is used.

STRATEGIES FOR MAXIMIZING OUTCOMES AND MINIMIZING COMPLICATIONS

Polishing the Posterior Capsule

Polishing both the anterior as well as posterior capsule helps to prevent posterior capsular opacification, provides better visual quality, and reduces shrinkage of the capsular bag. Polishing the capsule also reduces postoperative inflammation. I rarely see cells or flare in the anterior chamber on the first postoperative day. While the use of steroids and NSAIDs postoperatively certainly contribute to a quiet eye, polishing the capsule is a significant factor as well (Figures 18-10A,B,C).

Minimizing Pupil Size for the First Postoperative Day

I like to occasionally reverse dilation following surgery so the patient's early vision is optimized, and glare is reduced as quickly as possible. We use Carbochol after completing the surgery and instill RevEyes in recovery to return the pupil to a normal size. Brow ache and discomfort are the only disad-

vantages with Carbochol. Quick-acting miotics may cause more discomfort than the surgery itself.

Same-Day Postoperative Exams

The first several hours after surgery is the most important time to examine the patients. Checking the IOP in the early postoperative period is better than the following day, as we can frequently uncover IOP spikes or hypotony.

We also frequently refract patients in the early postoperative period to verify correct lens power, especially in cases of extreme hyperopia or myopia. If there is an unexpected refractive error, the IOL is more safely exchanged as early as possible.

The patients are either followed by us or sent back to the referring physician for continued follow-up. Same-day examinations are very practical, and frequently saves patients an overnight stay.

Monovision

Our goal in cataract surgery is not only to improve our patients' vision, but to provide them with the best functional vision possible. We offer our patients the choice of monovision or near emmetropia in both eyes. We generally suggest a "modified" monovision in which one eye is –0.50 D and the other is –1.50 D. Normally the first eye is targeted for –0.37 D to provide the most functional range of vision for the patient's general needs.

The lens selection for the second eye is based on the 1 to 2 week postoperative refraction. The patient chooses the focal distance for the second eye. Most patients select near emmetropia (approximately –0.50 D) for both eyes, but the monovision contact wearers usually prefer monovision.

It is crucial that preoperative patients thoroughly understand their options, along with the advantages and disadvantages of both monovision and distance vision. Often the patients' expectations are based on the familiar or their current refraction. For example, hyperopes are usually thrilled with refractions of –0.50 D in both eyes, because for the first time they can see clearly at distance as well as read medium to large print. Myopes, however, frequently have higher expectations and want clear distance vision, but are disappointed when they discover they cannot read fine print. For this reason, we are even more cautious when counseling the myopic patient, and often monovision is an excellent option in these cases. Monovision is also an excellent option for professionals who work at a computer, cashiers, musicians, and public speakers, or for anyone whose vocation or avocation requires good near vision. I generally recommend distance vision in both eyes for patients who play sports, or do a great deal of driving.

BEVEL-DOWN PHACO

Cavitation flows from the direction of the phaco tip. This cavitation radiates in the direction that the bevel is pointed. The cavitation then grabs hold of the lens material, pulls it, and destroys it. This process, along with the vacuum, sucks the lens material into the needle. The cavitation can be directed by pointing the bevel. Thus the bevel of the phaco tip should be pointed where the cataract is to be phacoemulsified.

Usually the bevel should be pointed down (Figures 18-11A&B). Dr. Robert Martin first described his bevel down technique in 1985. With the bevel down, there is less chance of damaging the endothelium. Since the phaco tip is usually on top of the cataract, rather than under it, a bevel down technique increases the efficiency.

A smaller bevel of 15° produces the most efficient suction. A larger angulated aperture will not perch as well on many lenses, particularly those that are soft and of median density, and will end up just scratching across the surface.

STRATEGIES FOR MANAGING INTRAOCULAR PRESSURE

Air-Puff Tonometer

Frequently the eye pressure may rise in the very early postoperative period due to the use of viscoelastic. However, even without viscoelastics, approximately 4 to 5% of patients have pressure elevations. We believe measuring the pressure postoperatively in the first half hour following surgery is critically important.

We use an air puff tonometer (Figure 18-12) to check the pressures rather than other contact methods to reduce the possibility of epithelial damage. The epithelium is very delicate postoperatively because of the preoperative drops used, the BSS during surgery, and topical anesthesia. Many of these patients have a history of keratitis sicca, which is aggravated by medication and surgery. In these delicate corneas, abrasions can occur easily. Accordingly, we use air puff tonometry because it is safer to the immediate postoperative cornea, although we realize the air puff method is less accurate. If the pressure recorded is not between 5 and 30 mmHg, we verify the measurement with applanation tonometry.

Our studies have demonstrated that hypotony or pressure spikes may occur in the early postoperative period and then return to normal when the pressure is checked the following day. By using this early check of IOP, we have found evidence of hypotony, suggesting leaky wounds, which may possibly be the etiology of endophthalmitis that has been documented with clear corneal incisions. We routinely pressure patch the eyes with well-formed anterior chambers when the IOP is 5 mmHg or less, and recheck the pressure after 15 to 30 minutes. If the IOP remains low, the anterior chamber is reformed with BSS. A bandage contact lens is inserted if no suture is needed. Pressure patches are never used for patients with anterior chamber IOLs or shallow anterior chambers.

Conversely, we have found many cases of elevated IOP that could have caused dilated pupils, damage to the optic nerve, or unexplained vision loss with no known etiology. Since many surgeons do not routinely check the pressure, the fixed pupil or visual loss that can occur in these cases is often incorrectly attributed to inflammation or some other cause. By routinely checking the pressure early postoperatively, we can ensure safer cataract surgery in a very simple way.

Paracentesis of the Anterior Segment

If a significant IOP spike occurs in the early postoperative period, a paracentesis can be performed at the slit lamp to lower the IOP. A 27-gauge needle is used to express aqueous and possible residual viscoelastic by pressing the incision site or the paracentesis port from surgery. If the trabecular meshwork is filled with viscoelastic, the pressure will usually spike again approximately an hour after the paracentesis. Therefore, it is important to recheck the pressure about an hour later. The paracentesis can be repeated as necessary if the IOP remains elevated. Immediately after the paracentesis, the eye is hypotonous, so it is important for the patient and technician to avoid touching the eye.

This technique is more effective than treating the IOP with medications such as Diamox and topical beta blockers. Iopidine and Eserine used in conjunction with the paracentesis is very effective in lowering the IOP.

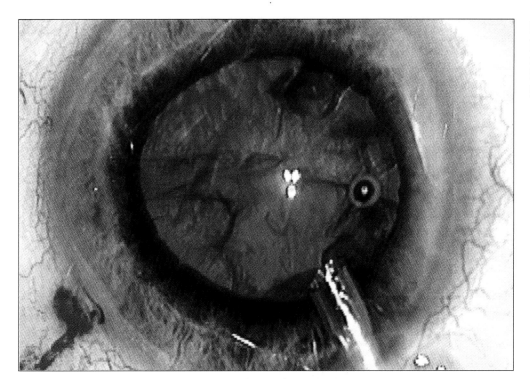

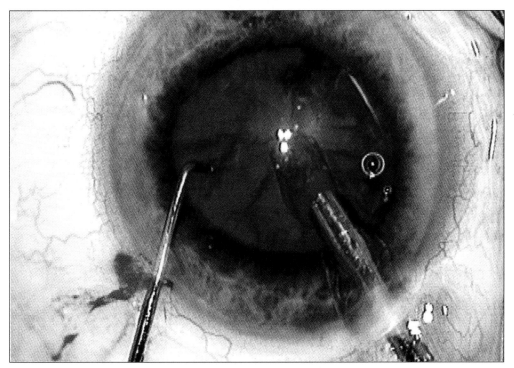

Figure 18-11. Bevel-down phaco. (A) Tip turned bevel up for entry. (B) Tip turned bevel down once inside the eye.

Arden Test

The Arden test can detect subtle central nerve fiber layer defects before they would appear on a threshold visual field test. The central nerve fibers are the first to be affected by glaucoma. The test enables me to identify which patients should be treated medically, surgically, or left alone. A low score with a slightly elevated pressure suggests the patient probably does not need medical intervention. Conversely, a patient who scores high and has an elevated pressure should be treated. This test also helps to identify those patients who are statistically at a greater risk of progressive glaucoma defects, who may require surgical intervention at the time of cataract surgery.

Figure 18-12. Air puff tonometer.

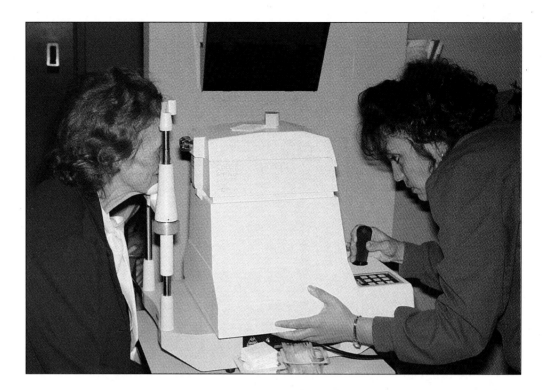

To Filter or Not to Filter

At one time we performed many combined cataract and filtering procedures. Approximately 60% of our patients with co-existing cataract and glaucoma received a filter. Now less than 5% of these patients are filtered at our practice.

At one time cataract surgery had the potential for worsening co-existing glaucoma, prompting us to perform a trabeculectomy in many cases. However, the clear-corneal and the SLiC incisions do not disrupt the trabecular meshwork or cause synechiae as the larger scleral incisions did. We now agree with many glaucoma specialists who believe that the cataract surgery actually improves the glaucoma in many narrow-angle cases, as the anterior chamber deepens following cataract removal.

If the Arden test scores are reasonably low to medium, we do not perform a filtering procedure. Gonioscopy is also performed, and I rarely proceed with glaucoma surgery if the angles are narrow. However, if the patient presents with disc loss, field loss, and/or high Arden scores, we do perform a filter.

This protocol reduces the risks of complications associated with filtering surgery, such as latent endophthalmitis, by avoiding the procedure in those patients who may not require it. Moreover, patients who do not receive a filter appreciate the faster recovery of vision. With many of the new procedures for treating glaucoma, such as the glaucoma wick and endoscopic laser treatment (see Chapter 17), if the glaucoma does become a problem at a later date, treating it is becoming easier and less invasive.

STRATEGIES FOR IMPROVING OUTCOMES WITH EXTRA PROCEDURES

Cataract surgery may be combined with many other procedures to provide a double benefit to the patient. A patient presenting with two complaints can thus be helped with one surgical procedure. Accordingly, we perform many types of combined and special procedures with our cataract surgery, including corneal transplantation, vitrectomy, glaucoma procedures, muscle procedures, and correction of astigmatism.

However, all these combined procedures may or may not work for the good of the patient. The physician must make an individual evaluation of each patient with strict care, to be certain that the risks are justified by the potential benefit.

Intentional Vitrectomy of the Posterior Capsule

Patients whose vision is limited from dense asteroid hyalosis can be helped with a vitrectomy during cataract surgery. This procedure is reserved for those patients who are as symptomatic from the floaters as from the cataract. The procedure has the greatest potential success and the lowest risk when the patient already has a posterior vitreous detachment.

An intentional, round posterior capsulotomy is made by sucking the posterior capsule into the I&A tip, and then cutting it with a cyclodialysis spatula (Figure 18-13A), which creates a perfectly round posterior capsulotomy through which to perform a vitrectomy (Figure 18-13B). The procedure involves minimal risk as long as a core vitrectomy is performed.

My observation is that over 95% of the patient feel they have significantly benefited from the procedure.

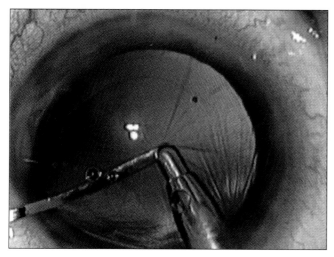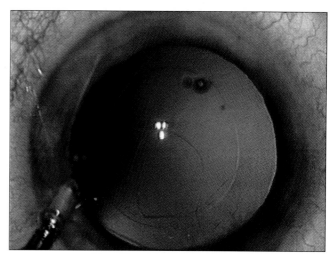

Figure 18-13. Intentional vitrectomy to reduce floaters. (A) The I&A tip is used to create gentle suction on the posterior capsule. The capsule is cut with a cyclodialysis spatula. (B) Note the round posterior capsulotomy.

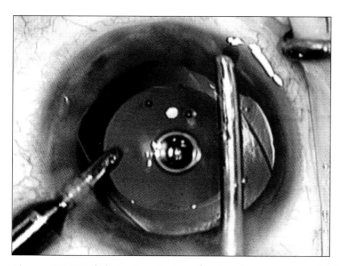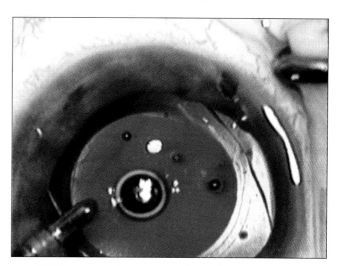

Figure 18-14. (A) A vitrector can be used to create an iridectomy. (B) Iridectomy that was made with a vitrector.

Occasionally, a patient may be unhappy if a floater still remains, so preoperative education is important. The patient must understand the risk of retinal detachment, so they are well educated about the symptoms and instructed to be evaluated immediately if any symptoms occur.

Iridectomy With the Vitrector

It is difficult to perform an iridectomy through a self-sealing incision. Normally, an iridectomy is made at the incision site. However, that location is not the best when using temporal small, self-sealing incisions. The iridectomy is more simply made with a vitrector and an anterior chamber maintainer (Figure 18-14A), creating a small, full-thickness superior iridectomy (Figure 18-14B) which can be performed without an additional incision and with minimal manipulation or reaction in the eye.

Correcting Strabismus With Cataract Surgery

Strabismus correction can be performed at the time of cataract surgery. Recession/resection can be done in conjunction with sutureless surgery. A simple myotomy is easy to perform and provides excellent results. A myotomy does not require sutures because of muscle adhesions so there is less inflammatory response.

Approximately 18 to 20 prism diopters of correction can be obtained by a full myotomy of the lateral rectus (Figures 18-15A&B). If less effect is desired than that of a full myotomy, a "Z" myotomy is done by cutting both sides of the muscle so it can stretch. The amount of effect can be titrated by adjusting the depth of the cut. This procedure provides excellent results for the patient and causes less inflammatory response than traditional recess/resect procedures.

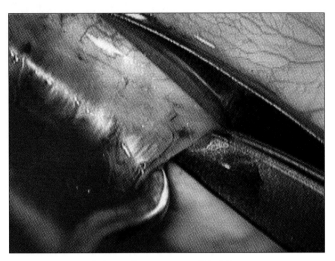 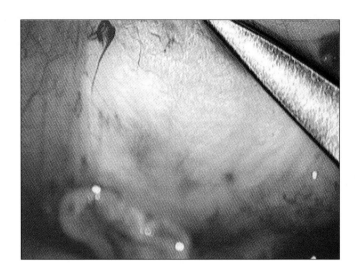

Figure 18-15. (A) Total myotomy. (B) After myotomy.

If done on the medial rectus, a full myotomy would produce between 30 to 40 diopters of effect, so a more conservative approach must be taken when correcting esotropia. The results are also more variable. Overcorrections are more likely to occur because there are fewer adhesions medially than laterally. I proceed cautiously with my surgical plan for esotropia, and I often initially perform a marginal myotomy rather than a full myotomy. If there is still an undercorrection, I can then perform a total myotomy. Frequently, the medial rectus responds more to the initial surgery.

In the case of a particularly large deviation (35 prism diopters or more) that is more pronounced in one gaze than another, a full myotomy can be combined with suturing the eye in the desired direction. For example, for a patient with a 35 prism diopter right exotropia, I would perform a full myotomy and suture the eye in. I follow these patients closely and usually remove the suture within 24 to 48 hours. The effect of the myotomy is increased by 50% if the suture is left in place for one day; the effect increases to 100% or more if the suture is left in 2 or more days. In this way, less surgery can create a greater effect. It may take time for the patient to fuse, and the patient may be aware of diplopia until able to fuse.

When a smaller deviation is present such as a vertical deviation (hypertropia), a marginal myotomy (cutting the muscle 90%) can be performed. I use this procedure to correct 2 to 4 prism diopters of vertical deviation. A Z-myotomy gives more effect depending on the depth of the cuts into the muscle. Certainly 8 prism diopters of vertical deviation can be corrected with a Z-myotomy of the culprit muscle. About half of the effect is achieved when correcting a horizontal deviation versus a vertical.

It is much more difficult to achieve the desired correction on post-retinal detachment patients because of complex factors. Many factors may contribute to the tropia such as: the use of Marcaine for the surgery, trauma of pulling on the muscles during surgery, and general postoperative inflammation from retinal detachment. Thyroid myopathies can also be very difficult to treat and may vary greatly in their response to this procedure.

SUMMARY

Knowing and using state-of-the-art techniques will bring a high level of patient satisfaction. However, maximizing the outcome to bring the highest satisfaction possible requires more. It requires an attention to detail and the commitment to go the extra step, to do everything possible in the patient's best visual and psychological interest.

EXTENDING THE BENEFITS OF MODERN SURGICAL TECHNIQUE TO THE THIRD WORLD

Juan F. Battle, MD, Robert G. Martin, MD

The ultimate goal of the cataract surgeon is to prevent blindness through a curative operation. In fact, cataracts are the leading cause of blindness worldwide and the fight against this curable disease has become the focus of most international organizations dedicated to blindness prevention, including Christoffel Blindenmission and Medical Ministries International.

In the recent meeting of the International Agency for Prevention of Blindness held in Cancun, Mexico, cataracts were declared the number one enemy in the efforts to reduce blindness in Latin America. The International Lion's Club Organization has focused their SightFirst program on the sponsorship of massive cataract surgery campaigns or Megaprojects throughout the world. The results of these efforts are encouraging, but it seems as if the final outcome depends on a profound knowledge and understanding of the complex socioeconomic problems of the underdeveloped countries. It is really in these underdeveloped areas where most of the curable cataracts now prevail. Phacoemulsification and other advanced cataract techniques are likely to become widely used, but only if they become affordable and accessible, and the ophthalmologists in the field can acquire these procedures with a minimum learning curve.

PREVALENCE OF BLINDNESS

There have been very few community-based population surveys on the prevalence of blindness in Latin American countries in recent years. The 1987 World Health Organization (WHO) figures for Latin America estimate that for a population of 397 million people, there are a minimum of 1,760,000 blind people and a maximum of 2,315,000 blind people. An average round figure would therefore be 2 million blind people in Latin America, alone.

Table 19-1 gives information on estimates for the number of blind people in South American countries. Table 19-2 details the problems of blindness for Central American countries and the Caribbean.

The first National Survey on Blindness was done in the Dominican Republic in 1995. This small nation in the Caribbean Sea shares an island with Haiti and a population of 7.5 million people. 0.45% of the inhabitants of the Dominican Republic suffer with blindness. Approximately 33,000 people are bilaterally blind and nearly half of them are blind from cataracts. The graph in Figure 19-1 shows the distribution of causes of blindness found in this stratified, random-sampling survey of more than 17,000 people.

The situation for most Latin American countries and also countries of the Third World are similar, with prevalence rates illustrated in Table 19-3. The prevalence rates for blindness are directly correlated with the socio-economic status of the nations in question. Higher rates occur in India and Africa, and the lowest in Europe and North America.

The four major causes of blindness are cataracts, glaucoma, diabetic retinopathy, and corneal scars for most of Latin America, as was shown in the Dominican Survey. In Africa and the East, onchocerciasis and trachoma are leading causes as well. Most authorities agree that cataracts represent half of the cases with blindness worldwide, and their cure and strategies to eliminate them remain a major goal of all blindness prevention programs.

EYE HEALTH FOR ALL

The World Health Organization ALMA ATA declaration of 1977 aimed at health for all by the year 2000. This objective would naturally include eye health for all and their immediate goals were:

TABLE 19-1
PREVALENCE OF BLINDNESS IN SOUTH AMERICAN COUNTRIES

Country	Pop. (Mill)	% Rural	No. of Blind	
Brazil	135	30	500,000 -	1,000,000
Colombia	28	30	100,000 -	150,000
Peru	20	30	80,000 -	120,000
Ecuador	9	55	35,000 -	50,000
Chile	12	20	40,000 -	60,000
Bolivia	7	60	25,000 -	40,000
Argentina	29	20	100,000 -	150,000
Venezuela	15	15	50,000 -	70,000
Uruguay	3	15	10,000 -	15,000
Paraguay	3.5	60	10,000 -	15,000
TOTAL			950,000 -	1,670,000

TABLE 19-2
PREVALENCE OF BLINDNESS IN CENTRAL AMERICAN AND CARIBBEAN COUNTRIES

Country	Pop. (Mill)	% Rural	No. of Blind	
Mexico	79	40	300,000 -	500,000
Guatemala	8	60	30,000 -	50,000
Haiti	6	75	30,000 -	50,000
Dominican Republic	7	45	30,000 -	50,000
Honduras	5	60	20,000 -	35,000
Nicaragua	4	45	15,000 -	25,000
Costa Rica	3	55	10,000 -	15,000
Cuba	10	35	30,000 -	50,000
El Salvador	5	55	15,000 -	25,000
Panama	2	45	5,000 -	10,000
Jamaica	2.5	55	5,000 -	10,000
TOTAL			490,000 -	820,000

1. There should be no unnecessary blindness from cataract, glaucoma, or diabetic retinopathy.
2. To prevent eye disease at all levels of health care, to diagnose, treat, and cure eye diseases, including eye infections and minor injuries.
3. To provide affordable spectacles.
4. Develop community awareness about eye health.
5. Provide specialized tertiary care services for complicated and more unusual causes of blindness.

This ALMA ATA declaration remains in the hearts of the people and organizations involved with blindness prevention. However there are major obstacles that must be eliminated to reach the ultimate goal of health for all.

PRESENT SITUATION OF COMMUNITY EYE SERVICES—LATIN AMERICA

The experience in Latin America is typical of the developing world in general. At the present time, more than 80% of the available eye services in most Latin American countries are confined to the 2 or 3 *largest cities* in each country. The services provided in these situations are mainly in the hands of ophthalmologists and optometrists and are by their very nature sophisticated in the use of modern equipment and technology which is expensive in terms of resources and manpower.

By contrast, 40 to 60% of the population of Latin America live in *rural areas*. There is an increasing literacy in the pop-

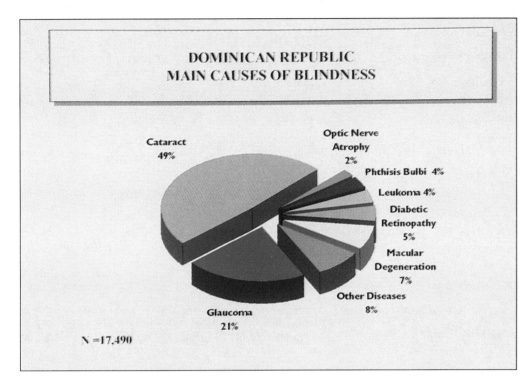

Figure 19-1. Main causes of blindness in the Dominican Republic (Battle).

ulation resulting in a greater demand for correction of refractive errors. There are also more people driving motorized vehicles requiring good distance and near vision.

Life expectancy is increasing in Latin America from 4.3% of the population being over 65 years in 1990 to 5.2% of the population by the year 2000, resulting in 30 million people being over the age of 65 years in Latin America by the year 2000, with a consequent increase in the number of people suffering with cataract, glaucoma, and retinal disease.

Latin American countries are going through a period of rapid urbanization. The structure of most countries can be divided into:

1. Highly educated/rich minority of the population concentrated in a few large cities. This segment represents 5 to 10% of the total and has access to private eye care.
2. Middle or working class population mainly living in the large cities and provided with eye services through the social security and government health care systems, representing between 10 to 40% of the population.
3. Poor people living in the marginal zones/barrios/periurban slum areas of the large cities. There is limited provision of eye care for these people because of economic and social barriers. This segment represents 10 to 40% of the total and is increasing in many countries as people move from the rural to the city environment.
4. The rural population consisting of 20 to 50% of the total population. There is very little provision of eye care for this sector with geographical barriers also being added to the economic and social barriers already mentioned for the poor urban population.

TABLE 19-3
PREVALENCE OF BLINDNESS IN SELECTED COUNTRIES

Country	Prevalence
Ethiopa	1.90%
Ghana	1.70%
Gambia	1.40%
South Africa	1.10%
Kenya	0.70%
Saudi Arabia	0.70%
Dominican Republic	0.45%
Italy	0.43%
China	0.24%
United States of America	0.20%

Categories 3) and 4) have been the focus of most charitable and non-governmental organizations and unfortunately represent the majority in most underdeveloped countries.

Distribution and availability of eye care is not only an issue of cost and geography. There is also a manpower limitation expressed in Table 19-4 as the ratio of ophthalmologists to population for various countries is illustrated. There are also countries in Africa where one or two ophthalmologists provide eye care for the entire population.

TABLE 19-4	
RATIO OF OPHTHALMOLOGISTS TO POPULATION	
Country	Ophth/Pop.
Haiti	1/230,000
Mexico	1/158,000
Ecuador	1/129,000
Guatemala	1/114,000
Costa Rica	1/85,000
Bolivia	1/70,000
Peru	1/67,000
Colombia	1/56,000
Chile	1/40,000
Dominican Republic	1/40,000
Brazil	1/27,000

TABLE 19-5	
ESTIMATED COST OF CATARACT SURGERY IN 1997	
Country	Cost
Africa	$8.00 to 12.00
India	$12.00 to 20.00
Haiti	$15.00
Honduras	$70.00
Dominican Republic	$110.00
Venezuela	$200.00
Colombia	$300.00
Canada	$100.00

AFFORDABLE, ACCESSIBLE, APPROPRIATE TECHNOLOGY

The meeting on Prevention of Blindness held in Berlin in 1994 stressed the importance of appropriate technology that is affordable and accessible to the countries where the technology is to be applied. Cataract surgery has a cost which varies according to the socio-economic development of the different countries. Table 19-5 demonstrates how this approximate cost varies widely from the poorest to the wealthiest nation.

The fact is that cataract patients from any country in the world are willing to spend up to one month of their salary on a cataract operation. When the cost of the operation surpasses that amount, the individual is unlikely to make the personal commitment. This variable cost of surgery is fully understood by many of the large pharmaceutical companies that produce disposable materials for cataract surgery. Unfortunately, the issue is always addressed from a marketing point of view, stating that: "Why should we sell an IOL for US $5.00 in India when we can get US $300.00 in Japan?" The answer is obvious from a business standpoint, but from the standpoint of blindness prevention programs should be completely different.

That is why prevention of blindness is not a money or a business issue. It is a discipline that takes all the social, geographic, political, economic, educational, psychological, and religious characteristics of a community into consideration in order to achieve the ultimate goal of curing those that are blind from a reversible cause.

BARRIERS TO CATARACT SURGERY

In various communities around the world there are different obstacles to the delivery of cataract surgery. These obstacles are not the same in every country or in every community. Generally speaking these obstacles are money, fear, distance, and ignorance. In the survey of blindness recently completed in the Dominican Republic, money was the main reason quoted for not having a cataract operation (Figure 19-2). However, there are people who have an inherent fear of the outcome of the cataract procedure, generally because of known adverse results or outcomes of the procedure, or because of psychological fear of the operating room, anesthetics, or medical facilities.

Ignorance plays a major role in the high prevalence countries, which is particularly true in countries with large rural populations where information about new cataract surgery technology is not easily received. Finally, conformity or acceptance of the state of blindness is a major factor, especially in countries where disease and death are viewed as a part of life that must be accepted and not something to be prevented or avoided. Other obstacles include the distance that must be traveled to a cataract surgery center. There are elderly people who do not like to travel far away from home to receive their care, and cataract surgery is not an exception.

Most cataract campaigns and successful cataract clinics try to minimize these obstacles. Insurance programs have been created and transformed to provide eye care for the elderly and the very young. Same-day surgical facilities without hospitalization, and the simplification of the follow-up examinations also have the purpose of minimizing the fear and complexity of the cataract procedure. In this regard, phacoemulsification has become the leading technology worldwide. Phacoemulsification has simplified the intraoperative and postoperative regimen in many ways.

Phacoemulsification can be performed with topical or peribulbar anesthesia. The intraoperative time has been reduced to less than 10 minutes. Sutures are not necessary, and with the new incisions, postoperative astigmatism is minimized. The postoperative visits are reduced and the time out of work or pleasure is likewise minimized during the recovery.

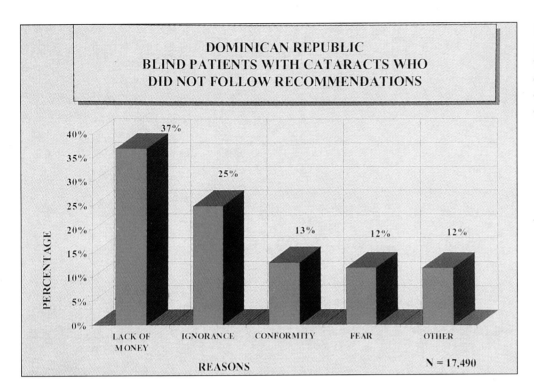

Figure 19-2. Reasons blind patients with cataracts in the Dominican Republic did not follow recommendations to have cataract extraction (Battle).

IS PHACOEMULSIFICATION AN APPROPRIATE, ACCESSIBLE AND AFFORDABLE TECHNOLOGY?

The real challenge in the Third World is to make the new phacoemulsification techniques affordable and accessible. There is no question about the excellence of the results in expert hands, but are the results reproducible in the hands of a loupe-trained intracapsular surgeon? The new incisions that permit insertion of foldable lenses are a definite advantage over the previous technology requiring 4 to 7 sutures. However, would foldable lenses be made available with the necessary viscoelastics at a price that would be affordable in Africa, India, and Latin America?

The new phacoemulsification instruments are programmable with variable power, adjustable vacuum and flow rates. However, will they be easily implemented in communities where power failures are the rule or in a rural community where service or maintenance is difficult? Again, the challenge would be to place these very sophisticated instruments in highly specialized tertiary centers. However, will doing so respond only to the needs of those that are wealthy and able to afford the new technology or will the technology also be made available to the poor and indigent who represent the vast majority?

These are the relevant issues and questions facing the introduction of phacoemulsification into the Third World. The solutions to many of these problems are not easy and require a generous spirit. If phacoemulsification can be intro-

duced as a safe, reproducible technology that can be used at an affordable price, it will become an instrument that can break down the economic barriers that now exist. If it cannot be made affordable, it will simply become one more obstacle in the current state of blindness by making money, or the lack of it, a limiting obstacle to cataract surgery.

In the meantime, North American surgeons are being trained in phacoemulsification techniques, and extracapsular surgery is becoming a technique of the past. There is a global challenge for these surgeons as they enter into the mission field finding themselves in situations where phaco machines are not available. Will there be phaco machines that can be easily packed for transportation to the mission field, and will there be microscopes with excellent coaxial illumination and resolution to allow capsulorhexis?

The real challenge is to train surgeons in the Third World in the new phacoemulsification techniques. Microscopes and phaco machines are rapidly evolving to make them more affordable and easily transported. Disposable material such as IOLs, viscoelastics, and anesthetics are becoming less expensive and the companies that manufacture them are more sympathetic to the worldwide problem. Surgeons in Latin America have accepted and adopted the blindness prevention campaigns and the governments are more willing to accept responsibility for their health problems. As these changes take place, phacoemulsification will become the gold standard of modern cataract surgery and the history of cataract surgery is unlikely to go back. A cataract operation will always become better and simpler.

Figure 19-3. Model of facility in Hangzhou, China (Martin).

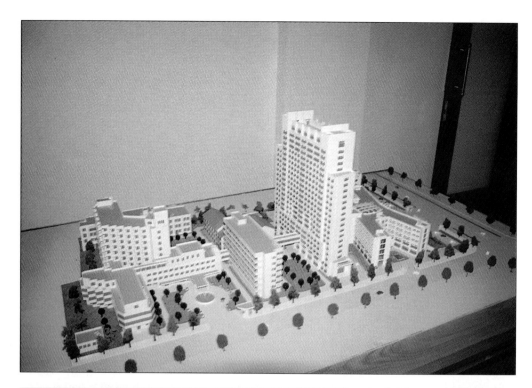

Figure 19-4. Opening ceremonies of new facility in Hangzhou, China (Martin).

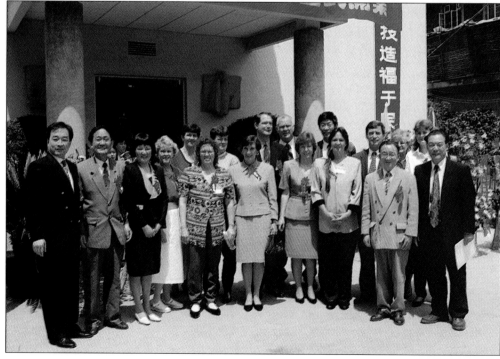

EXPERIENCE IN CHINA

State-of-the-Art Cataract Surgery Training in the Third World

We have some experience in addressing these issues in a developing country. Mr. Jim Marshall, President of International Business Consulting (IBC) approached me

(RGM) in 1994 about establishing a center in China for doing eye surgery. Basically, the idea was to transfer our clinical and surgical experience at Carolina Eye Associates to China. We had worked on the design and construction of the facility (Figure 19-3) and worked on procuring the equipment for approximately two years. Six Chinese doctors, three of whom were scheduled to do cataract surgery and three administrators came to Carolina Eye Associates in Southern Pines, NC

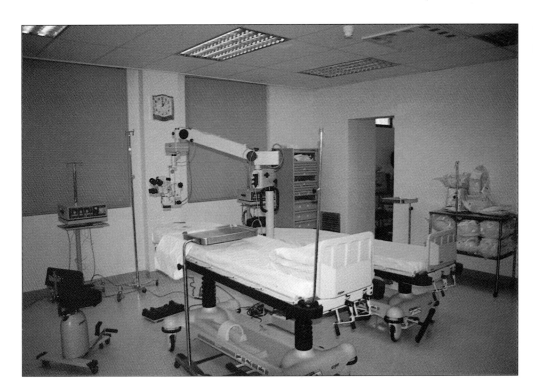

Figure 19-5. Operating room in Hangzhou facility (Martin).

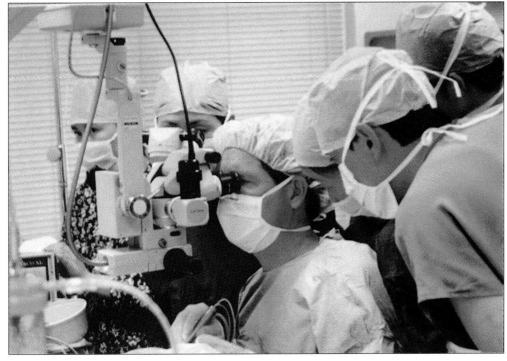

Figure 19-6. Chinese surgeons observing phacoemulsification technique (Martin).

on November 27, 1995. They stayed with us until December 17, 1995, observing clinical, surgical, and administrative procedures and processes on a day to day basis, meeting regularly to assimilate what they had learned.

A crew of 6 Carolina Eye Associates personnel plus various family members left on May 8, 1996, for the opening of the new center in Hangzhou, China (Figure 19-4). For about 4-5 days prior to the opening, we spent our time assembling

our A-scans, EyeSys corneal topographical unit, and other clinical and surgical equipment (Figure 19-5). After opening ceremonies, the clinic and surgical center began to function on May 13, 1996.

During this first week, approximately 112 cataract cases were done. Unfortunately, the Chinese wanted to again observe primarily me doing the surgery and the Chinese only did about 22 of these cases (Figure 19-6). All the cases performed were done using a bevel occlusion technique under topical anesthesia, except for two procedures which were done extracap. The Chinese performed the extracaps under peribulbar anesthesia. The patients essentially required no sedation and they had no intraocular lidocaine. The results were outstanding on both sides of the fence—the American surgeon and the Chinese surgeons. Though the Chinese said they had done phaco before and they knew how to fracture the nucleus, apparently their experience was non-existent with phacoemulsification at this point in time. Their only experience was in the weeks of observing at Carolina Eye Associates in North Carolina and the week that I had spent in surgery with them in China.

When I returned to China in July, 1996, the Chinese were doing approximately 30-40% of their surgeries topical, sutureless, using the STAAR lens. They were routinely using the diamond keratome for making their incisions. By this time, many of the diamonds had been damaged and had to be refurbished. Within three months of this trip, probably 5-6 months total time, the Chinese had converted approximately 90% of their cases to the topical anesthesia, sutureless corneal technique using the bevel occlusion instrument.

The thing that impressed me most about the Chinese doctors in Hangzhou at the Zheyi Eye Center is that they were all extremely eager to learn. Although they were not really aggressive operating in front of an American doctor, they were aggressive at adopting quickly to the techniques that they saw in private and advancing with these techniques. I believe the center has moved ahead two decades in less than 6 months. They are now moving forward with refractive surgery and retinal surgery. Prior to our arrival, diabetic retinopathy and angle closure glaucoma were not treated surgically. They have now begun to do a lot more surgical treatment of both these conditions.

The productivity of the Chinese surgeons has improved ten-fold probably within six months. Before our arrival there, the Chinese doctors were operating in a socialistic system where they were paid whether or not they performed surgery. One of the key changes we made was to make a system in which they are paid a certain amount per case. When their income increased with productivity, the productivity and efficiency have significantly increased and is projected to increase in the second year.

SUMMARY

As surgeons in the developed world rapidly move toward the advanced cataract techniques presented in this book, the next challenge will be to extend the benefits of these techniques to the developing world. Phacoemulsification, sutureless surgery, and topical anesthesia can not only improve outcomes but can make cataract surgery less expensive as surgical time and the need for follow-up care and spectacles are reduced. If surgeons within the developing world can be trained in these advanced techniques, the tremendous backlog of cataract surgeries can be effectively reduced, particularly in the urban centers where electricity and equipment may be more reliably available. Our experience shows that given motivated surgeons, training can be rapid and the learning curve short.

BIBLIOGRAPHY

Blindness Prevention Congress held in Bucaramanga, Colombia, 1989.

Blindness Prevention Congress held in Berlin, Germany, 1994.

National Survey of Diabetes and Blindness, Dominican Republic, February-March 1995, pages 26-27, 34.

Index